APHASIA
AND
ITS
THERAPY

APHASIA
AND
ITS
THERAPY

Anna Basso

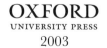

OXFORD
UNIVERSITY PRESS
2003

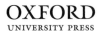

Oxford New York
Auckland Bangkok Buenos Aires Cape Town Chennai
Dar es Salaam Delhi Hong Kong Istanbul Karachi Kolkata
Kuala Lumpur Madrid Melbourne Mexico City Mumbai
Nairobi São Paulo Shanghai Taipei Tokyo Toronto

Published by Oxford University Press, Inc.
198 Madison Avenue, New York, New York, 10016
http://www.oup-usa.org

Library of Congress Cataloging-in-Publication Data
Basso, Anna.
Aphasia and its therapy / Anna Basso.
p. cm. Includes bibliographical references and index.
ISBN 0-19-513587-3 (cloth)
1. Aphasia. 2. Aphasic persons—Rehabilitation.
3. Speech therapy.
I. Title.
RC425 B378 2003
616.85'5–dc21   2002025037

2 4 6 8 9 7 5 3 1

Printed in the United States of America
on acid-free paper

Εἰ δὴ τισ ἐξ ἀρκῆσ τὰ πράγματα φυόμενα βλέψειεν, ὥσπερ
ἐν τοῖσ ἄλλοισ, καὶ ἐν τούτοισ κάλλιστ᾽ ἂν οὕτω
θεωρήσειεν.

It is by looking at things as they evolve from their origins that
we can best see them, here as anywhere else.
—Aristotle, *Politica*, II, 1

TO ARTHUR BENTON

During the autumn and winter of 1961 I was in Paris, at the Hôpital de la Salpêtrière, in the neurological service headed by Monsieur François Lhermitte. The Algerian war, one of the cruelest to ever take place, was raging. The French did not want to leave Algeria, which was one of their colonies, and the Algerians were fighting for their independence. The number of dead, wounded, and tortured soldiers and civilians was unimaginable. Before going to Paris, I had never heard of aphasia or so much as seen an aphasic person, but during my stay several jeeps arrived daily, bringing young French soldiers from the military hospital Val-de-Grâce to la Salpêtrière. They had all suffered head trauma and were aphasic. I was usually shut up in a room with them and asked to test them and draw up their neuropsychological profile. I was young and unprepared, and although I found it hard and taxing, the job fascinated me.

Once back in Italy, I started working at the Neurological Clinic of Milan University and began looking for some formal courses in neuropsychology. At that time, none existed at any level of formal education. Nor were there any professional courses for speech therapists. So I continued to learn by my own efforts.

In 1965 Professors Ennió De Renzi and Luigi Vignolo, both of whom were at the Neurological Clinic of Milan University, invited Professor

Arthur Benton to give a course in neuropsychology. I attended it and had the pleasure of meeting Dr. Benton, to whom I owe my only formal training in neuropsychology. Since then, Arthur and I have always kept in touch.

Nearly 40 years later, it is to Arthur Benton that I owe the idea of writing this book, and it is he who has encouraged me throughout the writing process. It is to Arthur Benton, a highly refined neuropsychologist, a good friend, and a wonderful person, that I dedicate this book.

PREFACE

Aphasiologists are generally interested in theoretical research, while clinicians are oppressed by the practical problems they have to face daily. The result is that the relationship between theory and practice is very loose; research on the nature of the deficit underlying language impairment and the practice of aphasia rehabilitation have sometimes diverged. In 1983 Marie-France Beauvois and Jacqueline Dérouesné hypothesized three categories of researchers. Asked whether they would ever do research on aphasia therapy, researchers in the first category would respond, "Never! I am a researcher, not a speech therapist," those in the second category would respond, "No, most of the time aphasia therapy is not effective," and those in the third category would respond, "Yes, of course I am interested in aphasia therapy. I try to evaluate its effectiveness."

Nowadays the outlook is brighter, and many researchers are interested in therapy, mostly because the results of a detailed therapeutic program can be used to verify the underlying hypothesis about the location of the functional damage in a predefined model. Expected findings confirm the original hypothesis; unexpected findings offer counterevidence and may be used to suggest new hypotheses about the structure of the damaged function.

However, it is still the case that few researchers read the literature on aphasia rehabilitation and few practicing clinicians read the literature on aphasia research, which is ever richer and more specialized. Attempting to straddle these two fields is a difficult matter.

The aim of the book is to help bridge the gap between aphasia research and therapy by pointing out their relationship. The book is addressed mainly to clinicians because its main thesis is that theoretical knowledge is necessary for treating patients. But it is also intended for researchers because it endeavors to give an idea of how therapy takes place in clinical settings. Experimental treatments offer interesting and new ideas about how a therapeutic intervention is related to specific functional damage and about its effectiveness. For treatment to be relevant to the patient's language capacities in daily living, however, it must go beyond the confines of experimental treatment in range and duration.

Having run an aphasia rehabilitation unit at Milan University for some 40 years, I have been directly involved in and fascinated by aphasia therapy and research, and I hope that this book will open lines of communication in both directions by making the domain of research accessible to clinicians and by giving researchers a taste of what clinical rehabilitation really is like. I have tried to avoid the use of specialized jargon and the minutiae of theoretical discussion, but I hope that the end result is a reasonably comprehensive overview of the two fields. The basic idea of the book is that knowledge of the past promotes understanding of the present.

The book is divided into three parts. The first part is dedicated to the first 100 years of aphasiology. Chapter 1 is historical and traces the history of aphasia from Broca's discoveries in 1861 and 1865 to the 1970s. During the second half of the nineteenth century and the first part of the twentieth century, the debate between the associationists and the holists was heated. The main question was whether aphasia was a unitary disorder varying only in severity or whether there were different types of aphasia, related to damage to different cerebral areas. In the twentieth century the holistic school gained support and the associationist view was more or less abandoned until, in the 1970s, the Boston school relaunched the associationist approach. Geschwind's work on disconnection syndromes and on the classic authors rekindled interest in their writings and in the Wernicke-Lichteim model (Geschwind, 1965, 1974). Anatomical–clinical correlations were now based on a more accurate study of the relationships between brain damage and language disorders and a more accurate linguistic analysis of the language impairment.

Somewhat outside the Western tradition, the Russian psychologist Luria argued for an intermediate position between associationists and holists: he rejected the idea that language is a function of the whole brain but also the idea that it is possible to relate directly a function to a specific brain area. His approach to the study of aphasia has come to be known as *functional* because he maintained that each function, such as comprehension or writing, is related to many areas in the brain and that damage to any of these areas impairs the function in different ways.

Chapter 2 describes Luria's and the Boston school's classifications of the aphasias. Many other classifications have been proposed, but none has gained wide support. Luria's classification is still used in some Eastern countries, and the Boston classification is still widely used by clinicians in the Western countries. Both of them have stood the test of time.

Chapter 3 describes the main approaches to aphasia rehabilitation from its beginnings to the 1970s and tries to relate them to their theoretical underpinnings. Before World War II, aphasia therapy was based on pedagogic principles and techniques of second language learning, with no reference to the disorder to be rehabilitated, namely, aphasia Language rehabilitation became common practice after World War II with the classic or stimulation approach, which was inspired by the holistic school. Successively, aphasia therapy took advantage of behavior modification theory (which inspired the behavior modification approach) and linguistics (which inspired the neurolinguistic approach), and it became increasingly sophisticated and tailored to specific language disorders. The last to be described is the neoassociationist approach, which brought together the basic principles of the stimulation approach and the syndrome-based approach; its theoretical basis was, however, still scanty.

Chapter 4 reviews the clinical studies on aphasia therapy effectiveness, regrouped according to the methodology used: studies on chronic patients, on groups of rehabilitated patients, comparison between groups of treated and untreated patients, and comparison of different therapeutic methods. Results of these studies have been criticized on methodological grounds, and it has been argued that the evidence in support of aphasia therapy effectiveness is unconvincing. Some meta-analyses have been carried out that generally support the efficacy of aphasia therapy. Finally, the relative importance of group studies and single case studies for the study of the efficacy of aphasia therapy is discussed. I conclude that there is sufficient experimental evidence that aphasia therapy in general is effective for aphasic patients in general, and that it is now time to pose more specific questions.

The second part of the book is devoted to cognitive neuropsychology. The classic aphasia syndromes have remained descriptive; they are unreal in the sense that it is not possible to delineate for any syndrome an invariant pattern shared by all patients classified under the same heading. With the advent of cognitive neuropsychology in the past 30 years, studies on aphasia have undergone a real revolution, and aphasia (as well as other cognitive functions) has been studied from the point of view of the structure of the processing components that define normal cognitive systems. An explicit theory of normal language processing allows one to deduce the possible patterns of language deficits and to relate the observed symptoms to the disruption of one or more components of the underlying functional structure.

Chapter 5 illustrates the basic assumptions of cognitive neuropsychology and reports on some of the most widely discussed topics: the use of single case studies, the relevance of dissociation and association of symptoms and of error analysis for the theory, and the possibility of distinguishing access and storage disorders. Finally, to illustrate the difference between the classic neuropsychological approach and the cognitive neuropsychological approach, the classic and cognitive dyslexia and dysgraphia syndromes are illustrated.

Chapter 6 presents a widely accepted model of lexical processing based on data from brain-damaged patients. Cognitive neuropsychologists have devoted much time and attention to the study of the lexicon, and models of the lexical system are fairly detailed and well illustrate the cognitive neuropsychological approach. They have also been frequently used as a theoretical basis for treatments of lexical disorders.

Chapter 7 reviews cognitive studies on the rehabilitation of language disorders. The aim of the chapter is to compare the theoretical assumptions described in Chapter 6 with the practical implementations reportedly inspired by the cognitive neuropsychological approach. I argue that the initial evaluation is more accurate than it used to be in classic neuropsychology. The actual implementations, however, are generally not new and have already been used in classic clinical neuropsychology. At the sentence level, however, therapy is more innovative and theory-directed.

The so-called classic and cognitive approaches both have advantages and drawbacks, and are useful in different ways in aphasia rehabilitation. The classic syndromes are clinically relevant and can dictate the choice of rehabilitation in severely aphasic patients. A cognitive neuropsychological diagnosis, on the other hand, tends to single out one phenomenon; while it helps identify the functional damage that causes the symptom (thus allowing for a more rational intervention), it generally fails to give the whole picture of the language disorder.

The third part of the book is concerned with aphasia therapy. Chapter 8 is devoted to a discussion of the theory of aphasia rehabilitation. A theory is a reasonable interpretation of the data and should be able to predict novel outcomes. I argue that it is not possible, for the time being, to sketch a theory of aphasia rehabilitation but that a conscious effort toward the systematic collection of data and toward the creation of a common starting point can and should be undertaken. Merely collecting data with no idea of where they can lead is useless.

Chapter 9 deals with specific intervention procedures for functional damage at the lexical and sentence levels. An effort is made to suggest tasks that are rationally derived from what is known about the structure and processing of the damaged component. The importance of cognitive neuropsychology for the treatment of aphasia does not lie in the contribution of new methods but in constraining the choice of rational interventions. Since therapy must be directed to the damaged process, the more detailed the diagnosis, the more constrained the choice of possible treatments.

Chapter 10 is devoted to therapy for severe aphasia. I argue that when the functional damage is severe and impairs all (or most of) the components of language processing, no constraint on the choice of logically linked interventions can be derived. A more general conversation-based intervention is suggested that takes as a starting point the patient's handicap—difficulty in communication—and not the functional damage. Conversation is the fundamental and primary type of language use and the form in which we all learn our native language. The structure of conversation is briefly sketched, and I argue that the therapist should create a communicative situation and maintain an *ecological* conversation with the patient, conversation similar to one sustained with a friend in daily living.

Finally, in Chapter 11, some concluding and general remarks are presented.

I am grateful to Alfonso Caramazza, Stefano Cappa, Guido Gainotti, and Luigi Vignolo for their helpful comments on a preliminary version of the book.

Milan   A.B.

CONTENTS

CHAPTER 8. IN SEARCH OF A THEORY OF APHASIA THERAPY, 185

CHAPTER 9. REHABILITATION OF LEXICAL AND SENTENCE DISORDERS, 203

CHAPTER 10. SEVERE APHASIA AND PRAGMATICS, 235

APHASIA
AND
ITS
THERAPY

1

A HISTORICAL OVERVIEW

THE IMPORTANCE OF THE PAST is frequently played down, but our concepts about aphasia have developed in the course of the last two centuries, and our current understanding and way of thinking about aphasia have been shaped by classic research. Chapter 1 retraces the history of aphasia from the discoveries of Broca in 1861 and 1865 to the 1970s.

Eighteenth-century localization of functions in the brain was conducted only in broad concepts, such as perception, intelligence, and memory. With Franz Joseph Gall the question radically changed. Gall (1825) argued that the brain contains separate organs located in the cerebral cortex and that each organ subserves a specific intellectual, moral, or spiritual faculty. Gall's ideas were revolutionary for his time and were opposed by many of his contemporaries, who rejected the idea that mental faculties could be localized in separate parts of the brain. In addition, Gall's phrenology and his bizarre list of 27 faculties rapidly threw discredit on his doctrine, and he is now remembered more for these aspects than for his undeniable merits. According to Benton, "a quantum leap to another mode of thinking was introduced by Franz Joseph Gall in the first decades of the 19th century" (Benton, 1988, p. 5). The claim that somehow survived and that played an important role during the following decades was that the language faculty was located in the frontal lobes.

The debate initiated by Gall on whether different parts of the brain were responsible for different mental faculties or whether, as it was then often held, the brain was unitary in function went on for approximately a century, with alternate ups and downs. It is generally agreed that the scientific study of language–brain relationships began a few decades later with the well-known discoveries made by Broca (1861, 1865), who was the first to demonstrate, by careful anatomo-clinical studies, that speech may be disrupted by a lesion localized in a specific area of the brain, the posterior part of the third frontal convolution of the left hemisphere (for reviews, see Hécaen & Lanteri-Laura, 1977; Caplan, 1987; Goodglass, 1993; Gainotti, 1999).

During the first 13 years of the "scientific" era, three major discoveries were reported: first, that loss of articulated speech follows a lesion of the foot of the third frontal convolution (Broca, 1861); second, that language impairment follows a lesion of the left (but not the right) hemisphere in right-handed people (Broca, 1865); and, third, that a different form of expressive aphasia with comprehension disorders follows a lesion of the (left) posterior first temporal gyrus (Wernicke, 1874). These discoveries laid the foundation for the associationist doctrine.

The labels *localizationist* and *associationist* are sometimes used interchangeably, but they refer to different theoretical positions. Broca believed that speech can be localized; he was a localizationist. Wernicke, an associationist, believed that language is the result of the collaborative work—or association—of various brain centers, each of which has a specialized function. He claimed that complex functions are built up by associating simple components, and he described the first associationist model of language functioning.

The opposite viewpoint rejected the idea that the language faculty could be localized to specific areas of the brain; followers of the *holistic* view argued that aphasia is a unitary disorder varying only in severity. For a time, the study of aphasia appeared to have come to an impasse. The two alternative positions—the associationist and the holistic—were periodically reproposed without any substantial change.

In both schools of thought, aphasiology was the preserve of physicians with an interest in brain diseases, whose knowledge of the nature and structure of language was rather primitive. Although distinct clinical patterns of language impairment were described, the analysis of the language behavior of aphasics was rather coarse, and no reference was made to the functional structure of language. Linguistics was a young science. It was only with Saussure (1916) that it became a scientific discipline, and it would take a few more years before the basic principles of linguistics were incorporated into the study of aphasia and the rehabilitation of aphasics.

In 1965, Norman Geschwind, a neurologist in Boston, published a two-part paper, "Disconnection syndromes in animals and man," in which he reviewed the contributions to neuropsychology of many classic authors. He attempted to explain in a more systematic and differentiated way than the classic associationists how particular aspects of language function may break down. His writings caused a resurgence of interest in aphasia and started the neoassociationist school.

Another important figure in the history of aphasia was Alexander R. Luria, a Russian neuropsychologist. For historical reasons, Luria's contribution to the study of aphasia and brain functions became known in the Western countries only in the 1960s when his books were translated into English.

Chapter 1 describes the views of the main representatives of the associationist and holistic positions and briefly outlines the neoassociationist approach heralded by Geschwind. It ends with the description of Luria's theoretical position.

ASSOCIATIONIST MODELS

Advocates of the associationist position considered language an autonomous function and thought it was made up of various capacities, such as the *faculty of articulate language*. They referred to the principles of the anatomo-functional organization of the brain and claimed that aphasic persons could have selective deficits of a single verbal faculty. The position of Broca, Wernicke, Lichtheim, and Dejerine are reported here.

Paul Broca

In the first half of the nineteenth century, there was great opposition to the view that language could be localized in the brain. Broca was drawn into the controversy between the localizationists and antilocalizationists almost by chance. In April 1861, at a meeting of the Société d'Anthropologie de Paris, Ernest Auburtin, a supporter of localization of functions in the cerebral cortex, reported the case of a patient who, in a suicide attempt, had extirpated his frontal bone, exposing the frontal lobes. He had normal language and intelligence but became unable to speak whenever his frontal lobes were compressed and recovered his speech when they were released.

Auburtin considered this a quasi-experimental case and declared that he would abandon his claim for localization of language function in the brain when shown an aphasic patient without lesion of the frontal lobes.

A few days later, Broca saw at his clinic in Bicêtre a patient who had become aphasic many years earlier. The patient was known as Mr. Tan, as he was only able to say "tan," generally repeated twice, "tan tan," and this had been his only oral production for the last 20 years. When first admitted to the hospital, Mr. Tan was considered to be physically healthy, with normal intelligence and good verbal comprehension. Ten years later he developed a right hemiplegia, and his intelligence slowly deteriorated. When examined by Broca, Mr. Tan appeared to understand what he was being told, and his behavior was considered adequate to the situation. Shortly after this examination the patient died and, in August 1861, Broca presented an extensive neuroanatomical report on the patient to the Société d'Anthropologie. He argued that convolutions of the brain—contrary to what was generally held—are relatively constant from subject to subject, and he stressed the idea that the lesion must be indicated by reference to the lobes and particularly to the damaged convolutions. In Tan's case the lesion was located in the postero-external part of the left anterior lobe, but in 1861 Broca had not yet realized the importance of the left side of the lesion.

In 1865, after studying eight consecutive cases of aphasia, Broca (1865) declared that we speak with the left hemisphere, contradicting the previously held biological law that symmetrical organs have identical functions. All eight patients had a rather similar language disturbance; their spontaneous speech was very poor, at times limited to a single expression ("tan," "lelo"), but their comprehension appeared relatively spared. Broca had examined Mr. Tan carefully and considered that his nonlinguistic communication was unimpaired and his comprehension intact, at least as far as could be inferred from the patient's nonverbal behavior.

The same was true of the patients he examined in the following years, which led him to the conviction that the third frontal convolution was the repository of 'motor word images' and the left hemisphere was dominant for articulate speech (not language). A lesion in this area (now known as *Broca's area*) would therefore cause loss of speech without impairing speech comprehension. Broca did not consider that the small differences in the pattern of convolutions between the left and the right hemispheres were responsible for the functional asymmetry. At the time, it was already known that in fetal development the left sulci are formed before the right, and, according to Broca, the basis for predominance of the left hemisphere was to be found in the precocity of the left over the right hemisphere. He also argued that in the rare cases in which the right hemisphere matures before the left, dominance for language and handedness shifts to the right hemisphere.

Broca's contribution to the study of brain–behavior relationships was important in many respects. He insisted that localization must be made by reference to the lobes and convolutions, which have a relatively constant pattern, and he established the fact that the two hemispheres are functionally different. Finally, he was the first to hypothesize a specific and localized center for one of the language faculties—articulate speech. However, even though he outlined major differences in aphasia, he did not localize them, and one had to await Wernicke for the first neurological model of language processing.

Carl Wernicke

After Broca's publications, interest in aphasia grew rapidly. Broca had proposed a theory that linked language disorders to existing neurological knowledge. Wernicke developed a scientific approach to the study of aphasia. It was the theoretical aspect of his approach that made it so fruitful. In 1874, Carl Wernicke published an extremely influential monograph (*Der aphasische Symptomencomplex*) that laid the basis for a theoretical framework for the interpretation and classification of the aphasias. He began by maintaining that both the idea of the equipotentiality of the brain and the arbitrary assignment of individual areas of the cortex to mental functions by phrenologists were untenable. Following both his teacher Meynert and recent physiological and anatomical observations, Wernicke pointed out that the parts of the brain lying anterior to the Rolandic central fissure are motor regions and the posterior parts are sensory in function. The memory for movements lies in the frontal lobes, and Broca or motor aphasia follows lesions of Broca's area, which is near the motor area for the tongue and mouth. Similarly, a posterior lesion located near the acoustic projection area where the auditory images for words are held should give rise to sensory aphasia with comprehension and production disturbances.

Wernicke did not conceive of the disorders in comprehension and production as being separable. He asserted that since language is learned by imitating heard language, transmission from the auditory receptive area to the anterior language motor area is necessary for production. In the usual act of speaking, the auditory memory traces in Wernicke's area are forwarded to the center for motor memory traces in Broca's area and thereby exercise continuous correction of the articulatory movements. The connection within these two centers is necessary for correct speech production and is mediated, according to Wernicke, by the cortex around the Sylvian fissure located between the anterior and posterior language zones. A disturbance of auditory word-memory images would disturb speech production, but the errors would not be in the actual production of sounds, as occurs in Broca aphasia. Loss of control of the motor speech area by the auditory receptive area prevents correct production of words. Instead of saying a particular word, a patient with a lesion in the temporal lobe might produce a phonologically or semantically related word. When the produced word was so different from any German word that it could not be understood, it was called a *neologism*, namely, a new word that does not exist in the vocabulary of the language.

Wernicke went on to postulate the existence of a third form of aphasia, which he called *conduction aphasia*, caused by the interruption of the pathway between Wernicke's and Broca's centers that mediates between the heard and the spoken word. In conduction aphasia the two language centers are unimpaired, which explains why motor speech and auditory comprehension are preserved. According to Wernicke, destruction of the association fibers provokes an alteration of speech in the same way as in sensory aphasia because the preserved sound images cannot control the choice of words. The patient, however, is capable of understanding and of judging whether or not what he or she says is correct. (Wernicke failed to mention the repetition disorder that was first noted by Lichtheim 10 years later.)

In the final part of his 1874 monograph, Wernicke described two patients with sensory aphasia. Both had very impaired comprehension and difficulty with spoken language, which was, however, different in nature from the speech output of Broca aphasics. Speech was not scarce, halting, or effortful; articulation was fluent, and the intonational patterns were normal but the speech did not make sense. The patients made errors in the selection of sounds and words that often made it difficult for the examiner to understand what the patient intended to say. One of the patients died. At autopsy, her brain showed an infarct in the posterior part of the first left temporal gyrus. Wernicke noted that it was near the cortical primary auditory cortex and that this could well be the area responsible for the comprehension of auditory language.

Wernicke's work introduced the deductive method in the study of aphasia, succeeded in spreading knowledge on sensory aphasia, and drew attention to the fact that all of its symptoms originate from a single lesion in what came to be called *Wernicke's area*, in the superior temporal gyrus.

Ludwig Lichtheim

In Wernicke's interpretation of the relationships between language and the brain, only the sensorimotor aspects of language were considered, as if language were a simple sequence of heard and produced sounds. His model included the primary auditory cortex, Wernicke's area, the connection between Wernicke's and Broca's areas, and the primary motor cortex. Language, however, is more than a sensorimotor activity; it conveys meanings and thoughts. Lichtheim proposed an expansion of Wernicke's model and introduced the idea of a concept area where concepts are formulated and stored. He argued that the concept area is not, in a strict sense, a language center, and he claimed that it is diffusely represented in the brain. At the same time, he argued that information flows from the auditory center to the concept area and from this to the motor center, and that the concept center is connected to both Wernicke's and Broca's areas. Disconnection of the concept center from Wernicke's area causes comprehension disorders. This is clearly a limit of Lichtheim's model: if there are, as his model presupposes, anatomical connections between the motor center, the auditory center, and the concept area, it could seem to follow that the concept area itself has a definite, though possibly widespread, anatomical localization. Lichtheim's expansion of Wernicke's model provides the basis for other forms of aphasia. In 1885 he published an important paper in the journal *Brain* (Lichtheim, 1885) reporting a complete enumeration of the seven aphasic syndromes he claimed to exist. In addition to those described by Wernicke (motor or Broca aphasia, sensory or Wernicke aphasia, and conduction aphasia), Lichtheim asserted the existence of four other forms of aphasia caused by the lesion of connecting pathways. These are (*1*) *subcortical sensory aphasia*, due to the interruption of the pathway from the primary auditory area to Wernicke's area; (*2*) *subcortical motor aphasia*, due to the interruption of the pathway from Broca's area to the articulatory musculature; (*3*) *transcortical sensory aphasia*, due to the interruption of the pathway from Wernicke's area to the concept area; and (*4*) *transcortical motor aphasia*, due to the interruption of the pathway from the concept area to Broca's area. In keeping with the idea that the concept area is not localized, conceptual deficits could not be related to a single specific area. Lichtheim maintained that he had observed all the seven types of aphasia predicted by his model, and in his paper he presents examples of each, but descriptions of the patients' disorders are scanty and insufficient to confirm his interpretation of the data. Figure 1–1 depicts Lichtheim's schema.

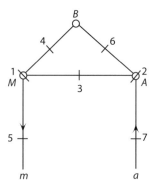

Figure 1–1. Lichtheim's diagram representing Broca's area (M), Wernicke's area (A), the concept center (B), and the pathways connecting them.

Lichtheim provided theoretical explanations for the aphasic syndromes he described. If one knows the nature of the language centers and the information flow, the symptoms in each form of aphasia are easily identified. In subcortical sensory aphasia due to damage to the connecting fibers from the primary auditory area to Wernicke's area, for instance, the auditory stimuli cannot be correctly processed. Comprehension, repetition, and writing to dictation are impaired since they all require a correct analysis of auditory inputs; all the tasks that do not need an auditory analysis, such as speech production, reading aloud, spontaneous writing, and so on are unimpaired.

In Lichtheim's view, the main psycholinguistic language functions (reading, writing, speaking, and understanding) are separate entities, each related to a specific site in the brain. His relatively simple model became more complicated when he added two more centers concerning written language: the center for the memory of the visual form of words and the center for the memory of the motor sequences involved in writing.

Lichtheim's model did not go unchallenged. The most obvious problem concerns the relationships between the various aphasic syndromes and specific loci of the brain. Some of his centers and pathways (in fact, those already described by Wernicke) are clearly related to anatomical sites, but the anatomical location of others is either denied (namely, the concept area that cannot be subject to lesions causing aphasia) or ignored. In fact, it is not clear to what degree Lichtheim was committed to an anatomically based model; it seems that although parts of the model are purely psychological, the model still retains a neuroanatomical basis.

Notwithstanding its limitations, Lichtheim's model had a great clinical and theoretical impact and still is a reference point for many aphasiological schools.

Jules Dejerine

Many other researchers followed in the lines of associationism (e.g., Charcot and Kussmaul, to cite but two), but they generally produced only variations of the Wernicke-Lichtheim's model and too often their schemes were completely unconnected to any neuroanatomical substrate.

Charcot systematically supported the associationist model and graphically represented the different forms of aphasia in a fanciful diagram that has become widely known as *Charcot's bell*. His writings on aphasia were never published in French; they were published in Italian, based on the notes taken by one of his students—Rummo—during his lessons at the Salpêtrière in 1883 (Charcot, 1884).

Kussmaul (1877) argued that language cannot be dissociated from thought and proposed a schema with four centers of images of words—acoustic, optic, phonic, and graphic—under the control of a concept center. He distinguished six forms of aphasia and identified *amnesia for words*.

Kussmaul's and Charcot's models are represented in Figure 1–2. As it can be seen, they are completely divorced from any neuroanatomical basis. This, however, was not the case for Dejerine, who clarified the neuroanatomical basis of alexia with agraphia and of pure alexia. He described a man who suddenly developed an inability to read and write, whose only neurological sign was a right hemianopia (Dejerine, 1891). The postmortem neuropathological examination, performed 8 months later, disclosed an infarct of the left angular gyrus extending inward to the occipital horn of the lateral ventricle. In Dejerine's view, the lesion had destroyed the visual memories for words, making it impossible for the patient to understand written language and to write.

A year later, Dejerine published the case history of a patient with pure alexia without agraphia and no sign of aphasic disorders. The patient could not read visually, but he could recognize letters and words when he traced the outlines of the letters with his hand (Dejerine, 1892). The only neurological symptom was a right hemianopia. Four years later and 10 days before his death, the patient suffered a second stroke with aphasia. At autopsy, the brain showed a recent lesion in the angular gyrus and an old infarct of the left occipital lobe (in the distribution of the posterior cerebral artery) and of the splenium of the corpus callosum.

A

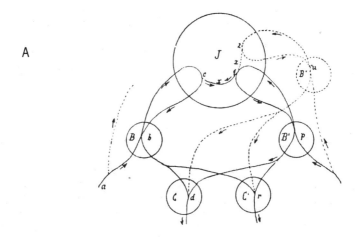

B

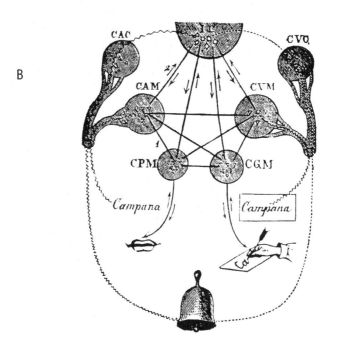

Figure 1–2. Diagrams of the functioning of language, according to (A) Kussmaul (from Moutier, 1908) and (B) Charcot (from Charcot, 1884).

Dejerine interpreted the syndrome of pure alexia as a disconnection syndrome because the visual stimuli, which could be perceived normally by the right occipital lobe, could not be transferred to the left language area because of the lesion of the corpus callosum and could not be recognized as letters or words.

HOLISTIC OR NOETIC MODELS

At the beginning of the twentieth century, associationist theories became quickly unpopular and serious objections were advanced by clinicians who denied the existence of separate anatomical centers and interconnections, each related to a specific language faculty. Objections to associationist theories came from different sources, but critics are generally referred to by the cumulative label *holists*.

Proponents of the holistic school denied the idea of the autonomy of language and argued either that language disorders are the expression of an underlying more central function, such as general intelligence, or that language is the result of the processing of the whole brain. According to the authors of the holistic school, everyday clinical evidence demonstrated how aphasic persons had across-the-board language disorders. Jackson's, Marie's, Goldstein's, Bay's, and Schuell's positions are summarized below.

John Hughlings Jackson

Although Jackson was aware of Broca's work, he does not seem to have been influenced by the associationist model. He was an early proponent of a more unitary psychological approach to the study of aphasia and applied evolutionary principles to its study. According to Jackson (1878), behavior results from the superimposition of increasingly complex functions: from more automatic, involuntary functions to more voluntary and intentional functions. Automatic functions are performed by more primitive structures of the nervous system, and voluntary, stimulus-free functions are performed by evolutionarily advanced structures. Language can be used at various levels of intentionality; swear words and memorized speech lie at the most automatic end and *propositional* language at the most intentional. Based on the observation that severely aphasic persons with large lesions of the left hemisphere could still swear or recite a prayer, Jackson believed that the automatic use of language is supported by the right hemisphere and that only its intentional use is supported by the left hemisphere.

Jackson also denied that words are the principal units of language; according to him, the basic unit is the meaningful proposition. A proposition has a structure and expresses a relationship among things; it allows us to convey new information or express our thoughts. The main defect in aphasia, according to Jackson, consists in the loss of the higher levels of language use, namely, the capacity to *propositionize*; the aphasic person may still swear or say "goodbye" in the appropriate situation, but cannot convey his or her intentions or thoughts independently of the actual external situation. Jackson underlined that what is important in the study of aphasia is the situation in which a patient can use language and not, as maintained by the associationists, what language behavior is impaired. Jackson, however, was not the first to observe a dissociation between voluntary/propositional and automatic uses of language, which had already been described by Baillarger (1865).

To illustrate the automatic–voluntary dissociation in the use of language, a beautiful example frequently recounted by Alajouanine is reported. He had asked an aphasic patient the name of her daughter, who was sitting beside her. After vainly struggling for her daughter's name, the lady turned toward her daughter and said in a very distressed voice, "Ma pauvre Jacqueline, voilà que je ne sais plus ton nom!" ("My poor Jacqueline, I don't even know your name!") (Alajouanine, 1968, p. 250). Answering Alajouanine's question required an intentional search for her daughter's name, but addressing her by her name was automatic.

As we will see, one of the cardinal principles of the stimulation approach to aphasia therapy is based on Jackson's and Baillarger's observation of dissociation between automatic and voluntary use of language. The dissociation has been considered as evidence that language is not lost but in certain situations it is inaccessible, and therapy has aimed to create situations that allow the patient to retrieve some language.

Jackson's writings were fated to be appreciated late; they were relatively neglected until relaunched by Head in 1926.

Pierre Marie

A very provocative challenge to the associationist view came from Pierre Marie, whose writings, unlike Jackson's, received almost immediate attention and fueled a heated debate. In his first paper on aphasia, Marie (1906) denied that Broca's area is the site of expressive speech and cited cases in support of his thesis: patients with a lesion in Broca's area without Broca aphasia and patients with Broca aphasia with no lesion in Broca's area.

Arguing that there are no subtypes of aphasia, Marie viewed aphasia as a single disorder due to the disintegration of the linguistic code, which damages all verbal behaviors more or less equally. A disorder of comprehension is always associated with aphasia and is, in fact, the core of the aphasic disorder itself. The comprehension disorder, however, can be relatively mild, and Marie suggests that it is manifested only if the patient is required to accomplish a complex act, such as the well-known three-paper test devised by Marie himself ("Of the three pieces of paper that I have put before you, take the largest one and crumple it into a ball, put the smallest one in your pocket, and take the middle one and fasten it to the window"). According to Marie, true aphasia is Wernicke aphasia, which is not due to the loss of the auditory images of words, as hypothesized by associationists, but consists in the loss of a specialized form of intelligence, where intelligence refers to the whole set of notions and procedures learned through instruction. This "true" aphasia is always due to a lesion in Wernicke's area but can be accompanied by other symptoms caused by other lesions, such as *anarthria* (a specific disorder of articulatory control), due to an anterior extension of the lesion into the deep white matter and the lenticular nucleus.

Marie's thesis was supported by the work of one of his students, Moutier, who published a review of 387 published cases and 44 personal cases (Moutier, 1908). All cases supported Marie's theory that a lesion limited to Broca's area does not cause aphasia.

The 1908 Debate

Marie's view did not go undisputed, and another debate between holists (championed by Marie) and associationists (championed by Dejerine) took place in 1908, similar to that of 1861 (Lecours et al., 1992). Three meetings of the Société de Neurologie de Paris chaired by Klippel were held in June and July (Klippel, 1908). Dejerine argued that there are several forms of aphasia with lesions at different loci, Marie that there exists only one form, Wernicke aphasia. The discussion was guided by a questionnaire prepared by Dejerine, and the first question was "Are motor aphasia and sensory aphasia clinically different from one another, or is motor aphasia a mere association of sensory aphasia and anarthria? What are the differences if any?" As often happens, after a lively and heated discussion, each participant remained convinced of his own ideas and no compromise was reached. None of the contenders abandoned their views, and the debate remained open. Marie had battled long and hard against classic views, but years later he published with Foix (Marie & Foix, 1917) a diagram of the lesions that produced different aphasic syndromes.

Kurt Goldstein

Goldstein (1948) was one of the strongest supporters of the holistic approach to the study of aphasia. To quote Geschwind, "he is often regarded as the greatest influence in the revolt against the classic school of thought about aphasia" (Geschwind, 1964, p. 214). Goldstein's work on aphasia was influenced by the principles of gestalt psychology. Two of the basic assumptions of gestalt psychology are that the organism reacts in a global, integrated way and that it actively contributes to perception. We do not perceive the isolated stimuli we see; rather, we perceive their relationships, and we immediately and unconsciously extract the figure from the background.

Goldstein introduced the concept of *abstract attitude*, which is the most critical human integrative capacity for the highest intellectual function. The ability to assume the abstract attitude is ascribed to the integrated activity of the brain. A brain lesion interferes with this general capacity. The aphasic patient has lost the capacity to use language in an abstract way and can only use it concretely. This is most evident in naming tasks. The aphasic patient cannot name a picture using the name of the category (to say, for instance, that a knife is a knife) because he or she cannot abstract from the specific picture to be named and consider it as a member of a category. A woman asked to name as many animals as she could, for instance, kept silent for a while and then started to give the names of some animals. Asked how she had found them, she answered that she could not find any animal's name until she imagined that she was at the zoo strolling around and looking at the cages. In this way, she could report the names of the animals as she came across them in their cages. What she had done, Goldstein argued, was to shift from an abstract to a concrete situation and name, instead of the category, the specific animals in the cages. However, naming a visualized animal requires abstraction and categorization processes, as does naming items of a predefined category.

Goldstein described other aphasic symptoms as due to an impairment of the abstract attitude, such as, for instance, agrammatism (see Chapter 2), which is associated with the abstract nature of grammatical morphemes. However, in Goldstein's view, the loss of abstract behavior is not an explanation for all aspects of aphasia: specific components of language can be disrupted by damage to different areas independently of the abstract attitude. Disturbances of the sensorimotor processes of language can be attributed to a precisely localized lesion. Subcortical motor aphasia, for instance, is argued to follow from lesion of the classic Broca's region.

More generally, Goldstein agreed with the correlation of symptoms and lesion sites established by earlier associationists.

In 1964, Geschwind wrote a paper about Goldstein's contribution to the study of aphasia with the intriguing title "The paradoxical position of Kurt Goldstein in the history of aphasia," where he states that "His contribution as a localizer in the classic sense is in fact highly significant although rarely taught" (Geschwind, 1964, p. 223).

Eberhard Bay

More recently, the view that aphasia is one entity has been sustained by Bay and Schuell. Bay (1964) was a strong advocate of the holistic approach. He rejected the sensorimotor dichotomy and argued that aphasia is an indivisible entity. It can vary in severity and accompanying symptoms, but it always entails impairment of conceptual thinking. Like Goldstein, Bay argued that the essence of the aphasic breakdown is a naming disorder, which is due to the disorganization of the underlying concept. In support of his interpretation of aphasia as an impairment of conceptual thinking, he cites the fact that when aphasic persons are asked to make models of plasticine objects, they frequently leave out some characteristic and necessary parts. They may leave out the wheel in modeling a wheel barrow or a giraffe's long neck.

Today such behavior would be considered typical of patients with damage to the semantic system (see Chapter 6) and not a defining characteristic of aphasia in general.

Hildred Schuell

Between World Wars I and II, aphasia, while still studied by clinical neurologists, also attracted the interest of experimentally minded psychologists, such as Weisenburg and McBride, who in 1935 introduced quantitative assessment measures. During World War II, therapy for aphasia became a priority because of the numerous and relatively young brain-injured patients who suffered from aphasia. Hildred Schuell was an American speech pathologist and director of an aphasia rehabilitation program, whose views on the nature of aphasia and on rehabilitation are still influential in the United States. Like Marie, Goldstein, and Bay, she believed that aphasia is a unitary disorder, but in contrast to them she did not believe that it is due to a more general disorder, such as a breakdown of abstract attitude or conceptual thinking. According to Schuell, aphasia is a language disorder, but a single general language factor accounts for almost all of the aphasic impairments. In 1955 she published a comprehensive battery, the Minnesota Test for the Differential Diagnosis of Aphasia (MTDDA; Schuell, 1955), for the evaluation of aphasic persons, and a few years later she conducted a factor analysis of the performance of 155 patients on 69 subtests of the MTDDA (Schuell et al., 1962). Results of the factor analysis led the authors to conclude that there is a general language deficit in aphasia and that there is no support for the hypothesis of the existence of two main forms: a motor or expressive aphasia and a sensory or receptive aphasia. In Chapter 3, we will see that her therapeutic approach is perfectly coherent with her views about aphasia.

NORMAN GESCHWIND AND NEOASSOCIATIONISM

It is to Norman Geschwind that we owe the revival of associationism in the 1960s. A century had passed since Broca's and Wernicke's first publications, and anatomical and physiological studies had greatly advanced knowledge about brain structures. Geschwind challenged the then predominant holistic orientation and reasserted the importance of knowledge of the anatomo-clinical correlations for a better understanding of aphasic symptoms. He reconsidered the work of previous associationists and came to the conclusion that they were generally correct. In his 1965 paper "Disconnection syndromes in animals and man," he presented his conception of a *disconnection syndrome* (Geschwind, 1965). He argued that the different aphasic syndromes are most fruitfully studied as disturbances produced by anatomical disconnection between language areas or between these areas and motor and sensory areas. To illustrate his concept of disconnection, his interpretation of the naming capacity in humans will be briefly described.

Object naming is, according to Geschwind, the simplest aspect of language and becomes possible in humans because of the existence of a new, evolutionarily advanced association area, the angular gyrus. This area is not directly connected with any primary receiving area, but it receives most of its afferent fibers from adjacent association areas. It is "an association area of association areas." The ability to form cross-modal (e.g., vision–audition) associations is, in Geschwind's view, a prerequisite for the acquisition of language, and left hemisphere dominance for language depends on its ability to make rapid cross-modal associations. Naming and concept formation depend on associations between auditory stimulation and other types of stimulation, namely, somesthetic, visual, or tactile. A child acquires the capacity to name a spoon, for instance, by hearing its name and associating it with the visual and tactile stimuli he or she receives from the spoon. Naming disorders depend on damage to this area. According to this view, the reason no subhuman species have language is that they have not developed the necessary association area. In no animal species in fact are direct intermodal associations possible. Geschwind and his colleagues (Goodglass & Kaplan, 1972; Benson, 1979; Albert et al, 1981; Benson & Ardila, 1996) once again proposed the Wernicke-Lichtheim classification. The classic syndromes of aphasia were revived, but they were slightly modified and improved on the basis of a more refined knowledge of neuroanatomy and the use of standardized batteries for the evaluation of language disorders. The next chapter describes the neoassociationist aphasic syndromes, as illustrated by Benson and Ardila (1996).

THE LURIA SCHOOL

In the Eastern European countries, Luria was the most influential figure. In 1947 he published in Russian an important book, *Traumatic aphasia*, based on the observation of traumatic patients. Luria took an intermediate position between the associationist and holistic approaches. According to him, attempts to solve the problem of the relationship between language and brain have all led to dead ends. The associationists' attempts to solve the problem of the cerebral localization of language involved a search for a direct localization of distinct language capacities, such as comprehension, reading or writing, in definite brain centers. The idea of direct localization of complex linguistic abilities in specific cerebral areas was rejected by researchers of the holistic camp, who believed that the pathological condition does not depend on the site of the lesion but rather on the quantity of cerebral tissue damaged. In Luria's view, both positions must be rejected. He argues that the relationship between language and brain is an indirect one and that an isomorphic relation between language and brain does not exist. According to Luria, pathological conditions of the brain cannot produce a direct disintegration of a specific aspect of language, and attempts to correlate a given cerebral area directly with a given language task only have the value of an initial summary of clinical observations. Nor, he argues, can the idea of mass action of the human brain hold and, indeed, the idea that the brain is a homogeneous and undifferentiated mass of tissue conflicts with known clinical facts and studies of brain morphology.

Luria thus rejected both the associationist and the holistic approaches and argued for a functional representation distributed over widespread areas. His basic concept is that the brain is divided into three basic functional parts: the anterior part for programming and controlling human actions; the posterior part for reception, elaboration, and storage of information; and the limbic system responsible for vigilance. Language, as well as any other human behavior, requires coordination of all three functional units. In order to understand the relationship between language and the brain, one has to single out the basic components of language, find the factors needed for its realization, and locate the different parts of the brain that play a role in these factors. Normal articulation, for example, requires an acoustic analysis of the phonemes, a precise kinesthetic organization of the oral movements, and a smooth transition between them. The acoustic analysis is carried out by the temporal region, the kinesthetic organization by the parietal region, and the smooth transition by the premotor cortex. Any lesion in this functional system impairs articulation, but in different degrees and in different ways.

Functional systems are based on a network of neurological structures, which are linked in the execution of a common task. A brain lesion can damage a link in this functional system, but the system enjoys a certain degree of plasticity and the damaged link can be reorganized. When this happens, it is again possible to perform the damaged task.

Luria published "Traumatic aphasia" in 1947 and "Restoration of function after brain injury" in 1948 in Russian. His views on aphasia rapidly became known and appreciated in Eastern Europe and by a small group of Western colleagues but remained unknown to the majority of researchers in the field of aphasia. Only 20 years later were his books translated into English (Luria, 1963, 1970). A renewal of interest in the work of Luria is demonstrated by various recent publications, among which are the book *Contemporary neuropsychology and the legacy of Luria*, edited by Goldberg (1990), and two special issues, one in *Journal of Neurolinguistics* (vol. 4, n. 1, 1989) and one in *Aphasiology* (vol. 9, n. 2, 1995).

CONCLUSIONS

After a period of glory in the second half of the nineteenth century, associationist theories were largely abandoned. The early classification of syndromes was discarded and more general principles were proposed to explain language disorders. The holists generally claimed that the variety of the clinical pictures was not intrinsic to aphasia, although it was recognized that aphasic patients differ in many respects, not only the severity of the language disorder. The associationists considered language the sum of a number of faculties—comprehension, production, reading, and writing—that can be separately damaged. They emphasized the aspects that differentiate one form of aphasia from the others, relating them to damage of different cerebral areas. By contrast, the holists emphasized the common aspects of the language breakdown in aphasic patients.

It seems reasonable to describe the history of the first decades of aphasia research as marked by the important question of the psychological nature of language and its neuroanatomical correlates, but it is somewhat misleading simply to oppose associationists and holists. The dichotomy is oversimplified, and various positions can be recognized in both camps. Among the authors generally referred to as associationists, Geschwind, for instance, makes a distinction between the associationists and the *mosaicists*, who multiplied specific centers (Geschwind, 1967). Notwithstanding the internal differences, it is, however, possible to recognize a certain degree of homogeneity in the associationist camp and, perhaps more significantly, a certain accumulation of knowledge. Broca stated that a lesion in a specific area of the brain causes a certain language impairment. Wernicke offered the first model of language functioning that incorporated Broca's discovery and was enriched by Lichtheim. Finally, Dejerine added more precise knowledge about reading processes.

On the holistic side, positions differed more widely and critics of the associationist school came from a variety of positions. Jackson viewed language in hierarchical terms, each level of language processing corresponding to the function of a phylogenetic successive level in the nervous system. Marie denied that aphasia was a language disorder; he considered it to be the expression of damage to a more general capacity, such as general intelligence. Goldstein argued that a single impairment (loss of abstract thinking) is at the core of the aphasic disorder, although it cannot explain all the different manifestations of aphasia. Schuell, more pragmatically, performed a factorial analysis of aphasic patients' test results and identified a common general factor that she interpreted as being the essence of aphasia.

However, the two positions are not as irreconcilable as could be expected, and the clinical observations reported by authors of the two camps are very similar.

CHAPTER

2

CLASSIFICATION OF THE APHASIAS

THE FIRST 80 YEARS OF STUDIES IN APHASIA produced many interesting findings, such as the discovery that lesions in specific parts of the brain may produce selective cognitive disorders of language, perception, and praxis. Yet, the classic anatomo-clinical method had some limitations connected to the paucity of studied cases and the necessary presence of a striking defect, with the obvious consequence that *negative cases* (patients with damage in a given area without the expected symptoms), were not taken into consideration. The classic anatomo-clinical correlation method inferred the neural basis of a cognitive function from the clinical analysis of the damaged behavior and the subsequent (generally postmortem) localization of the lesion. However, if only *positive cases*, namely, patients in whom a given area is damaged and the putative corresponding symptoms are present, are considered, it is not possible to demonstrate whether a lesion in a given area always damages a specific function. In addition, it is always risky to extrapolate from a single case. One should wait for replications before reaching a conclusion about a relationship between a given impaired function and a specific cerebral area. Finally, many patients die long after having been examined; they may survive for many years, and when they undergo autopsy, it is not always easy to identify the exact lesion that produced the symptoms of interest.

On the clinical side, an important limitation of the clinical methodology concerns the clear definition of the symptoms. It is generally agreed that a patient with severe and pervasive language disorders is aphasic, but what about a patient affected by only subtle comprehension disorders or very mild word-finding difficulties? In these cases, it is indispensable to have some norms against which to compare the subjects' results.

A new era in neuropsychology began at approximately the same time as the associationist theory was relaunched by Geschwind in 1965. The major difference between the associationist and the modern neoassociationist approach to the study of aphasia lay in the methodology adopted. In the modern era, clearly defined and standardized methods largely replaced the classic clinical evaluation. The advantages of such a method are obvious. Studies were performed on groups of patients chosen for the presence of a lesion rather than the presence of a symptom. This allowed negative cases, if any, to be observed. Another nonnegligible advantage was the opportunity to compare the performance of two or more patients; this is not possible if the patients have not been examined in the same way. Furthermore, the patient's performance could be compared with that of normal subjects if data from a normal control group were collected in constructing the battery. Finally, the main aim of a standardized test is to compare results among the groups studied (namely, controls versus aphasics, right- versus left-hemisphere-damaged patients, or groups of patients with different intrahemispheric lesions). This requires the use of statistical analyses, which are, with all their limitations, the most reliable way to compare results of different groups or results among subjects in the same group.

It was approximately in these same years that Luria's writings began to be widely known in the Western countries.

Chapter 2 briefly describes two classifications of aphasic disorders: Luria's classification and the neoassociationist classification of the aphasias generally accepted in the Western countries. The two classifications differ both in the types of patients studied and the methodology used. Luria's approach is based on a precise theoretical position and detailed clinical observations Two assumptions are fundamental in Luria's neuropsychological theory. First, a function such as reading, for example, is not directly connected with a single and specific cerebral area. Lesions in different parts of the brain can damage the function. Second, the observed damage is qualitatively different according to the location of the lesion. Luria studied patients with head trauma and did not make use of quantitative and standardized measures. By contrast, the neoassociationist approach studied patients with vascular lesions, had as a starting point the assumption that

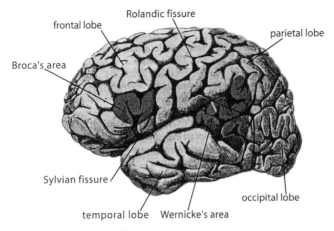

Figure 2–1. Lateral view of the left hemisphere.

language behaviors are related to specific areas of the brain, and used standardized tests for the evaluation and diagnosis of aphasic patients.

Many other classifications have been proposed, but none has gained wide support or stood the test of time. Luria's classification, by contrast, is still used in some Eastern countries, and the neoassociationist taxonomy is still very popular among clinicians, notwithstanding severe critics, the growing use of single-case studies, and the fact that the very idea of a taxonomy of aphasic disorders has been criticized (e.g., Caramazza, 1984; Schwartz, 1984, Chapter 5, this volume).

In describing the neoassociationist aphasic syndromes Benson and Ardila's (1996) taxonomy, which is very close to the nineteenth-century classification, will be followed. (For a more detailed description see Albert et al., 1981, and Benson and Ardila, 1996.) To help visualize the anatomical loci named, a lateral view of the left hemisphere is presented in Figure 2–1.

Three aphasia examinations based on different interpretations of aphasia will also be described and some limits of the neoassociationist syndrome approach pointed out. Goodglass's (1993) proposal, which takes into account the criticisms raised against the syndrome approach even though it remains in the classic tradition, closes the chapter.

LURIA'S CLASSIFICATION

Luria was concerned with how language function can be disturbed in different tasks rather than with the relative impairment of various language behaviors, which is the basis of the associationist and neoassociationist classifications. He isolated six aphasic syndromes, which will be briefly described together with the basic factor that, according to Luria, lies at their root. His taxonomy was based on relatively young patients with brain trauma, and the clinical pictures he describes, although similar to the neoassociationist syndromes mainly based on older patients with vascular disease, are not identical. One reason for that is the difference in etiologies. Moreover, no description is totally objective; it reflects the influences of its author's views. The six clinical forms are dynamic aphasia, afferent motor aphasia, efferent motor aphasia, sensory aphasia, acoustico-amnestic aphasia, and semantic aphasia (Luria, 1964, 1970).

Dynamic Aphasia

Patients with dynamic aphasia do not have naming or comprehension disorders but are unable to develop narrative speech. This defect is most evident when they have to produce spontaneous connected speech or answer questions. They repeat the question echolalically or respond with a cliché. If the question requires the formulation of structured and connected sentences, the patient is unable to do it. Luria quotes the example of a patient who, asked to talk about the North, said, "The North. In the North there are bears" and, after a long delay added, "That's what I must tell you" (Luria, 1964, p. 159). The defect in dynamic aphasia cannot be explained by a memory disorder because the patient can answer questions about a narrative he or she has just read but cannot report it without being prompted by questions. Luria acknowledges that the basic deficit is not clearly identified but argues for a disturbance of the "predicative function of speech." According to Luria, we cannot directly transform a thought into an extended sentence; there is an intermediate state, *inner speech*, which is the transitional link between thought and language. "This inner speech is supposed to be a mechanism used by the subject for a transition from a preliminary idea to the extended verbal proposition. We hypothesize that this inner speech with its predicative function, which takes part in forming the structure or scheme of a sentence, is disturbed in cases of dynamic aphasia" (Luria, 1964, p. 103). As a rule, dynamic aphasia arises as a result of a lesion involving the frontal lobe just anterior to Broca's area.

Afferent Motor Aphasia

In afferent motor aphasia the lesion is located in the lower part of the post-central region, and it impairs the afferent basis of articulatory movements.

The complex realization of delicate articulatory movements requires continuous afferent correction. The patient with afferent motor aphasia does not differentiate among similar articulatory positions and substitutes similar phonemes in speech production. This is the primary defect, which inevitably causes secondary disturbances in comprehension, reading, and writing. As far as writing is concerned, the patient is generally unable to write the letters representing sounds that he or she is unable to produce since, according to Luria, articulation participates actively in writing. In reading, the patient has great difficulty blending the sequences of letters because he or she cannot categorize them into variants of particular phonemes, thus producing errors similar to those found in speech and writing. Finally, acoustic speech processes are altered and phonemes cannot be easily differentiated, causing a comprehension disorder.

Efferent Motor Aphasia

This form of aphasia corresponds to classic Broca aphasia with damage to Broca's area. The ability to articulate individual sounds is preserved, but the smooth transition from one sound to the next is impaired. The serial organization of the spoken word is disturbed, and this shows up in writing as well. The difficulty in transition is also evident in whole sentences, especially during recovery, and the patient exhibits "telegram-style" speech that more or less corresponds to agrammatic speech (see infra). According to Luria, the grammatical structure of language is based on internalized dynamic schemata that are lost in efferent motor aphasia. In this form of aphasia, words retain only their static designative function and can be used to name objects, but the patient is unable to string them together to form grammatically correct sentences. The patient utters series of unrelated words, generally nouns, in spontaneous production and in repetition.

Sensory Aphasia

A lesion in the posterior part of the first left temporal convolution causes impairment of auditory analysis and a deficit in the analysis and synthesis of phonemes. Disintegration of phonemic hearing is an unavoidable consequence. This primary disturbance is the source of all the symptoms of sensory aphasia: disturbances in speech production, repetition, comprehension, reading, and writing. Naturally, disintegration of phonemic hearing prevents the patient from distinguishing sounds in the flow of speech and thus leads to comprehension and repetition disorders. Naming and

speech production in general are impaired because the sound structure of
the words is disturbed. The writing disorder is similar to the speech
production disorder and is due to the loss of the sound structure of words.
Reading is less affected than writing; reading impairment is most evident
when the patient has to read an unfamiliar word on the basis of its
phonetic structure; reading of familiar words that can be performed in an
ideogrammatic way can be spared. Reading of numbers, which does not
require auditory mediation, is also spared in sensory aphasia.

Acoustico-Amnestic Aphasia

Lesions of the temporal lobe, in an area just below that causing sensory
aphasia, produce a similar but less severe form of aphasia. Phonemic hearing may be relatively intact since the auditory association area is not
destroyed. The impairment may be evident only in special situations that
require stable retention of auditory traces, as when the patient, for
instance, is required to repeat three words that are similar in sound structure, such as *table, cable, stable*. When the acoustic load is great, acoustico-
amnestic patients may have difficulty understanding the meaning of
uncommon words.

Semantic Aphasia

In afferent motor aphasia, efferent motor aphasia, sensory aphasia, and
acoustico-amnestic aphasia, the articulatory-acoustic organization of
language is impaired. This level is preserved in semantic aphasia, in which
the semantic organization of language is defective. According to Luria, the
meaning of a sentence is not given by the simple summation of the meanings of the isolated words; it requires a complex simultaneous synthesis of the
words that compose the sentence. Patients with semantic aphasia do not have
problems understanding isolated words, but they have difficulty comprehending such constructions as "the brother's father" or "the father's brother"
or spatial relations as "the circle under the square" or "the square under the
circle." The primary underlying deficit is impaired simultaneous synthesis
that is associated with damage to the parieto-temporo-occipital junction.

NEOASSOCIATIONIST CLASSIFICATION

As argued before, the neoassociationist syndromes are still very popular
among clinicians. Even when patients are not explicitly classified, the

information given can easily be traced back to such a taxonomic approach. The most recent detailed description of the classic syndromes is Benson and Ardila's (1996), which will be summarized here.

Benson and Ardila argue that "although limited and imperfect, the syndrome classification originally developed by the nineteenth-century continental investigators remains basically accurate, replicable, and clinically useful" (Benson & Ardila, 1996, pp. 111–112). However, within many of the classic syndromes Benson and Ardila recognize the existence of two symptom clusters sufficiently constant and different to be separately classified.

Benson and Ardila's idea of a syndrome is something defined by a cluster of symptoms plus a specified brain lesion. As we shall see, there is no absolute relationship between the type of aphasia and the site of damage, but it is difficult to understand which of the two criteria, in Benson and Ardila's view, is predominant. Sometimes the symptom cluster seems to predominate, as when they write that "In keeping with the clinical style of the present volume, however, the features will be discussed as symptom clusters, not as general clinical–anatomical correlates" (p. 168). But at other times the predominant role appears to be played by the site of the lesion. This can be inferred from statements such as "the classification of aphasic syndromes based on cortical involvement that will be followed in this volume" (p. 119) or "the marked variations in the locus of lesions producing the symptom cluster cast doubt about the reliability of anomic aphasia as a clinical entity" (p. 165).

Leaving aside the question of what Benson and Ardila exactly mean by an aphasic syndrome, their classification starts from two primary anatomical divisions: pre- and postrolandic and perisylvian and extrasylvian. Common to all perisylvian lesion syndromes is impaired repetition, whereas in all extrasylvian syndromes repetition is preserved. The prerolandic–postrolandic dichotomy closely corresponds to the nonfluent/fluent dichotomy proposed by the Geschwind school. Nonfluent or prerolandic speech is sparse and effortful; fluent or post-Rolandic speech is well articulated and paraphasic. In the description of the clinical types of aphasia, the perisylvian and extrasylvian dichotomy will be taken as starting point.

Perisylvian Syndromes

The perisylvian syndromes are Broca aphasia, Wernicke aphasia, and conduction aphasia, the three forms of aphasia described by Wernicke. According to Benson and Ardila, these syndromes are "supported by a great deal of corroborating anatomical and clinical data" and "represent the most stable material available for brain–language correlation purposes" (p. 145).

Broca aphasia. In Broca aphasia speech output is nonfluent, sparse, effortful, and consists of short phrases. Overlearned series, such as counting or reciting the days of the week, usually can be well articulated. The articulation deficit (the *anarthria* of Marie) is now generally regarded as an *apraxia of speech* (Rosenbeck et al., 1989); the term *apraxia* underlines the fact that articulation can be more or less preserved in automatic series, while it is damaged in more intentional speech. Repetition and reading aloud are difficult. *Anomia*—a general term for almost any condition in which an aphasic patient has difficulty finding words—is always present, and the majority of Broca aphasics have a more or less severe agrammatism. Agrammatism is hard to define because of the great variability of symptoms among patients. Clinically, patients are defined as agrammatic if they speak in short phrases, with loss of subordination, and omit function words; verbs tend to be used incorrectly, with omission of tense and person designations, and there is a relative abundance of nouns with respect to verbs.

Comprehension in Broca aphasia is relatively good in a conversational situation but can be shown to be impaired whenever comprehension of syntactic structures is necessary. Broca aphasics have difficulty comprehanding reversible sentences (such as "John is following Mary"), which require them to grasp the word order, and difficulty comprehending the passive construction, in which the grammatical subject is not the same as the logical subject. In the sentence "The apple was eaten by John," *apple* is the grammatical subject but it is John who does the eating. Reading comprehension generally parallels auditory comprehension. Writing is impaired, with misspellings and letter omissions; spontaneous writing is very poor and frequently agrammatic.

Broca aphasic patients generally have oral and ideomotor apraxia and right hemiplegia or hemiparesis. The lesion is located in the frontal lobe.

According to Benson and Ardila, two subtypes of Broca aphasia can be distinguished, depending on the severity of the disorder and the amount of recovery. In Broca aphasia Type I, defects of articulation are mild, agrammatism is rarely total, comprehension is good, hemiparesis is minimal, and recovery is rapid. This restricted form of Broca aphasia occurs when damage is limited to Broca's area and the immediate subcortical structures. The full-blown picture of Broca aphasia—Broca aphasia Type II—is more severe and long-lasting, and it is caused by more extensive lesions that affect the operculum, the insula, and the periventricular white matter.

Wernicke aphasia. In this form of aphasia, verbal output is fluent and frequently abundant; articulation, prosody, and phrase length are normal. Verbal output is characterized by the presence of paraphasias (at the phonological or lexical level) and empty words (such as *thing, affair*) with a relative paucity of semantically rich content words. Writing is always impaired and qualitatively similar to verbal output; that is, it is very rare to find letter distortions in the same way as there are no articulatory disorders in speech. Furthermore, misspellings appear in writing if phonemic paraphasias are frequent in oral production, and spontaneous writing is laden with paraphasias if verbal paraphasias are frequent in speech. Repetition and reading aloud are also impaired, but the defining feature of Wernicke aphasia has always been considered the comprehension deficit, and many authors (for instance, Albert et al., 1981) argue that comprehension is always severely impaired in Wernicke aphasia.

However, patients with all the characteristics of Wernicke aphasia but whose comprehension is only moderately impaired are common; aphasia can be moderate from the onset or patients can partially recover, and auditory comprehension is the first verbal behavior to improve in most patients (see infra). One can either do without the constraint of "severely" impaired comprehension and classify these patients as Wernicke aphasics or choose to consider these patients "unclassifiable" due to their relatively preserved comprehension.

Ideomotor apraxia is common in Wernicke aphasia. Routine neurological examination will frequently disclose a visual field defect—a quadrantanopia or hemianopia—but motor disorders are rare.

Since the first description by Wernicke, there has been general agreement about the locus of the brain pathology in Wernicke aphasia: the posterior-superior temporal region in the left hemisphere.

Benson and Ardila describe two types of Wernicke aphasia. What distinguishes the two types is the relative impairment of auditory and reading comprehension. In Wernicke aphasia Type I, reading comprehension is better preserved than auditory comprehension, while the reverse is true in Wernicke aphasia Type II.

Conduction aphasia. In conduction aphasia speech output is fluent, that is, it is not scarce and there is no apraxia of speech. Speech flow is, however, frequently interrupted by phonemic paraphasias and *conduites* *d'approche*—successive phonemic variations of the target word, which are produced by the patient as self-corrections—a phenomenon typical of conduction aphasia. The *conduites d'approche* can end up with the correct word or a phonemic paraphasia. Comprehension is only moderately or mildly impaired. The third basic characteristic of conduction aphasia is severely impaired repetition; errors in repetition are mainly at the phonological level and very much resemble errors in naming and spontaneous production. The repetition deficit has classically been explained in terms of the disconnection of language comprehension from speech output (Lichteim, 1885; Geschwind, 1965; Damasio & Damasio, 1980). Reading comprehension is relatively well preserved, but reading aloud is clumsy because of the ubiquitous phonemic errors. Writing, either spontaneous or to dictation, is impaired.

The defining symptoms of conduction aphasia (relatively preserved comprehension and more impaired repetition in a fluent aphasic) define a dissociation, whose degree is undetermined. This allows for highly subjective criteria, and patients classified as conduction aphasics can be highly heterogeneous with respect to the defining characteristics of conduction aphasia. Resorting to the localization of the lesion to identify a more homogeneous group of patients is of no great help because there is no clear agreement about the locus of damage in conduction aphasia. It was originally considered a disconnection syndrome, with damage in the left arcuate fasciculus that runs from Wernicke's to Broca's area (Wernicke, 1874; Geschwind, 1965; Damasio and Damasio, 1980). More recently, a wide cortico-subcortical area has been considered important in the genesis of conduction aphasia. This area, which can be variably destroyed, comprises the primary auditory cortex, the insula and its subcortical white matter, and the supramarginal gyrus (Damasio, 1991). Ideomotor apraxia is common, and motor and/or sensory deficits can also be present.

Extrasylvian Syndromes

The extrasylvian syndromes comprise anomic aphasia and the transcortical aphasias. In all these cases, repetition is normal or nearly so.

Transcortical motor aphasia. This is a rather infrequent form of aphasia. Benson and Ardila identify two subtypes. Common to both are nonfluent speech, good comprehension, and preserved repetition. Naming is also good, but spontaneous verbal output is almost absent. Patients tend to speak very little, do not start a conversation, and respond with incomplete sentences, although grammar is generally correct. Reading comprehension is also good, but reading aloud can be defective.

The main differences between Type I and Type II are the locus of the lesion and the accompanying neurological symptoms. According to Benson and Ardila, in Type I the dorsolateral prefrontal area is damaged and in Type II the supplementary motor area. As for the accompanying neurological symptoms, in Type II there is mild dysarthria and motor and sensory disorders of the contralateral lower extremity. Extra-aphasic neurological signs can be absent in Type I. Praxis is normal in both forms of transcortical motor aphasia.

Transcortical sensory aphasia. This too is a rare syndrome. It is due to damage in the posterior language area. Benson and Ardila's Type I closely resembles the commonly described form of transcortical sensory aphasia. Language is fluent but lacks communicative value because of the presence of frequent verbal paraphasias, which can sometimes render the patient's production totally unintelligible; in this case we speak of *verbal jargon*. *Echolalia*, a patient's tendency to repeat what has been just said to him or her, may be present. Writing, spontaneous and to dictation, is impaired. Comprehension of oral and written language is severely impaired. Reading aloud can be relatively well preserved, but the salient characteristic of this form of aphasia is preserved repetition of words and sentences.

Two studies (Whitaker, 1976; Davis et al., 1978) have shown that transcortical sensory aphasics do sometimes correct grammatical errors (such as gender or number agreement) in repeating sentences that they do not understand.

Ideative apraxia is frequently associated with this form of aphasia; ideomotor apraxia is less common but can also be present. Routine neurological examination generally discloses a visual field defect—quadrantanopia or hemianopia.

According to Benson and Ardila, the lesion is "usually located at the junction of the temporal, parietal, and occipital lobes (roughly, the lower angular gyrus and upper portion of Brodmann area 37)" (1996 p. 158).

Their Type II is a less severe form of aphasia. Speech is fluent, with frequent circumlocutions and rare content words. Comprehension is sufficient for conversational purposes. The patients, however, fail to comprehend complex sentences and do not grasp the meaning of relationships. Repetition is preserved, but reading and writing are impaired.

Praxis is generally impaired. The lesion lies approximately in the parietal-lobe angular gyrus, but there is no general agreement on the specific locus of the lesion, which also explains some variations in the clinical picture.

Anomic aphasia. Anomia in confrontation naming tasks and spontaneous speech is the main symptom in anomic aphasia. Word-finding difficulties can be equally present for all grammatical classes of words or can be more evident for nouns than verbs (e.g., Miceli et al., 1984, 1988b); other errors, such as phonemic and verbal paraphasias, can also be present but are rare. Comprehension is preserved, as is repetition. The main difference with the above-described transcortical sensory aphasia Type II is that in anomic aphasia reading and writing are not or only mildly impaired.

Classically, anomic aphasia was related to damage to the posterior language areas (Brodmann areas 37 and 39) (Brain, 1961; Newcombe et al., 1971). However, it is now generally held that anomic aphasia is the endpoint of many recovered aphasics (Kertesz & McCabe, 1977), and as such it has no localizing value. Even when anomic aphasia appears in the acute stage it cannot be reliably localized. Separate brain areas are, in fact, activated in confrontation naming tasks, depending on the type of stimulus to be named (Damasio et al., 1996).

Global Aphasia

Benson and Ardila mention global aphasia only as the syndrome resulting from total occlusion of the middle cerebral artery; they do not include it when describing the various aphasic syndromes. However, global aphasia is a fairly frequent occurrence in which all aspects of speech and language are severely affected. Oral production is nonfluent and scarce and may be limited to a stereotypic utterance ("tan," "lelo") or to a few different syllables. Reading and writing are totally abolished, and the patient may even be unable to trace his or her signature. When tested, comprehension is nil but the patient can sometimes understand some context-related personal question or commands ("Are you married?" "Close your eyes"). Global aphasia is generally associated with apraxia—oral, ideomotor, and ideative—and with motor and sensory disorders; sometimes visual field defects are also present.

In most cases, the lesion destroys large portions of the anterior and posterior language zone.

Subcortical Aphasia

All the syndromes so far described were already known and discussed in the nineteenth century. Subsequently there was a more detailed clinical observation that led to the distinction of different types in many aphasic syndromes and more precise neuroanatomical localizations. In addition, specificity of subcortical aphasia has been recognized. The notion that aphasia can ensue from subcortical lesions is not new (e.g., Henschen, 1922). Yet, the introduction of computed tomography (CT) and magnetic resonance imaging (MRI) in clinical practice has allowed investigators to identify lesions of the subcortical white matter and the striato-capsular region and to study the relationship between language disturbances and damage in these areas in series of patients. Patients with aphasia from established purely subcortical lesions, however, are fairly rare since the locus of the lesion can be identified only by means of neuroradiological studies that are not always available. Besides, negative cases are frequent; many patients with subcortical lesions identified by a CT scan have no signs of aphasic disorder (Vignolo et al., 1992). The physiopathological mechanisms underlying subcortical aphasia are also unclear. Whether language disorders are the direct result of subcortical damage or the result of hypoperfusion of or disconnection from cortical areas remains an unsolved issue.

Benson and Ardila describe three different subcortical syndromes: striato-capsular aphasia, thalamic aphasia, and aphasia associated with white-matter disease. However, there is no general agreement about the possibility of distinguishing with sufficient certainty different symptom clusters related to the site of the subcortical lesion. The main character- istics found in subcortical aphasia will be described without trying to differentiate them, depending on the locus of brain damage.

As a rule, in subcortical aphasia repetition is preserved but hypopho- nia—a reduction in voice volume—is a frequent finding. Speech produc- tion is fluent but rather scarce; word-finding problems are present, and writing is impaired. Oral and written comprehension is relatively preserved; so is reading aloud. The language disorder is generally mild or moderate, and recovery can be rapid. Following the development of a left thalamic lesion, transcortical-like symptoms are frequent (Cappa & Vignolo, 1979). Depending on the site of the lesion, neurological impairments such as hemiparesis or hemisensory loss can be present.

APHASIA EXAMINATIONS

By the end of World War II, many aphasiologists were aware of the limitations of the clinical method and of the necessity for more objective evaluations. Also, in response to the growing demand for rehabilitation, various standardized tests for aphasia based on statistical analyses were published. These tests allow comparison of patients' results with those of normal controls as well as among patients and groups of patients with similar lesion. Three of these tests, which were among the first to appear in the literature and which are based on different theoretical positions and aims, will now be described.

The Minnesota Test for Differential Diagnosis of Aphasia (MTDDA; Schuell, 1955) is the result of numerous revisions of an original experimental version and was administered to hundreds of patients. The test reflects Schuell's belief that language is unitary and aphasia is one, and that all aphasic disorders involve a unitary loss of language, which may vary in severity or because of accompanying disorders. Accordingly, the MTDDA identifies five syndromes: simple aphasia, aphasia with visual involvement, aphasia with sensorimotor involvement, aphasia with generalized brain damage, and irreversible aphasic syndrome. It is composed of five sections evaluating auditory disturbances, visual and reading disturbances, speech and language disturbances, visuomotor and writing disturbances, and numerical and arithmetic disturbances. Each section comprises a sizable number of subtests, generally organized from the easiest to the most difficult, where the degree of difficulty is mainly evaluated by phonological complexity and length. The evaluation can be started at any level according to the patient's impairment.

To Schuell, the most important goal of evaluation is to guide therapy, which the MTDDA does with ease. In Schuell's view, treatment for aphasia does not vary qualitatively from patient to patient, but according to the severity of the language impairment and to the accompanying disorders, which are clearly reflected by the test results.

The Boston Diagnostic Aphasia Examination (BDAE; Goodglass & Kaplan, 1972; 2nd edition, 1983) has as its primary focus the diagnosis of classic anatomically based aphasic syndromes. This diagnostic goal is easily attained because the BDAE has been standardized on a sample of 207 aphasic patients with well-defined aphasic syndromes and distinct lesions. Characteristic profiles of the various syndromes have been drawn and permit comparison of individual results with these typical profiles. Many patients do not fall into any of these clearly separated syndromes and are considered unclassifiable. The test comprises five sections, each composed of many subtests, evaluating comprehension, production, reading, writing, and repetition. Scores on each subtest are transformed into standardized z-scores.

An important aspect of the BDAE is its careful analysis of conversational and expository speech. A speech characteristics' profile is derived that allows the examiner to make a differential diagnosis between fluent and nonfluent aphasics.

The Neurosensory Center Comprehensive Examination for Aphasia (NCCEA; Spreen & Benton, 1977) is guided neither by a preconceived theoretical interpretation of the nature of the aphasic disorder nor by a therapeutic goal, as are the BDAE and the MTDDA. It is composed of 20 subtests that focus on language comprehension, language production, reading, and writing, and of four control subtests of visual and tactile processing that allow the examiner to differentiate deficits on other tasks as either linguistic in nature or due to other dysfunctions. Normative data are based on the results of 206 unselected aphasic patients. Individual results, corrected for the influence of age and education, are converted into percentile scores. These can be compared to three different profiles based on results achieved by normal controls, aphasic patients, and nonaphasic brain-damaged patients.

The NCCEA provides a comprehensive assessment of language function, but the low ceiling of some of the subtests (naming, for instance) does not permit the recognition of subtle disorders. Other tests are sufficiently complex to avoid a ceiling effect in normal controls.

In the following years, further aphasia batteries appeared in other countries and in different languages, and numerous methods are now available for assessing language disorders. Each battery is based on an explicit or implicit interpretation of the nature of aphasia, and each has a main goal. When aphasiologists began to think that the most important impairment in aphasia was the loss of communicative competence, for instance, batteries aimed at evaluating the patient's communicative capacities were developed. Among these are the Functional Communication Profile (FCP; Sarno, 1969) and the Communicative Abilities in Daily Living (CADL; Holland, 1980). When cognitive neuropsychologists directed their attention to normal models of language processing and the underlying functional damage that caused the aphasic symptoms, tests aimed at assessing the various components of the model of language processing were devised. One such test is Psycholinguistic Assessment of Language Processing in Aphasia (PALPA; Kay et al., 1992).

No single existing aphasia battery can answer questions about classification, functional diagnosis, treatment, and recovery. It is up to the examiner to select the best one for his or her goals, but it must not be forgotten that no battery can answer questions that were not foreseen in its development.

SOME LIMITS IN THE NEOASSOCIATIONIST THEORY

The syndrome approach based on correlating language processing disorders with focal brain lesions has been criticized by cognitive neuropsychologists, who denied the usefulness of this approach for the study of the functional structure of normal cognitive systems (see Chapter 5). Even within the sphere of the classic approach, however, it has become evident that there is no absolute relationship between the locus of the cerebral lesion and the pattern of cognitive impairments. For some populations, such as left-handers and children, it has long been known that the classic anatomo-clinical relationship does not hold. For other groups, women and illiterates for example, it has recently been argued that the intrahemispheric organization is different from standard teaching. Moreover, in determining the relationship between the locus of a lesion and a specific syndrome, etiology is also important. In addition, postacute aphasic patients can be more reliably classified than chronic patients because the clinical picture evolves and the patient partially recovers with time. Finally, the aphasia batteries are not neutral, and patients can be classified differently if examined with different aphasia batteries. These factors, which must be taken into consideration in the study of antomo-clinical correlations, are briefly illustrated.

Population

From the very first assertion that the left hemisphere is dominant for language, it was also argued that this is not true for everybody. Broca (1865), in fact, stated that left-handers have right hemisphere dominance for language.

In 1949, Wada (1949) described a procedure for anesthetizing one hemisphere by injecting a short-acting barbiturate into one carotid artery. Data obtained by Milner et al. (1964) with the Wada test did not confirm a strong link between handedness and dominance for language. However, they demonstrated that for about one third of left-handers, the left-hemisphere dominance for language is reversed or incomplete. In addition, it has been argued that from a clinical viewpoint, aphasia in left-handers with left hemisphere dominance for language is not identical to aphasia in right-handers and that it has a better prognosis (Subirana, 1969; Luria, 1970; Gloning et al., 1976).

Different brain–language relationships have also been suggested for other populations. In children, the degree of hemispheric dominance for language was argued to develop with advancing age, and major clinical differences between the early and adult forms of aphasia were claimed to exist by the majority of investigators until the 1980s, as well as a much better prognosis for children than adults. The better prognosis was explained by the degree of bilaterality of the representation of language and the clinical differences by a different intrahemispheric organization of language (Basser, 1962; Collignon et al., 1968; Loonen & van Dongen, 1991; Martins & Ferro, 1991). A difference in organization has also been claimed for women (McGlone, 1977, 1980; Basso et al., 1982a; Pizzamiglio et al., 1985) and for illiterates (see Coppens et al., 1998b, for review). Without going into detail about the peculiarity of brain–language organization in each of these populations compared with the standard teaching of language organization, it is clear that the syndromes described above and their corresponding locus of the lesion are considered valid for a relatively limited part of the world's population (see Coppens et al., 1998a, for a recent view of aphasia in atypical populations).

Etiology

A significant determinant of aphasic syndromes is etiology. The classic aphasic syndromes are based on patients with vascular disease whose lesional localization is partially circumscribed by the vascular system. Traumatic lesions, which are the second most frequent cause of aphasia, are not identical to vascular lesions, and the same syndromes cannot be expected. This is evident if one considers Luria's (1964, 1970) classification of traumatic aphasia. Notwithstanding some obvious similarities between his and the classic taxonomy, some differences are evident. These differences can be traced in part to different theoretical interpretations of aphasia that lead investigators to emphasize the clinical features that best correspond to their personal theoretical interpretation. However, to understand the difference between the clinical pictures described by Luria and those in classic aphasiology, one has to take into consideration etiology as well, which is mainly vascular in classic aphasiology and traumatic in Luria's patients.

Another example of a pathology that clearly influences the resulting picture of the cognitive disorder is herpes simplex encephalitis (HSE). The majority of patients with HSE show selective damage to the semantic system (see Gainotti, 2000, for a review).

Time After Onset

Another important element to consider is the time that has elapsed since the onset of the disorder. Improvement from aphasia can initially take place because of changes at the neural level and later because of changes at the behavioral level, whether spontaneous or therapy-induced. In the first weeks following development of an acute brain lesion, perifocal edema and other complications may contribute to the severity of the disorder. Regression of the functional damage usually takes place in the following 1 or 2 months, and the clinical picture partially clears. Between approximately 1 and 2–3 months after onset, the clinical picture best corresponds to the anatomical damage. Further recovery of function takes place in the majority of patients, and in chronic patients it may become difficult to relate the clinical picture to a given lesion site.

Comprehension, for instance, has been shown to be the verbal behavior that recovers first and in the largest number of patients (Kenin & Swisher, 1972; Kertesz & McCabe, 1977; Hanson & Cicciarelli, 1978; Lomas & Kertesz, 1978; Prins et al., 1978; Basso et al., 1982b). The diagnostic difference between a global and a Broca aphasic is based mainly on the level of the comprehension disorder; thus recovery of comprehension in a global aphasic may result in the reclassification of the patient as a Broca aphasic. In addition, with the passing of time, the positive symptoms, such as verbal paraphasias, agrammatism, or jargon (totally incomprehensible fluent output), tend to disappear and to be replaced by negative symptoms such as word-finding difficulties or reduction of speech (e.g., Basso et al., 1996), making a diagnosis more difficult.

Aphasia Testing

As for the impact of the aphasia battery chosen for evaluating a patient, two considerations are in order. First, most of the existing examinations use subjective standards to judge the presence or absence of symptoms that vary on a continuum. The concept of *fluency*, which is fundamental to reaching a correct clinical diagnosis in the neoassociationist approach, is difficult to define because the fluency scale (Goodglass & Kaplan, 1972) does not measure a single well-defined dimension of speech production. It takes into consideration such heterogeneous criteria as phrase length, verbal agility, melodic line, articulation, and grammatical form. Furthermore, in the process of making a diagnosis, one can follow one of two routes: choosing the most probable syndrome and forcing each patient into a diagnostic category or diagnosing the patient as unclassifiable if he or she does not fit well in any of the diagnostic categories. The first is the approach taken by the Western Aphasia Battery (WAB; Kertesz, 1982), the second by the BDAE. Secondly, no examination for aphasia is neutral. It is based on a more or less explicit interpretation of the nature of aphasia, and it can only show what it was constructed to elucidate. For example, if a naming test has not been constructed to measure selectivity in naming disorders, it will probably not comprise items of different semantic or grammatical categories and will be unable to demonstrate a specific naming disorder.

Exceptions

Even in right-handed literate adult patients with vascular disease, a well-defined aphasic syndrome does not determine with certainty the location of the lesion. Although the correlation between the classic syndromes and the expected locus of the lesion has been roughly confirmed by many CT studies, many exceptions to the classic doctrine on language–brain relationships have been found.

Basso and colleagues (1985), for instance, studied the frequency of exceptions to classic aphasia localizations in 267 right-handed literate Italian aphasic vascular patients with a left-hemisphere CT lesion. The most striking exceptions were six cases of fluent aphasia and anterior CT lesions and six cases of nonfluent aphasia and posterior CT lesions, illustrated in Figures 2–2 and 2–3, respectively. The probabilistic nature of the relationship between locus of damage and aphasia type is now widely accepted. An updating of the classic neoassociationist doctrine has been suggested by Goodglass, who, in 1993, proposed an alternative view to the classic one of an invariant relationship between a specific lesion locus and an aphasic syndrome.

AN ALTERNATIVE CLINICAL APPROACH

Goodglass asserts that the variability in lesion site for any aphasic syndrome is such that the standard accepted relationship between a given pattern of language disturbances and brain damage in a given area has only a probabilistic and not a fixed value. According to him, there are "common or modal self-organizing tendencies towards which many brains gravitate" (1993, p. 218), and the classic aphasic syndromes are viewed as "modal patterns of language breakdown" (p. 229). "The anatomical basis of language is constrained by the hard-wired sensory input and motor output systems and by certain essential connecting fibers" (p. 230), but within these boundaries considerable individual variation in the use of resources of the association areas is possible and "each maturing brain finds its own specific, most efficient neural organization for carrying

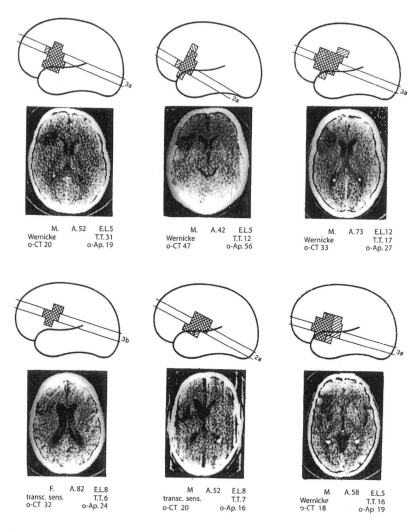

Figure 2–2. CT scans of patients with anterior lesions and fluent aphasia (from Basso et al., 1985). M = male; F = female; A = age; E.L. = educational level (years); T.T. = Token Test's score; o-CT = onset-CT (days); o-Ap = onset-aphasia examination (days).

out the operations of language production and comprehension" (p. 218). For example, Goodglass states that two children acquiring the same language may rely differently on semantic or phonological associations to letter strings in learning to read. Following brain damage, they could therefore develop different reading disorders. Deep dyslexia is a reading disorder characterized, among other errors, by semantic paralexias, such as reading *skirt* for *dress* or *window* for *door* (see Chapter 5). The child who relied more heavily on semantic association in learning to read may

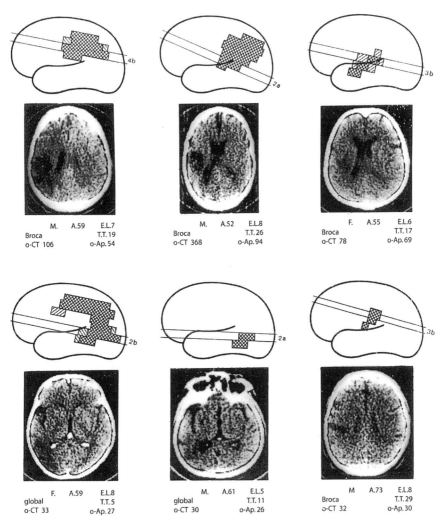

Figure 2–3. CT scans of patients with posterior lesions and nonfluent aphasia (from Basso et al., 1985). Abbreviations: see Figure 2–1.

become a deep dyslexic and produce semantic paralexias if he or she suffers from brain damage in adulthood. The other child, who relied more on phonological associations in learning to read, may not be prone to becoming a deep dyslexic and may make only phonological errors in case of brain damage.

Based on these considerations, Goodglass proposed an alternative method to substitute the classic syndrome-based taxonomy. His approach is clinical in so far as it is based on clinical symptoms; it is hierarchical in that it consists of a decision tree for the first few steps. The examiner bases his or her decisions on some salient differences among patients. The first decision to make is about fluency, but three categories of fluency are now proposed—fluency, nonfluency, and intermediate fluency. The second step varies in the three categories: with or without paraphasia in the fluent category and a severity rating of fluency in the nonfluent and intermediate fluency categories. Successively, a severity rating must be assigned to some important features of the patient's performance. This process ends up with a description of the patient's performance that in some cases can easily be translated into the classic neoassociationist taxonomy, but the clinician is not forced to classify all patients. Figure 2–4 illustrates the decision tree for fluent aphasia.

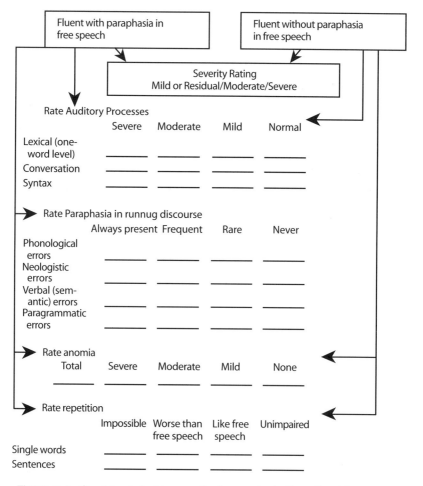

Figure 2–4. Goodglass's decision tree for fluent aphasia (from Goodglass, 1993).

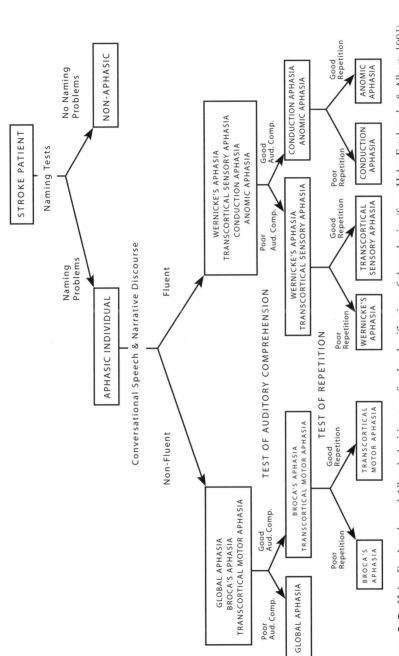

Figure 2–5. Helm-Estabrooks and Albert's decision tree for the classification of the aphasias (from Helm-Estabrooks & Albert, 1991).

This less rigid view of the relationship between the brain structures and the aphasic syndromes in no way diminishes the pragmatic validity of the symptom clusters. At the same time, it acknowledges the existence of some variability among patients classified as having the same syndrome and links it to interindividual variability in the organization of language processes in the brain. An important question that remains unanswered refers to the extent of possible structural variation. If very limited, it would not help explain unexpected brain–behavior relationships; if too large, the whole enterprise of studying brain–behavior relationships would become trivial.

A decision tree for the classification of aphasia also has been suggested by Helm-Estabrooks and Albert (1991). They argue that 80% of vascular patients with aphasia can be reliably classified on the basis of their performance in four language areas: naming, conversational speech, comprehension, and repetition, to be assessed in this same order. Evaluation of naming permits the examiner to distinguish aphasic from nonaphasic patients, assessment of conversational speech in aphasic patients differentiates between fluent and nonfluent aphasics; assessment of comprehension and repetition allows one to reach a specific diagnosis. Figure 2–5 outlines the diagnostic tree for aphasia in vascular patients.

CONCLUSIONS

A parallel between Luria's and the neoassociationist classification of the aphasias has frequently been drawn. It has been maintained that efferent motor aphasia, for example, corresponds to Broca aphasia, afferent motor aphasia to conduction aphasia, acoustico-amnestic aphasia to transcortical sensory aphasia, and so forth (e.g., Benson & Ardila, 1996).

Actually, as argued before, the two classifications have widely different origins. Firstly, the patients studied differ. Luria based his classification on traumatic patients, whereas vascular patients are at the basis of the classic neoassociationist classification. Secondly, Luria's interpretation of the aphasia started from a neurolinguistic process model concerned with the qualitative nature of the language breakdown. The associationists' and neoassociationists' primary interest lay in anatomical–clinical correlations. This does not mean that there are no similarities between the two classifications, but the resemblance is superficial. Luria did not provide any standard tools to evaluate aphasia, and he created testing tasks on the spot and followed his clinical intuition. By contrast, as noted when discussing it, the BDAE was standardized on a large sample of aphasic

TABLE 2–1. Comparison of Different Classifications

Benson (1979)	Broca (1865)	Lichtheim (1885)	Head (1926)	Weisemburg & McBride (1935)	Goldstein (1948)	Gloning et al. (1963)	Bay (1964)	Wepman & Jones (1964)	Luria (1964)	Kertesz & Phipps (1977)	Hécaen & Albert (1978)
Broca	Aphemia	Cortical motor	Verbal	Expressive	Central motor	Motor	Cortical dysarthria	Syntactic	Efferent motor	Broca	Pure motor
Wernicke	Verbal amnesia	Cortical sensory	Syntactic	Receptive	Wernicke sensory	Sensory	Sensory	Jargon, pragmatic	Sensory	Wernicke	Sensory
Conduction		Conduction			Central	Conduction	Sensory		Afferent motor	Efferent and affernt conduction	Conduction
Transcortical motor		Transcortical motor			Transcortical motor		Echolalia		Dynamic	Transcortical motor	Transcortical motor
Transcortical sensory		Transcortical sensory	Nominal		Transcortical sensory				Acoustic amnestic	Transcortical sensory	Transcortical sensory
Mixed transcortical					Mixed echolalia					Isolation	
Anomic			Semantic	Amnestic	Amnesic	Amnestic	Pure	Semantic	Semantic	Anomic	Amnesic
Global		Total		Expressive-receptive						Global	
Alexia with agraphia											Alexia with agraphia
Alexia without agraphia											Pure alexia
Aphemia		Subcortical motor			Peripheral motor						
Pure word deafness		Subcortical sensory			Peripheral sensory	Pure word Deafness					Pure word deafness

Source: Adapted from Benson (1979).

patients, and characteristic profiles of the various syndromes permit a more objective classification. Moreover, when some of Luria's hypotheses were put to the test, they did not pass it. The idea that a deficit in the analysis and synthesis of phonemes is at the root of the comprehension disorder in sensory aphasia has been disproved (Blumstein et al., 1977a, 1977b; Miceli et al., 1988a; see Chapter 6).

Yet, not even the neoassociationist classification has gone uncriticized. Firstly, there is no such thing as a universally accepted classification of the aphasias. Benson (1979) defined 12 aphasic syndromes and tentatively related previous authors' classification to his own. Even a cursory glance at Table 2–1, adapted from Benson (1979), reveals how confusing the field of aphasiology can be.

Moreover, the anatomical–clinical correlations have proved to be less reliable than was initially expected and classification of the patients more subjective than desirable. Goodglass (1993) made an attempt to reduce the excessive reliance of the neoassociationist approach on anatomy, but his approach remains descriptive and we have to wait for cognitive neuropsychologists for a real renewal in the study of aphasia.

Many clinicians, however, still rely on patients' classification, though syndromes have lost their theoretical status. Wernicke's and Lichteim's models were supposed to capture the organization of language; Wernicke's area, for example, was supposed to be the center of sensory word images and disruption of this area to cause sensory aphasia with comprehension disorders. Today, nobody would seriously argue that all patients classified in any given syndrome share a necessary and sufficient characteristic of that syndrome. Classification is a useful tool for summarizing the patient's symptoms and for capturing some regularities of language disruption due to the regularities of brain vessels.

APHASIA THERAPY FROM WORLD WAR I TO THE 1970s

THIS CHAPTER RETRACES THE HISTORY OF aphasia rehabilitation and correlates it with contemporary interpretations of the nature of aphasia. Before World War I only sporadic and anecdotal treatment reports can be found. From World War I to World War II aphasia therapy remained a rather uncommon procedure, mostly developed in the German-speaking countries and essentially based on didactic principles (Howard & Hatfield, 1987). After World War II it gained popularity and began to be regularly practiced in other countries as well.

Retracing the history of aphasia rehabilitation is a difficult task. Neuropsychology lies at the intersection of many disciplines—among which are neurology, psychology, linguistics, and psycholinguistics—and has benefited from scientific progress and new ideas in each of these disciplines. Hence, in reporting on changes in aphasia rehabilitation, one must also comment on new ideas in these fields. Furthermore, the history of rehabilitation is closely interwoven with the history of the studies on its effectiveness, and many researchers have been more interested in demonstrating the efficacy of language rehabilitation (independently of how it was carried out) than in the rehabilitation process itself. For their part, speech therapists have not been very keen to publish the results of their experience. The published studies, therefore, often assume more importance than is warranted by the results since they may not reflect the clinical reality but only personal opinions and unshared techniques. However, apart from personal experience, the published studies are the only sources of knowledge. Fortunately, however, the last 20 years have witnessed some attempts at organizing and describing the history of aphasia rehabilitation (see, e.g., Seron, 1979; Howard & Hatfield, 1987; Paradis, 1993).

Any classification presents both advantages and drawbacks: the most evident merit of any classification is the attempt to give some sort of order to a disorderly field, and an obvious drawback is the necessary simplification it implies. Furthermore, any attempt at taxonomy reflects in a more or less transparent way the author's personal point of view and hence is in partial disagreement with other classifications. The following attempt to give a structure to the history of aphasia rehabilitation is no exception.

FROM WORLD WAR I TO WORLD WAR II

Before World War I, aphasia rehabilitation was only occasionally practiced. Some aphasiologists interested in the matter suggested potential strategies for the rehabilitation of aphasic patients (e.g., Broca, 1865; Bastian, 1898). On the whole, however, nineteenth-century associationist theory did not pay much attention to rehabilitation.

The interest in aphasia rehabilitation grew very slowly, and the need for a special approach to aphasia therapy was ignored for a long time. The methods used between the end of the nineteenth century and the beginning of the twentieth century were much the same as those used for teaching children with delayed or defective speech. It was only after World War I that the problem of aphasia rehabilitation was approached in a more organized way. Gutzmann ran a clinic for voice and speech problems in Berlin, and Froeschels ran one in Vienna. Poppelreuter worked in a rehabilitation center in Cologne during World War I, and Goldstein directed a rehabilitation clinic for a few years shortly after the war (Howard & Hatfield, 1987).

Gutzmann (1896) and Froeschels (1914, 1916) distinguished between motor and sensory aphasias, proposing different types of intervention. The reeducation of articulatory disorders in motor aphasics was similar to the technique used with deaf children. Articulatory movements were retaught following the order of acquisition. Vowels, for instance, are the first phonemes to be acquired by children, and so they were the first to be taught to motor aphasic patients. Gutzmann and Froeschels also suggested taking into consideration the relative visibility of the movements, visible movements being more easily reproduced by aphasics than less visible ones. Production of more complex syllables and words followed. In sensory aphasia the main problem was held to be difficulty in comprehending the word sounds. To overcome this problem lip reading and the use of diagrams representing the positions of the articulators for the various phonemes were suggested.

In 1935 Weisenburg and McBride published their book *Aphasia: A clinical and psychological study*, which represents a cornerstone in the history of aphasia rehabilitation. They were the first to use standardized tests for the evaluation of the aphasic disorder; they describe verbal tests (for spontaneous production, naming, repetition, and comprehension), verbal intelligence tests (finding opposites, analogies, absurdities, etc.), and nonverbal tests, for which they give normal control data. With respect to rehabilitation, the most important change from what was suggested previously was a provision for active collaboration by the patient. The rehabilitation program was less didactic than earlier programs. Weisenburg and McBride suggested that it should be adapted to the individual patient, taking into account his or her personal interests. However, the exercises they proposed were not very different from those already used: confrontation naming, pointing, repetition, learning the articulatory movements, and so forth.

In conclusion, aphasia rehabilitation between the two world wars was based mainly on the idea that aphasic patients had to relearn lost language. Learning theories had still to be developed, and most exercises were based on repetition and drilling.

FROM WORLD WAR II TO THE 1970s

In the United States, aphasia therapy received great attention after World War II because of the dramatic situation of thousands of relatively young men with head gunshot wounds. These patients were admitted to Veterans' Administration hospitals, which became the first to include rehabilitation centers. At the same time, the need for rehabilitation for older patients with vascular disease increased.

For a long time, infirmity and its consequences were deemed to be an integral part of life. They were considered a natural component of the aging process and a necessary passage toward death. Slowly, with social and attitudinal changes, the idea that treatment is possible for every human infirmity gained ground. Rehabilitation developed and took root. In the same years, aphasia, which up to then had been largely ignored by the public, became a fashionable topic; newspapers reported that Winston Churchill had suffered a cerebrovascular accident and that President Dwight Eisenhower had become aphasic. The request for rehabilitation increased, and many new therapeutic interventions were devised (Sarno, 1991).

Analysis of the various approaches makes it possible to identify several main threads that, to a certain extent, appeared one after the other or developed in different countries. Their boundaries, however, are not very sharp, and it is not always clear where and when a given approach ends and another one starts. The stimulation approach (frequently referred to as the *classic* approach), the behavior modification approach, the Luria approach, the pragmatic approach, the neurolinguistic approach, and the neoclassic approach will be described. These approaches were based on different concepts of aphasia, but the relationship between the nature of the disorder and the proposed therapeutic intervention was rarely made explicit. For each approach, an effort will be made to relate the therapeutic intervention to the contemporary interpretation of the aphasic disorder and to the contributions from related fields, mainly psychology and linguistics.

THE STIMULATION APPROACH

Although rarely explicitly recognized (but see Darley, 1982), the stimulation approach evolved out of the holistic school. Many different and very heterogeneous interventions are generally grouped under this label. Followers of this school maintained that language is a complex, indivisible, psychological function, not represented in the brain by a number of discrete centers but a property of the total brain. The two cardinal properties of the holistic school are the idea that aphasia is a unitary disorder varying in severity but not in type, and the assumption that knowledge of language is not lost but cannot be accessed because of cerebral damage.

As far as the "unitariness" of the aphasic disorder is concerned, supporters of the holistic school could be found in Europe through the 1960s (see, e.g., Bay, 1964). In the United States, this view developed on a more practical level. As mentioned in Chapter 2, Schuell et al. (1962) examined a large number of patients with a series of standardized tests and performed a factorial analysis, which disclosed one main factor. According to Schuell, the main factor corresponds to the severity of the disorder and the other factors correspond to disorders in other cognitive, perceptual, or motor areas, such as visual, spatial, sensorimotor, and so on. In other words, two patients may differ because they have different accompanying deficits (e.g., verbal apraxia) or because of the different severity of the aphasic disorder but not because they have different types of aphasia.

The second common theme of the stimulation or classic school is the assertion that aphasia does not cause a loss of language knowledge but only a variable impairment in the access to it. This assertion is based on the common observation that aphasic patients can produce words or sentences in certain situations but not in others, the so-called automatic–voluntary dissociation first observed by Baillarger (1865) and Jackson (1878/1958). In addition to the automatic–voluntary dissociation, the observation of the variability of the responses given by aphasic patients who correctly name a picture one day and cannot find its name 10 minutes later, but name it again correctly after some time, is frequently taken as evidence that language is not lost but is inaccessible.

Variability of response has been demonstrated experimentally in a confrontation naming task (Howard et al., 1984). Moreover, a group of agrammatic patients were shown to be able to produce some grammatical structures that were not present in their spontaneous speech in a facilitating situation, such as story completion (Gleason et al., 1975). Variability of response and automatic–voluntary dissociation are regarded as evidence that language is not lost, for if it were it would be difficult to explain how in certain circumstances the patient can produce words, sentences, or grammatical structures that he or she cannot produce in other situations.

The two major representatives of the stimulation school were Schuell (Schuell et al., 1964) and Wepman (1951).

Schuell's methods are probably the most consistent with the holistic interpretation of the aphasic disorder. She claimed that rehabilitation can be essentially the same for all patients because aphasia is a unitary disorder, and recovery of any verbal behavior will cause recovery of all verbal behaviors. Stimulation must be mainly auditory because comprehension is at the root of language processing and must be repeated many times. Its length and complexity must be controlled because the aphasic disorder varies in severity and the intervention must be tailored to the individual patient; the stimulus is considered adequate when the patient, without being forced, can respond. The request that the stimulus be repeated many times is probably due to the dominance of behaviorist thinking, which in those days was still popular in the United States. According to behaviorist theory, the more frequently a response has been produced, the higher the probability that it will be produced again.

Wepman too was an advocate of the idea that there is only one form of aphasia, caused by the breakdown of a central mechanism for processing language. Language is viewed as a higher-level symbolic activity that exerts a form of control over thought since it is a tool of thought. In 1972 Wepman wrote, "the expression itself becomes part of the thought, effecting the thought process" (p. 207). According to Wepman, if an aphasic calls a square a circle, this will change his or her thinking about the square and make him or her think of the square, at least in part, as a circle.

In keeping with his interpretation of the nature of aphasia, Wepman's therapy is *thought centered*. The patient's attention must be diverted from the linguistic form and be directed to the thought content of what is said. To illustrate what he meant by thought-centered therapy, Wepman reported a successful therapeutic intervention with an aphasic patient who was a lawyer. "Each day began with one member of his staff discussing a particular case the office then had in litigation. His attention was diverted from any attempt to express himself to a greater understanding of the legal facts of the case in question" (Wepman, 1976, p. 135).

For Wepman, therapy must be based on three parameters: stimulation, facilitation, and motivation. The therapist must stimulate the patient when he or she is psychologically ready (motivated) and in such a way that the patient's effort are facilitated and the response is given. Unlike Schuell's approach, Wepman's approach to aphasia therapy is indirect because the therapist is explicitly asked not to strive to obtain a linguistically correct response but to direct the patient's attention to the content of what he or she wants to express, ignoring the linguistic form of the message. Wepman, however, had initially proposed a more traditional direct, language-centered therapy (Wepman, 1951), and only later did he develop his thought-centered therapy.

Darley's concept of aphasia and the therapy he proposed will be illustrated as a final example of the stimulation approach's intervention strategies. The first chapter in Darley's 1982 monograph on aphasia is entitled "Aphasia without adjectives," which clearly indicates his theoretical position on the nature of aphasia. He distinguishes aphasia proper from speech disorders such as dysarthria and apraxia of speech, which are often observed to coexist with aphasia but which are "not an integral part of the aphasia" (p. 21). A second distinction is between aphasia, a language-specific disorder, and more general disorders such as dementia. Finally and most importantly, aphasia is not a modality-bound disorder. In conclusion, Darley argues that he has "separated aphasia, a language disorder, from disorder of speech. We have differentiated aphasia, a language-specific problem, from disorders that may resemble it but in which other aspects of cognition and interaction are also impaired to significant degrees. We have distinguished aphasia, a multimodality disorder resulting from impairment of a central language process, from modality-bound disorders that result from impairment of given input or output transmission channels" (p. 41).

Darley's therapeutic program is in agreement with such an interpretation of aphasia. Like Schuell, he considers comprehension a central process of language processing and believes that it is always impaired in aphasia. He reports the results of successful interventions based on auditory stimulation (Wiegel-Crump & Koenigsknecht, 1973; Helmick & Wipplinger, 1975) and argues that priority of comprehension treatment is supported by these facts.

A second principle of rehabilitation is that the tasks should be of increasing difficulty. There is no discussion of what increasing difficulty means; it is only stated that it is based on the length and complexity of the linguistic message. The suggested tasks go from recognition of single words, to execution of one-step commands, to answering questions about paragraphs. When auditory comprehension is sufficient, reading comprehension tasks that parallel auditory comprehension tasks are introduced. Production tasks follow. The patient is not asked to produce words in isolation but always to retrieve them in meaningful units.

Beyond this rather vague description, it is very difficult to define the principles that guide the stimulation approach and describe its actual implementations. Therapists who claim to follow Wepman's and Schuell's methods use in fact different and extremely heterogeneous approaches, and rarely have they expressed their theoretical foundations.

THE BEHAVIOR MODIFICATION APPROACH

The behavior modification approach is not derived from a particular theory of aphasia. It stems from the application to aphasia therapy of the principles of operant conditioning and is a good example of the priority of theoretical concepts over their practical applications.

As is well known, behaviorism adopted the philosophy that only observable behavior can be studied; internal mental states are not considered appropriate for psychological study because they cannot be directly observed. According to Skinner (1957), verbal behavior is not qualitatively different from other human behaviors; it is ruled by the same principles and can be modified by them. Animals and humans interact with the environment, and the results of those interactions change their future behavior. In operant conditioning, whenever a subject gives a predetermined response, the response is reinforced; after a variable amount of reinforcement, the new response is learned.

An attempt to apply the work of Skinner to aphasia therapy was made, based on the idea that conditioning procedures can be effective in retraining language in aphasic patients because aphasia can be considered a maladaptive communication behavior. In a very loose sense, the operant conditioning approach encompasses all forms of aphasia therapy because they all aim to change the patient's verbal behavior. However, in a strict sense, *programmed instruction* refers to a systematically designed intervention program in which the behaviors of both the therapist and the patient are specified a priori and aphasia therapy aims at modifying the patient's verbal behavior by changing the antecedent or the following events.

One of the main research topics of the operant conditioning school concerned the learning process itself, and many questions about learning were investigated. The relative advantage of massed and distributed exercises and the best ratio between the number of stimuli and reinforcements were some of the areas of interest. As for aphasia therapy, an important question that was debated was whether aphasics could learn and, if so, whether qualitative differences between the learning capacity of aphasics and normal controls existed. A further question was whether these possible differences were confined to verbal material or related to visual material as well. The conclusions reached by those researchers were remarkably uniform and positive: most aphasic patients can learn, and they utilize adequate strategies, as do normal subjects, even if learning is less efficient (Tikofsky & Reynolds, 1962, 1963; Edwards, 1965; Brookshire, 1971).

Once it was established that aphasic patients can learn, it rationally followed that some therapeutic interventions could be based on principles of operant conditioning or, more precisely, on principles of programmed instruction, which represents an important application of the operant conditioning paradigm.

The programmed instruction approach views aphasia therapy as an education process and applies the methods of operant conditioning taken from learning theory. A psycholinguistic analysis should guide the choice of the content of the program. The therapist must then define the behavior that he or she wants the patient to produce; once a goal is identified, the therapist must program a series of perfectly controlled steps. The first step is the collection of baseline data, which should apply directly to the training program. A preestablished criterion of a given number of correct responses must then be set, and gradual steps within the program must be planned.

The two most important techniques used in programmed instruction are shaping and fading, and they both assume that the required behavior or a similar one exists in the patient's repertoire of responses. In fading, the required response is assumed to exist but the patient alone is unable to produce it. The therapist must select effective antecedent events (facilitation) that help the patient to provide the response. The facilitation is then faded away until the target response is given by the patient without any facilitation. Shaping is used when the required response is not available but a similar one is presumed to exist in the patient's repertoire. Starting from the existing response and manipulating the stimuli, it is possible to obtain responses ever more akin to the required one until the target behavior is obtained; this must then be positively reinforced. Treatment is generally based on memorization achieved through repetition; a stimulus is repeatedly presented to the patient until he reaches the preestablished criterion level, when a new stimulus is presented.

Principles of programmed instruction have been utilized in aphasia therapy by Pizzamiglio and Roberts (1967), Holland (1967, 1970), Sarno et al. (1970), Naeser (1975), and Seron et al. (1980). In addition, many therapists use less rigorous formalizations deriving from the programmed instruction principles. They generally have a specific goal, reinforce correct responses, and go in small steps from a first erroneous response to the correct required one without, however, strictly adhering to the theoretical justification of the behavior modification approach.

Compared to the stimulation approach, an intervention based on principles of programmed instruction is a step forward in aphasia therapy with regard to the reproducibility and rigor of the methodology, which requires that the treatment be programmed in fine detail, the collection of baseline data, and a standardized implementation. However, the approach is not based on a theoretically sound analysis of aphasia. The nature of language is not a matter of interest; only the surface level of language is considered and complexity is equated with length, namely, the number of words in a sentence. The lack of inquiry into the nature of the aphasic disorder is a serious drawback of the operant conditioning approach, which can at best be used for implementing other types of therapy.

THE LURIA OR FUNCTIONAL REORGANIZATION APPROACH

The Luria approach is a good example of unity of theory and practice and of a coherent therapeutic system. Luria (1963, 1970; Luria et al., 1969) distinguished functional disturbances due to the temporary loss of activity in some brain areas from the functional disturbances resulting from the destruction of brain tissue. In the first case, the temporary loss of activity in some brain area causes inhibition of function, which can rapidly resolve by itself and does not require treatment. If it does not resolve spontaneously, pharmacological or psychological treatment should be started.

By contrast, destruction of brain tissue is irreversible and the damaged function can never be restored to its previous form; however according to Luria, the patient should never be taught to adapt to his or her defects. Therapy must be directed toward the reorganization of the function by transferring it to other brain structures or functional systems, and the patient must be taught to perform the damaged operation through new roundabout methods by means of a partially new neural organization. The defective process must be reconstructed by creating new functional systems through the use of other undamaged links (intersystemic reorganization) or by transferring it to a different level of the same functional system (intrasystemic reorganization). In the case of intrasystemic organization, the defective process can be shifted down to a lower and more automatic level or up to a higher and more voluntary level. In aphasia therapy the damaged function is generally reconstructed at a more voluntary level, which, with time, should recover some automaticity. This is possible because "in man *almost any cortical area can acquire new functional significance and thus may be incorporated into almost any functional system*" (Luria, 1970, p. 382; emphasis in the original).

We can identify some general guidelines of the functional reorganization method. The first step, as in any other therapeutic program, consists in the identification of the basic impairment. A careful analysis of the inner structure of the function allows one to correctly identify the damaged level. The primary defect depends directly on the irreversible destruction of a given cerebral area. The original function cannot be restored, but it can be performed by calling into play other undamaged brain areas. The identification of exactly which links are damaged and which are preserved makes it possible to outline different training procedures.

The second step consists in identifying which of the other intact links should be utilized to reorganize the damaged function. In pure alexia, for instance, visual recognition of isolated letters is impaired because, it was argued, the lesion to the left occipital cortex and the splenium of the corpus callosum would cause a disconnection of the linguistic areas in the left hemisphere from the right visual areas. A frequently suggested strategy to overcome this problem was the use of proprioceptive feedback instead of the damaged visual recognition process. The patient was asked to trace the contour of the letters with a finger and to pay attention to the movements made. This maneuver is generally sufficient to enable the patient to recognize the letters.

A further example of the use of an intact link is the rehabilitation of a bilateral tactile aphasic by Beauvois et al. (1978). A patient is said to have tactile aphasia if he or she cannot name objects while exploring them tactilely but can show how they are used (which demonstrates that the identification of the object is correct) and can name them when seeing them, which demonstrates that he or she does not have a naming problem. Beauvois et al.'s patient had this pattern of behavior, and the authors suggested that the use of a visual relay would help the patient name tactilely explored objects. They therefore instructed the patient to form a visual image of the object before trying to name it. The suggested strategy was successful. Tactile naming improved, and the patient was better at naming objects that he could easily imagine visually than at naming objects that were difficult to imagine visually.

A third important suggestion of the reorganization method is to expand and perform the program in its entirety, step by step. No link of the reconstructive activity can be omitted without threatening its effectiveness. According to Luria, a complex psychological process follows a complex course in ontogenesis. When a child learns to read, for instance, reading is initially based on a complex chain of independent actions. Gradually the various actions are performed more easily and more quickly until reading becomes automatic. Brain damage destroys this automatization. The functional reorganization approach requires that the damaged operation (reading or naming, for instance) be subdivided into small sequential steps that correspond to the various operations performed in ontogenesis and that the patient is capable of performing in isolation. The patient is then asked to perform them one by one and to verbalize what he or she is doing. When necessary, external aids are provided that help the patient to carry out the process consciously and to compensate for existing defects. Repeated exercises allow the patient to do without the external aids, to abolish verbalization, to perform the sequential steps more quickly, and to achieve some automatization. However, the operation rarely reaches a high degree of automatism or unconsciousness and never results in a level of functioning identical to the lost one.

Finally, the reorganization approach stresses the importance of feedback, which must always be provided. Feedback allows the patient to make a comparison between the performed action and the planned action and to correct the former if necessary.

The therapeutic program for dynamic aphasia described by Tsvetkova (1972) illustrates the functional reorganization approach. In dynamic (or transcortical motor) aphasia, the major impairment consists in the lack of propositional language. The patient has relatively well-preserved comprehension, naming, reading, and writing but has difficulty initiating speech, and spontaneously generated verbal output shows poorly elaborated and incomplete sentences. The patient responds correctly to yes/no questions, but responses to open-ended questions are incomplete. In short, the patient is unable to express himself or herself fully.

The program comprises various levels and many steps at each level. At level one, the goal of therapy is to have the patient produce short sentences, and pictures are used as support. The patient is asked (*1*) to look at a picture, (*2*) divide it into meaningful parts, (*3*) indicate with arrows the parts of the pictures that are connected, (*4*) review all the preceding steps, (*5*) lay out a number of external markers (pieces of paper, for instance) equivalent to the meaningful parts of the picture, and (*6*) say the sentence aloud. These steps must all be carried out in a conscious way and repeated many times. When the patient has internalized all the necessary steps and is capable of describing a simple picture with a short sentence in a fairly automatic way, the same procedures are carried out with a more complex picture. The units that the patient has to single out at level two are not words but short sentences. When this second level is acquired, the program continues with the support of a written text instead of the picture.

Restoration of phonemic hearing disturbances can be briefly described as a further example of Luria's rehabilitation methods. The basic defect in sensory aphasia is considered to be impairment of word comprehension due to damaged phonemic hearing. Initially the therapist explains to the patient the difference between two phonemes (/p/ and /b/, for instance) and has the patient observe the articulatory difference by palpation of the throat. He or she then selects pairs of identical words differing only in the initial phoneme (such as *pill* and *bill*) and shows the patient the corresponding pictures with the words written underneath them. The patient has to associate the picture with the spoken word and pay attention to the difference in the initial sounds. The variants of a given phoneme should then be worked through in order to reestablish the phonemic generalizations because the patient is unable to pick out the phonemically important cues from heard speech. The phoneme /p/ in *pin*, for instance, is aspirated, but it is not aspirated in *spin*; in both cases, however, it is exploded but it becomes unexploded in *apt* because it is followed by a stop consonant.

Once the patient has mastered the stage of phonemic hearing, the constancy of the word meaning should be restored. This can be achieved by asking the patient to identify the root, the inflectional endings, and the prefixes and suffixes of a word and to use the same word in different contexts. In this way words slowly regain their constancy of meaning, and the patient's comprehension improves.

Luria's ideas are wide-ranging, and they will continue to influence aphasia research and therapy. Treatment of aphasia disorders, however, requires both therapeutic methods and diagnostic tools, but Luria was critical of standardized tests and quantitative methods. He emphasized the flexibility of the clinical approach and argued that knowing how a patient attempts to fulfill a task is more important than knowing whether or not he succeeds. The Luria-Nebraska Battery (Golden et al., 1980) is an attempt to standardize Luria's original approach to diagnosis, but it is too general to monitor recovery. This makes it difficult to evaluate the efficacy of Luria's therapeutic proposals. They remain interesting suggestions awaiting experimental confirmation.

THE PRAGMATIC APPROACH

The pragmatic approach, like the neurolinguistic approach described below, has evolved not from better knowledge of the nature of the aphasic disorder but from the application of linguistic knowledge to aphasia therapy. In the stimulation approach the patient was required to use very limited language in standardized situations, such as confrontation naming and picture description. Rarely was the patient required to produce something longer than one or two sentences joined by *and*; the sentences were mainly descriptive and affirmative and were devoid of any real informational content. In addition, the sentences had to be syntactically correct, with subject, verb, and direct object. The main change between the pragmatic and classic approaches lies in the shift of attention from syntactic correctness to exchange of communication by whatever means.

In the 1970s, linguistics became more interested in the pragmatic aspects of language, hitherto rather neglected. Pragmatics emphasizes the main function of language, namely, communication; it studies the use of language in context because a statement spoken in real life is never detached from the situation in which it is spoken. The context comprises the participants, the spatiotemporal parameters of the communication, and the participants' knowledge and beliefs. To define pragmatics is not easy. Yet, as far as it concerns aphasia rehabilitation, it is enough to say that pragmatics takes into consideration the relation between language and the entire situation in which it is used. To illustrate the effect of the situation on the use of language, one can think of two persons exchanging greetings. How greetings are expressed linguistically cannot be independent of the degree of acquaintance of the interlocutors and of their social roles. With the appearance of pragmatics, there has been a widening of the field of interest in aphasia rehabilitation. Therapists are no longer interested only in the linguistic message but also in the patients' capacity to communicate. A number of researchers demonstrated that aphasics' capacity to communicate is better preserved than their capacity to express themselves through language (Wilcox et al., 1978; Kadzielawa et al., 1981; Foldi et al., 1983), and a variety of formal functional evaluations were developed (Sarno, 1969; Holland, 1980).

As regards implementation of the pragmatic approach, the proposed techniques fail to live up to expectations. Let us consider the best-known and most widely used approach, PACE (Promoting Aphasics' Communicative Effectiveness; Davis & Wilcox, 1985). The two most innovative theoretical aspects of PACE are that the rehabilitation must give the patient the most efficacious communicative strategies, regardless of whether they are linguistic or not, and that therapy must always consist of a passage of new information between the therapist and the patient.

In practice, concealed cards are used and their content must be communicated. When it is the patient's turn to send a message, he or she must choose one of the cards and have the therapist understand what is represented in the picture. The patient is urged to use words, gestures, drawings, or any other communication device. If the patient succeeds in getting the message across, the roles are reversed, with the therapist sending a message and the patient identifying the picture.

In contrast with what happens in traditional rehabilitation, where the patient had to describe a picture seen by both interlocutors without any information exchange, in PACE the patient has to communicate something new to the therapist (or, alternatively, must understand it). However, the whole situation seems very distant from an *ecological* exchange. First, the patient cannot choose what to talk about because the topic of the "conversation" is predetermined by the pictures. In PACE the concept of new and shared information (see Chapter 10) is altered because the therapist, knowing the cards, can to some extent anticipate what the patient will try to communicate. This was also true in the classic approach, where the patient was generally asked to describe a picture in full view of the therapist. The aim of the stimulation approach, however, was to have the patient produce a syntactically correct sentence, and no importance was given to the factor of communication. The pragmatic approach, by contrast, stresses communication, but the patient is not given the chance to really communicate. Second, the production consists in a description of what is seen, and this is not a typical way of communicating. Except perhaps when speaking on the telephone, we rarely describe to our interlocutor what we are seeing; we talk of our feelings or beliefs, or of things that are not present, or have happened in the past or will happen in the future. Finally, this exchange takes place in a rather rigid and structured situation that has little to do with a conversational exchange in daily living.

The pragmatic approach originates from a well-grounded criticism of the stimulation school, which confined the patient to the use of declarative and affirmative sentences with very little communicative value. Its theoretical basis, however, is meager, if not totally absent. It is based upon one particular claim, namely, that the aphasic patient must communicate and that communication is more than speaking and understanding. As with the behavior modification approach, any idea about the nature of the aphasic disorder, as well as any notion that two aphasic patients may present different disorders and require different interventions, is abandoned. Notwithstanding these severe limitations, the new focus on communication is an important step forward in the history of rehabilitation; but it is a mistake to claim that communication is all that we should be interested in. No doubt, modern therapists know that aphasic patients can have different impairments, and are also aware that any rehabilitation method that fails to recognize this variability can be useful, at best, for some patients but not for all.

To conclude, the suggestion not to limit the therapeutic intervention to linguistically correct but only minimally communicative content is very interesting, but the actual implementations that can be found in the literature are inadequate. Moreover, it is certainly not true that this type of intervention can be useful for all patients; there are patients with specific aphasic disorders who do not have communication problems. To treat patients with an isolated disorder, word-finding difficulties for instance, with the pragmatic approach would be the same as teaching a second language to a normal person by asking him or her to use gestures or pictures without learning the second language's vocabulary. This may help to make the best use of what one already knows but not to learn more.

THE NEUROLINGUISTIC APPROACH

Neurolinguistics is a relatively recent term that came into use in the 1970s. It is the branch of linguistics that analyzes in terms of the principles of the language structure the language impairments that follow brain damage. The term *neurolinguistics* is neutral about the linguistic theory it refers to, but any linguistically based approach to aphasia therapy is based on the principle that language has an internal organization that can be described by a system of rules.

The first linguistically based typology of aphasic impairments appears to be that of Roman Jakobson (1964). He suggested that language processing is based on two fundamental and opposite operations: selection and combination. When we speak, we have to select each word from among possible alternatives along the similarity axis and combine the selected word with the preceding ones along the contiguity axis. Disorder in the similarity process causes selection of wrong words (paraphasias) and is typical of Wernicke aphasia; impairment of the contiguity axis causes errors in the sequencing of words and is typical of Broca aphasia. Two further dichotomies (encoding/decoding and limitation/disintegration) are suggested to explain the normal processing of language. Impairments along one or both of these axes allowed Jakobson to interpret the six types of aphasia described by Luria, as illustrated in Figure 3–1. This model is, however, too generic to guide therapeutic choices.

Many authors have underlined the importance of linguistic theory for aphasia therapy (Hatfield, 1972; MacMahon, 1972; Hatfield & Shewell, 1983; Lesser, 1989; Miller, 1989), but as long as aphasia was the neurologists' preserve, linguistic analyses were not carried out in great detail. The neurolinguistic approach to aphasia therapy stresses the role of language in aphasia and analyzes it according to principles of theoretical linguistics. It differs from the pragmatic approach, the main goal of which is the amelioration of all patients' communicative competence without previous analysis of their linguistic deficit, which is considered subordinate to the communicative competence impairment. In the neurolinguistic approach, the rehabilitation methods are based on neurolinguistic principles and are specific for each linguistic impairment. The therapist must first localize the

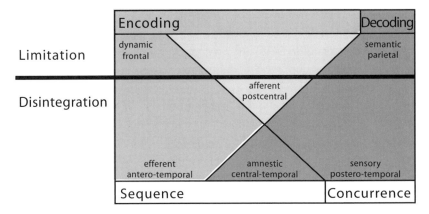

Figure 3–1. Jakobson's model of the language dichotomies underlying Luria's aphasia classification (modified from Jakobson, 1964).

patient's linguistic problem(s) and then devise a rehabilitation program specifically for that impairment. Procedures must vary for different impairments, but patients suffering from the same linguistic impairment can be rehabilitated with similar procedures. Weniger and colleagues suggested that "It is therefore possible to analyze the component deficits of a syndrome and to design specific therapy programs that only require slight modifications for the individual patient" (Weniger et al., 1980, p. 149).

By all appearances, it should be an easy task to single out the neurolinguistic treatments. Whenever a language disorder is analyzed according to some explicit linguistic principle and the treatment is consistent with the linguistic theory, the treatment can be considered to pertain to the neurolinguistic approach. However, it is not always easy to decide whether a given intervention should be considered neurolinguistic or not. Seron (1979), for instance, includes Weigl's deblocking method (Weigl, 1961) in the neurolinguistic approach. In deblocking, rehabilitation consists in first having the patient produce the correct response in a modality that is not too severely damaged and that is not blocked (repetition, for instance). Immediately after deblocking through repetition, the target response can be accessed in the previously inaccessible modality (confrontation naming, for example) because the first repetition response has deblocked the same response in the more impaired and inaccessible modality. The effect of deblocking is short-lived, and the target response will soon become inaccessible. The deblocking technique is based on a general principle and it utilizes the same intervention for all patients, choosing the modality to be deblocked and the modality to be used to deblock it. The therapist has to evaluate all the language modalities (repetition, comprehension, naming, reading, writing, and so forth) and arrange them from the least to the most impaired. The least impaired modality should then be used to deblock the most impaired.

It is not clear how this type of intervention can be related to a linguistic theory. It seems more appropriate to classify Weigl's deblocking method under the heading of the stimulation approach. The basic theoretical principle of the deblocking technique, in fact, is the assumption that language is not lost but cannot be accessed through all modalities, and the therapeutic method is the same for all patients. It may, however, be argued that the aphasic patient has not lost his competence but has damaged performance, and that the deblocking technique finds its rationale in Chomsky's (1957) distinction between competence and performance and thus legitimately pertains to the neurolinguistic approach.

Explicit reference to the distinction between competence and performance is made by Weigl and Bierwisch (1970). They argue that in Broca aphasia performance is disrupted and competence is preserved, as indicated by Broca aphasics' agrammatic production and preserved comprehension. Successive studies, however, (e.g., Caramazza & Zurif, 1976) have shown that comprehension in Broca aphasics is also impaired.

As for therapy, specific interventions for phonemic, lexical, and syntactic disorders have been described by Weniger et al. (1980). Naeser et al. (1986) have proposed a treatment for phoneme discrimination through the use of minimal pairs based on the theory of distinctive features. In a previous study, Naeser (1975) explicitly referred to Chomsky's theory of transformational grammar in describing a treatment program for syntax. Aphasic patients were asked to describe pictures and produce three types of sentences ("This is a house," "The woman opens the door," "The soldiers march") in response to questions that were standard for each type of sentence, for example, "What is this?" for the first type.

Wilk and Paradis (1993) review linguistic theories that underlie aphasia therapy and report treatments that have been based on theories about specific units of linguistic structure—phonetics, phonology, morphology, syntax, and lexicon. They argue, however, that "despite consideration by many authors of the importance of linguistic theory in aphasia therapy … there has been no systematic application of a specific linguistic theory to a rehabilitation programme for aphasic patients" (p. 103). Only very general and vague linguistic principles entered aphasia therapy, and to call this approach neurolinguistic is an appraisal of its intention rather than of its practice. Moreover, linguistics is a diagnostic tool that is useful in the assessment phase; it is not a theory of rehabilitation, and it does not provide indications about what to do. It helps to circumscribe the language impairment and probably to suggest a hierarchy of difficulty. Notwithstanding its limitations, the neurolinguistic approach, as well as the previously described approaches, has fostered some progress in aphasia therapy because therapists have been reminded of the necessity of a precise diagnosis and of a theoretically motivated intervention aimed at each patient's specific damage.

THE NEOASSOCIATIONIST APPROACH

Together with the stimulation school from which it derives, the neoclassic approach is the most heterogeneous among the various approaches described. As noted in Chapter 2, the neoassociationist school flourished in the 1960s and 1970s in Boston with a group of psychologists and neurologists (Norman Geschwind, Harold Goodglass, Frank Benson, Edith Kaplan) who have had a lasting and important influence on clinical studies in aphasia. The associationist aphasic syndromes were redescribed and reanalyzed in terms of more sophisticated linguistic analyses and anatomical knowledge. However, the neoclassic school, despite noteworthy progress in the clinical study of aphasia, failed to bring about great theoretical changes in rehabilitation.

As in the stimulation approach, the target response must be elicited, facilitating the patient's efforts by any possible means, but exercises are more varied than in the stimulation approach and are tailored to the various syndromes. Therapists are more concerned with the formal aspects of therapy (which could be a legacy of the behavior modification approach) and with the results achieved. The question of the efficacy of rehabilitation is considered very important, and many clinical studies sought to clarify the issue. Moreover, some linguistic principles are now familiar to the majority of therapists, although the linguistic analysis is still rather unrefined and the verbal behaviors are not analyzed in fine detail; only a hierarchy of difficulty based on linguistic units (phonemes, morphemes, words, and sentences) is generally taken into consideration.

To illustrate this approach, two comprehensive rehabilitation methods and some more detailed programs for a specific symptom or a particular aphasic population will be described. The first of the comprehensive methods that will be described is Ducarne's method, which has been widely followed in the French-speaking countries; the second is Shewan and Bandur's Language Oriented Treatment.

As clearly stated in the title of her book on aphasia rehabilitation, *Rééducation sémiologique de l'aphasie*, Ducarne's method is based on the detailed observation of the patient's linguistic behavior (Ducarne, 1986). Her proposed intervention is not prescriptive; she insists that intervention must be adapted to the patient by determining the most effective form of stimulation for each patient and the situation in which it is possible to cause the unleashing (*déclenchement*) of the language. Ducarne describes some guidelines for the rehabilitation of the main aphasic syndromes and also gives some more specific therapeutic instructions because she argues that patients presenting with the same syndrome vary widely both qualitatively and in the severity of the disorder. She also gives a very detailed account of the rehabilitation suggested in cases of verbal apraxia.

The basic principle of Ducarne's treatment is that the aphasic person must not be taught language (as is the case when a person learns a second language). The aphasic has known the language, which now must be "revived," making use of the patient's residual capacities without trying to teach the patient what he or she has lost. In addition, the proposed exercises should always follow a functional hierarchy, from easiest to most difficult. The hierarchy can be constructed either on linguistic principles or on the stages of reacquisition by groups of aphasics that vary in the different aphasic syndromes.

In general, Ducarne is more exhaustive for production than comprehension deficits. Reading and writing disorders are not treated at length because Ducarne maintains that they parallel disorders in oral production and comprehension. Except for very peripheral impairments, such as in motor agraphia, rehabilitation of reading and writing can be carried out along the same lines as rehabilitation of oral production and comprehension. For the rehabilitation of speech disorders in Broca aphasia, what is most important for the patient is to hear and to produce the target response many times in different verbal contexts. The same word must be heard and produced many times in different sentences, and the same linguistic structure must be produced and heard many times in different contexts. Dialogue and narrative speech are also used in therapy and are carried out with the help of an audiovisual series.

In cases of phonemic jargon (abundant and normally articulated production, with frequent neologisms that make it totally incomprehensible), the patient must learn to control phonology. This can be achieved by asking the patient to name to confrontation a picture whose name he or she can handle and respond to precise questions that suggest a specific response. In semantic jargon aphasia the patient's speech is made incomprehensible by the presence of numerous paraphasias. Language rehabilitation in these patients is preceded by a period of nonlinguistic therapy, the core of which would probably be considered today to be rehabilitation of the semantic system (see Chapter 6). Successively, the patient is asked to do some multiple-choice exercises such as finding the correct association for the sentence "I write with" among "a telephone," "a pencil," and "a handle."

In Ducarne's view, the family has a very important role in the rehabilitation process because the patient is required to repeat many times at home, with the help of a caregiver, the exercises proposed in the rehabilitation setting.

Ducarne also describes guidelines for the rehabilitation of acquired aphasia in children and older persons (over age 65).

Another example of a comprehensive and detailed therapy for aphasia pertaining to the neoclassic approach is Shewan and Bandur's Language Oriented Treatment (LOT; Shewan & Bandur, 1986). LOT is based on the idea that the language content of the treatment is very important. It divides language into five modalities (auditory processing, visual processing, gestural-verbal communication, oral expression, and graphic expression) that, to facilitate therapy, are considered to be nonoverlapping. Training in any modality is designed not to involve other modalities or, if impossible, to involve them at a very easy level so as not to interfere with the retrained modality. Each modality is in turn subdivided into areas, nine areas for auditory processing, seven for visual processing, five for gestural-verbal communication, nine for oral expression, and seven for graphic expression. The areas encompass the whole modality and, again, for practical purposes, are considered to be mutually exclusive. These areas are organized from the easiest to the most difficult. In auditory processing, for instance, they go from awareness of auditory stimuli, to monitoring speech, to comprehension of words, sentences, paragraphs, and discourse. Hierarchies of difficulty are based, when possible, on data from the literature. When these are not available, they are based on the authors' intuitions. LOT is presented in 10-item blocks of stimuli of comparable difficulty. The patient progresses to the next level of difficulty when he or she is 70% correct at the preceding level. If the patient fails on two consecutive blocks, the therapist returns to the preceding level. When the patient cannot produce a response independently, the therapist elicits the target response by cueing the patient. A hierarchy of cues drawn from data in the literature serves as a starting point; the therapist has to select the

Most Effective	Cue	Description
	Repetition	The target word is presented as a model for the subject.
	Delay	The subject delays before responding with name.
	Phonemic	The initial phonema or syllable is provided by the clinician.
	Sentence completion	A sentence is presented by the examiner with a blank for the subject to complete with the target word. The fewer the number of possible words that can complete the sentence the more efficient the cueing.
	Semantic association	A word that is semantically associated with the target word is presented by the clinician.
	Printed word	The printed target word is presented.
	Description	A description of the item is provided by the clinician.
	Rhyming word	A word that rhymes with the target is presented by the clinician.
	Situational context	A situation in which the item would be found is provided
	Spelled word	The target word is spelled orally for the subject.
	Functional description	The function of the target item is given by the clinician.
Least Effective	Superordinate	A superordinate term is provided by the clinician.
	Generalization	A general statement that provides little specific information is given by the clinician.

Figure 3–2. LOT's cueing hierarchy for naming disorders (from Shewan & Bandur, 1986).

most efficacious cue for the patient and elicit the response. Figure 3–2 illustrates the suggested hierarchy of cues for naming derived from an amalgamation of information from several sources. Cues should be progressively reduced, and eventually the patient should no longer need the therapist's help.

To illustrate LOT, word retrieval—area 6 in oral expression—will be described in some detail. Data from the literature indicate that many factors can influence word retrieval in aphasics. Accordingly, Shewan and Bandur suggest that the choice of stimulus words must take into account the characteristics of the referent to be named, the characteristics of the referent's name, the type of stimulus presentation, and the context in which naming is required, all of which have been shown to influence naming. The characteristics of the referent to be named refer to the semantic category (objects, actions, colors, and so forth) and the grammatical category (nouns and verbs) of the referent. The hierarchies are different for Broca and Wernicke aphasics because they have been shown to be differently influenced by these characteristics. Nouns, they argue, are easier for Broca aphasics and verbs for Wernicke aphasics. Frequency of use and length are two important characteristics of the referents' name, whereas real objects versus pictures refer to the type of stimulus presentation. Finally, the context in which naming is required can change, the easiest being sentence completion, confrontation naming being of intermediate difficulty, and naming to description being the most difficult.

The efficacy of LOT has been subjected to experimental investigation. Shewan and Kertesz (1984) compared recovery in 22 patients who underwent LOT treatment with a self-selected group of nonrehabilitated patients. The treated group improved more than the untreated group (see Chapter 4).

LOT is a comprehensive treatment for aphasia full of subtle clinical suggestions and based on an enormous wealth of data from the literature (Shewan and Bandur report approximately 400 references). It is, however, rather rigid. The clinician has to determine the modalities to be retrained and, for each modality, the areas that best correspond to the patient's needs. Once this is done, the application of the method is standardized and samples of 10-item series for each area are given in the text.

The neoclassic approach has also produced a wealth of therapy programs specifically designed for subgroups of aphasics or particular symptoms. Among those programs designed for specific aphasia types are the Helm Elicited Language Program for Syntax Stimulation (HELPSS; Helm-Estabrooks et al., 1982) and the Treatment for Wernicke's Aphasia (TWA; Helm-Estabrooks & Albert, 1991). Among those designed for particular symptoms are the Treatment of Aphasic Perseveration (TAP; Helm-Estabrooks et al., 1987) and the Voluntary Control of Involuntary Utterances (VCIU; Helm & Barresi, 1980). For a detailed description of these therapies see Helm-Estabrooks and Albert (1991).

The content of the program and the targeted patients change in each program, but the format is similar. Candidacy for the program is described, as are the scoring procedures, the content of the program, and the measurement of the responses. As an example of their general structure, HELPSS will be described. Candidates for HELPSS are left-hemisphere brain-damaged patients with agrammatism and good comprehension who display good attention and memory. The rationale for HELPSS came from a previous study by Gleason et al. (1975). In this study, eight agrammatic patients were asked to produce 14 syntactic constructions in a story completion task. They were shown to produce correctly some syntactic structures that were absent in their spontaneous speech, indicating that a story completion task has a facilitating effect. Moreover, results of the study made it possible to construct a hierarchy of difficulty among the 14 syntactic structures. HELPSS is based on these results; it uses 11 syntactic structures that go from imperative, to *wh*-interrogative, to declarative, to passive, to embedded sentences. Approximately 20 exemplars are given for each construction, and each exemplar is accompanied by a simple picture illustrating the story. There are two levels in HELPSS. At level A, the patient is required to produce a given construction that was previously uttered by the therapist; at level B, he or she is required to produce the same sentence as a logical completion of the story without its being previously produced by the therapist. When the patient reaches a 90% correct response rate for a given construction, the therapist proceeds to the following one. The purpose of HELPSS is not to teach specific syntactic constructions but to stimulate and facilitate the production of grammatically correct sentences.

A well-known method for the rehabilitation of nonfluent aphasics with severely reduced output is Melodic Intonation Therapy (MIT; Sparks et al., 1974), which exploits the right hemisphere's musical competence. Briefly, in MIT each word or phrase is intoned by the therapist; the patient should initially hum the melody pattern, then sing in unison with the therapist, and finally reach a stage when he or she can intone the phrase alone. At the third and final level the patient should be able to revert to normal speech prosody. Sparks et al. (1974) reported the results of eight patients who had already undergone therapy without improvement of verbal expression. After entering the MIT program, six patients showed marked improvement.

These therapies were all developed in Boston. Other programs have been developed in other centers, but the Boston studies have been published and are frequently referred to, and they are among the best known outside the United States.

To conclude, the main characteristics of the neoclassic approach are a more rigorous methodology, greater attention to the various aspects of the language disorder, the use of some linguistic principles, a wealth of therapeutic suggestions, and greater experimental rigor in the study of the effectiveness of therapy. Table 3–1 summarizes the six therapeutic approaches and their theoretical underpinnings.

CONCLUSIONS

So far, the main schools in the history of aphasia rehabilitation after World War II and the relationship between the contemporaneous concepts

Table 3–1. Approaches to Aphasia Rehabilitation and Their Theoretical
Underpinnings

Stimulation Approach

Stimulation of inaccessible language
mainly through comprehension
exercises that vary only according to
the severity of the aphasic disorder.

Holistic School

Language is a complex, indivisible
psychological function, a property of
the total brain. Aphasia can only vary
in severity; in aphasia, language is not
lost but inaccessible

Behavior Modification Approach

Applies to aphasia therapy the
principles of operant conditioning
and programmed instruction.
Shaping and fading are the most
important techniques. Stresses
methodology.

Operant Conditioning

Human behavior is determined by
external stimuli; verbal behavior is
not qualitatively different from other
behaviors. Only external stimuli and
responses can be studied scientifically.

Functional Approach

Analysis of all the steps underlying the
execution of the impaired task and
conscious execution of each step,
with external aids.

Conscious substitution of the impaired
link with one from an undamaged
system.

Luria

Language functions are based on a
network of neurological structures,
each playing a different role but all
contributing to correct processing.
Aphasia syndromes differ according
to the site of lesion, which interferes
with a basic component of a
language function.

Pragmatic Approach

The main goal of therapy is to restore
communicative competence by
whatever means: language, gestures,
mimic, drawing, and so forth.

Pragmatics

Stresses communication and studies the
use of language in context. Views
aphasia as a communication
disorder.

Neurolinguistic Approach

Scattered and rather vague suggestions
to base therapy on linguistic
principles.

Principles of Chomsky's
competence–performance dichotomy
and transformation grammar have
been used.

Neurolinguistics

Analyzes in terms of a linguistic theory
the language impairments that follow
brain damage.

Neoassociationist Approach

Therapy is still mainly based on
stimulation, but more attention is
given to the level of the linguistic
disorder (phonemic, lexical, or
syntactic) and therapy varies
according to the type of aphasia.
Much research on aphasia therapy
effectiveness.

Neoassociationism

Language is the sum of a number of
faculties—comprehension,
production, reading, writing. Damage
to different areas of the brain
differently affects verbal behavior.

about the nature of aphasia and the implementation of therapy have been illustrated. As noted in the introduction, any taxonomy is a simplification and constrains the observational data. This is even truer in this case because what actually goes on in the various rehabilitation settings is unknown. All one knows is the literature and personal observations. Another important limitation to what one can know about implementation of aphasia therapy is that it is highly probable that papers and manuals of aphasia therapy are published in the author's language and are unknown to people who do not speak that language. This is at least what Ducarne and I have done when writing about the methods of aphasia therapy (Basso, 1977; Ducarne, 1986; Basso & Chialant, 1992).

Actual rehabilitation is, however, far more heterogeneous than what can be appreciated from the above picture. Recently, Audrey Holland wrote in the preface of a book edited with Margaret Forbes that having had the chance in the past several years to visit many rehabilitation units in various countries, she had observed "how little I really know about the work of my colleagues in other parts of the world" (Holland & Forbes, 1993, p. ix). This drove her to publish a book that aims to describe the situation of aphasia rehabilitation in various countries, such as Germany, Italy, South Africa, Canada, Belgium, Japan, and so forth. The book is interesting because it offers a geographically vast view of rehabilitation. The therapeutic approaches described are extremely heterogeneous, and it is sometimes difficult to force them in any of the above-described approaches.

EFFICACY OF APHASIA THERAPY

I N CHAPTER 3, AN ATTEMPT WAS MADE TO OFFER a guide to the rich and varied treatments for aphasia by regrouping them into six different approaches. Before describing more recent changes in aphasic patients' management, it is worth considering whether aphasia therapy based on the approaches so far described has had any positive effects on recovery of language. The efficacy of the Luria approach will not be discussed because it has rarely been applied in Western countries and experimental data are scanty. Interested readers are referred to Luria's original work (Luria, 1970), where many follow-up cases are described in great detail. As for the other approaches, the type of aphasia treatment involved has rarely been specified and it is not possible to compare their relative efficacy.

I will argue that the efficacy of aphasia therapy *in general* has been demonstrated sufficiently, although no single experimental study is free from methodological limitations. Today, questioning the efficacy of aphasia therapy in general, for aphasic patients in general, without further specification, is meaningless because we now know more about aphasic disorders, diagnoses are more precise, and therapy is more tailored to the patient's deficits. We are now in a position to ask more specific questions about which treatments can be beneficial to which particular types of patients. To quote Robey, "having settled the basic issue, it is important now to expend resources in testing focused hypotheses" (Robey, 1998, p. 183).

The question of whether deliberate intervention can influence the course of recovery from aphasia is not new. During World War II several army hospitals in the United States started programs for brain-damaged patients, including programs for aphasia, and this furnished the database for the first studies with large samples of patients. The following attempt to organize the research on aphasia therapy efficacy while seeking to be sufficiently complete and as objective as possible will reflect my personal reading of the literature. Investigations will be regrouped according to the methodology used, which also reflects to some extent the period in which they were carried out. The effect of treatment was first studied in groups of treated aphasic patients; subsequently, results of a control group of untreated patients were compared to results of treated patients. Afterward, patients treated by speech therapists or nonprofessionals were compared. These clinical studies have been criticized, and a different methodology (the single-case approach) has been advocated by many. In this chapter, results of group studies and the criticisms of their use for the study of efficacy of aphasia therapy will be presented. They will be preceded by a short account of spontaneous recovery.

SPONTANEOUS RECOVERY

The functional behavioral disorders resulting from nonprogressive pathology of the nervous system undergo a variable degree of recovery in the first months following injury. Over the past 10 to 15 years our knowledge in this area has increased greatly, and the concept of *cerebral plasticity* has broadened. Experimental research in primates documents the existence of massive cortical reorganization after sensory deafferentation and motor exercise (Kaas, 1991). An interesting finding is that the somatosensory area of the left hand of violinists and cellists is larger than the corresponding area of the right hand (Elbert et al., 1995). It is conceivable that this difference is a direct consequence of the different use of fingers since the finger movements of the left hand in violin and cello players are subtler and more complex than those performed by the right hand.

Brain plasticity in brain-damaged patients has been less studied. We do not know whether rehabilitation can affect cortical reorganization, and the neurological basis underlying recovery remains little understood (see Chapter 8).

Two main hypotheses, not mutually exclusive, have been advanced: regression of diaschisis and functional takeover (see Cappa, 1998, for a review). *Diaschisis* (Von Monakow, 1914) refers to the functional impairment present in distant, structurally unaffected regions of the brain that are connected with the damaged area. Almost invariably, regression of functional depression takes place in the first months after onset. Functional takeover occurs for longer periods of time, either through the homologous contralateral areas of the right hemisphere or the undamaged areas within the left hemisphere. The relative contribution of the areas surrounding the damaged area in the left hemisphere and of areas of the right hemisphere remains to be assessed.

Whatever may be the neurological bases for recovery, what is very important for the evaluation of aphasia therapy efficacy is the time course of spontaneous recovery. This is a topic of continuing interest and has been the focus of several studies with aphasic patients (Sarno & Levita, 1971; Hagen, 1973; Pickersgill & Lincoln, 1983; Lendrem & Lincoln, 1985; Wade et al., 1986). The results of these studies are summarized in Table 4–1. There is general agreement about the spontaneous recovery curve: it is decelerating, steepest in the first 2–3 months after onset, when resolution of diaschisis also occurs, and flattening out in the following 3–4 months, when improvement in performance is not associated with obvious neurological changes. It is generally agreed that no spontaneous recovery occurs after 6 months, although a few patients have been described who showed significant spontaneous improvement for longer periods of time (see, for instance, Hanson et al., 1989).

Notwithstanding some agreement about its time course, the phenomenon of spontaneous recovery is still little understood. Many variables for the prediction of the outcome, such as age at onset, sex, handedness, etiology, and site and size of the lesion, have been investigated and been found (with the exception of lesion size) not to have a large effect on recovery (for a review see Basso, 1992; Cappa, 1998). Moreover, the meaning of the word *spontaneous* is not well defined. A really spontaneous recovery, independent of any language stimulation, probably does not exist. Aphasic patients do not live in a vacuum; they are more or less stimulated to listen to what other people tell them and to express themselves. It can be argued that the so-called spontaneous recovery is highly dependent on this ecological and broad stimulation. If this were the case, spontaneous recovery in severe aphasics would probably be less consistent than in moderate or mild aphasics. Severely aphasic patients, being unable to understand or say anything if the interlocutor does not take some measures to make himself

Table 4–1. Group Studies on Spontaneous Recovery

Authors	N of Patients	Tpo at Testing	Pre/Post-evaluation	Recovery
Sarno & Levita (1971)	14 (severely aphasic)	2 w, 3 m, 6 m	FCP	Greater in the first 3 m
Hagen (1973)	10 (hemiplegic)	3 m, 6 m, 12 m, 18 m	MTDDA	Takes place during the first 6 m
Pickersgill & Lincoln (1983)	20	mean, 3–4 m	PICA TT	Trend in the Token Test scores
Lendrem & Lincoln (1985)	52	4 w, 10 w, 22 w, 34 w	PICA FCP	Max within 10 w, slight between 10 and 22 w, none between 22 and 34 w, when more patients deteriorated
Wade et al. (1986)	545 stroke pts: 24% were aphasics and 28% unass.	7 d, 3 w, 6 m	MTDDA (short version)	At 3 w 9% were unass. and 20% aphasics; at 6 m. 3% of survivors were unass. and 12% were aphasic

N = number; Tpo = time post-onset; w = weeks; m = months; d = days; FCP = Functional Communication Profile (Sarno, 1969); MTDDA = Minnesota Test for the Differential Diagnosis of Aphasia (Schuell, 1955); PICA = Porch Index of Communicative Ability (Porch, 1967); TT, Token Test (De Renzi & Vignolo, 1962); unass. = unassessable.

or herself understood and obtain a response, are in fact scarcely stimulated. Less severely impaired patients, on the other hand, will be able to express themselves, even if only in familiar settings, and understand at least some of what is said to them and will undergo a greater amount of unspecified language stimulation than severely aphasic patients.

It is well known that the initial severity of the language disorder is an important determinant of the degree of recovery in treated and untreated patients, but this is insufficient evidence to confirm the hypothesis that severe aphasics recover less because they are less stimulated. To test this hypothesis, the relationship between spontaneous recovery and the amount of unspecified language stimulation given to the patient must be studied, if such a study is possible.

In brief, to summarize what has been said about spontaneous recovery, we know that some spontaneous recovery occurs in many patients and we have some knowledge about its time course, but we are unable to predict its amount.

CLINICAL STUDIES WITHOUT A CONTROL GROUP

Table 4–2 briefly reports the main clinical studies on effectiveness of aphasia therapy that did not control for spontaneous recovery.

Butfield and Zangwill (1946) followed the recovery course of 70 aphasic patients with different etiologies (mainly traumatic), most (59) under the age of 45. About two-thirds of the patients started treatment less than 6

Table 4–2. Group Studies on Treatment Efficacy in Rehabilitated Patients

Authors	N of Patients	Duration of Therapy	N of Sessions	Evaluation pre therapy	post therapy	Results
Butfield & Zangwill (1946)	70	n.r.	5 to 290	3-point scale	3-point scale	70–80% of patients recovered
Marks et al. (1957)	159	1 to 12 m	1 to 110	n.r.	4-point scale	50% showed poor recovery, 21% fair recovery, 29% good recovery
Leischner & Lynk (1967)	116	n.r.	n.r.	n.r.	6-point scale	5% showed no recovery, 40% slight to moderate recovery, 55% good recovery
Sands et al. (1969)	30	2 w to 32 m (mean: 7.5 m)	n.r.	FCP	FCP	Mean recovery: 10 percentile points; 3 patients showed no recovery
Sarno & Levita (1979)	34	3 to 12 m	3 to 5 weekly	FCP NCCEA	FCP NCCEA	Improved in all modalities

N = number; m = months; w = weeks; n.r. = not reported; FCP = Functional Communication Profile (Sarno, 1969); NCCEA = Neurosensory Center Comprehensive Examination for Aphasia (Spreen & Benton, 1977).

months postonset, and a third started it later. The patients were treated by speech therapists in two half-hour daily sessions until they reached a plateau or were judged to have only negligible disorders. The number of sessions varied widely among patients, ranging from a minimum of 5 to a maximum of 290. Before treatment the patients' impairments in speech, reading, and writing were separately rated as severe, moderate, and mild, and at the end of treatment they were rated as much improved, improved, or unchanged. About 20% of the patients were classified as unchanged in speaking (19%), reading (22%), and writing (28%); the remaining patients had variably improved. The percentage of "much improved" was higher in mild and moderate than in severe aphasics. Butfield and Zangwill also described some patients who started therapy more than 6 months postonset (when spontaneous recovery should no longer occur) and were judged to be much improved.

Marks et al. (1957) studied 159 mainly vascular patients rehabilitated for variable periods of time (1 to 12 months) with a wide range of therapy sessions (1 to 110). Improvement was judged by speech pathologists on a 4-point scale. Recovery was considered poor in 50% of the patients, fair in 21%, and good in the remaining 29%. No patient had worsened.

The 116 patients reported by Leischner and Lynk (1967) had aphasia of variable etiology and ranged from 14 to 70 years of age. The results of therapy were evaluated with a 6-point scale. No information was given about the duration or intensity of therapy. The highest levels of recovery were attained by 55% of the patients, who all started therapy within 6 months postonset; a further 40% of the patients, including those who started rehabilitation 3 years or more after onset, showed moderate or slight improvement. Only 5% of the patients did not improve. The percentage of nonimproved patients was higher among those classified at entry as "total aphasics."

The Functional Communication Profile (FCP; Sarno, 1969) was utilized to evaluate 30 poststroke patients at entry (2 weeks to 48 months after onset), at the end of therapy (median duration: 7.5 months), and at follow-up (median: 13 months after discharge) by Sands et al. (1969). All patients were rehabilitated but the duration of therapy was highly variable, ranging from a minimum of 2 weeks to a maximum of 32 months. At the end of treatment the mean gain for the whole group was 10 percentile points. At follow-up, a further gain of 5 percentile points was noted. Only three patients did not show any improvement. Patients with a high score on the FCP at entry recovered more than patients with a low score at entry.

Finally, Sarno and Levita (1979) explored the influence of time on recovery from aphasia. They tested 34 vascular aphasic patients at 4, 8, 12, 26, and 52 weeks postonset with the FCP and the NCCEA (Spreen & Benton, 1977). Patients received three to five therapy sessions weekly and were treated for 3 to 12 months. The greatest change for the whole group occurred during the third month postonset, but global aphasics showed the greatest improvement in comprehension more than 6 months postonset. Improvement on the FCP, which takes into account communication effectiveness, was more evident than improvement on the NCCEA, which is more linguistically based.

All these studies report improvement in treated aphasics, more evident in moderately and mildly affected patients (Butfield & Zangwill, 1946; Leischner & Link, 1967; Sands et al., 1969). However, they all have obvious methodological limitations. Their purported aim is to investigate the effects of treatment, but the amount of treatment varies widely among studies and, more importantly, among patients in the same study. Since it is unlikely that these researchers believed in some sort of miraculous effect of therapy, it is not immediately clear how patients who received 1 or 5 therapy sessions can be considered treated patients and grouped together with patients receiving 110 or 290 therapy sessions (Butfield & Zangwill, 1946; Marks et al., 1957). A second important drawback refers to the evaluation of improvement, which is generally subjective and reported with a 3- to 6-point nominal scale.

Each study presents other minor drawbacks, but what makes the results of all these studies useless for the demonstration of treatment efficacy is that they all fail to consider the effect of spontaneous recovery. Butfield and Zangwill (1946) described recovery in some chronic aphasic patients, and Sarno and Levita (1979) reported recovery, albeit less pronounced, between 6 and 12 months postonset, when spontaneous recovery is no longer expected. However, these data are anecdotal and not experimentally sound.

TREATMENT EFFECT IN CHRONIC APHASICS

The efficacy question can be addressed without employing a no-treatment control group by considering only chronic patients beyond the period of spontaneous recovery, thus obviating the main shortcoming of the clinical studies on recovery involving only treated aphasics. Table 4–3 reports the main results of these studies.

Table 4–3. Group Studies on Treatment Efficacy in Chronic Rehabilitated Aphasics

Authors	N of Patients	Tpo	Duration of Therapy	Treatment Regimen	Pre/Post-evaluation	Results
Wepman (1951)	68	minimum: 6 m	18 m	6 h/d 5 d/w	3-point scale	51% much improved; 35% improved; 14% unchanged
Broida (1977)	14	12 to 72 m	2–21 m (mean: 9 m)	3–5 h/w	PICA	mean recovery: 11 percentile points
Aten et al. (1982)	7	mean: 98 m	12 w	2 h/w group therapy	CADL, PICA	significant improvement in CADL but not in PICA scores
Mackenzie (1991)	5	minimum: 9 m	4 w	5 h/d group therapy	CADL, PNT, VET	good recovery in three patients; two patients unchanged

N = number; Tpo = time onset; w = week; m = months; h/d = hour/day; h/w = hour/week; d/w = day/week; PICA = Porch Index of Communicative Ability (Porch, 1967); CADL = Communicative Abilities in Daily Living (Holland, 1980); PNT = Picture Naming Test (Mackenzie, 1991); VET = Verbal Expression Test (Mackenzie, 1991).

Wepman (1951) studied the language rehabilitation of 68 young (age range: 19–38 years) traumatic patients. Language treatment started at least 6 months postonset and lasted for approximately 18 months; it was provided by skilled teachers for 6 hours a day, 5 days a week. Using Butfield and Zangwill's scale, Wepman reported that 51% of the patients were much improved, 35% were improved, and only 14% were unchanged. Retest showed that patients made a mean gain of five school grades compared to a mean loss following brain injury of six school grades.

A more traditional regimen of aphasia therapy was delivered to 14 male patients 1 to 6 years postonset (Broida, 1977). Patients were evaluated before and after therapy with the Porch Index of Communicative Ability (PICA; Porch, 1967). Therapy sessions were administered three to five times weekly for a period ranging from 2 to 21 months (mean treatment time: 9 months). Thirteen patients improved and only one worsened slightly; the mean overall PICA score before therapy was 60, and it rose to 71 posttherapy. Aten et al. (1982) reported the results of seven chronic aphasic patients (mean postonset time: 98 months) evaluated with the

PICA and Communicative Abilities in Daily Living (CADL) tests (Holland, 1980). Patients were given group therapy twice a week for 12 weeks; therapy was specifically aimed at functional communication in selected communicative situations derived from content areas sampled within the CADL test. No difference was detectable in the PICA scores posttreatment, but improvement in CADL scores was significant. Finally, five chronic aphasic patients, at least 9 months postonset, received 4 weeks of intensive group treatment, for a total of 85 hours (Mackenzie, 1991). Three patients showed widespread improvement, and two were virtually unchanged. At follow-up a month after termination of therapy, only one of the patients had fully maintained the gains achieved during treatment.

All in all, these studies demonstrate that aphasia therapy can also be effective in chronic aphasics long after the period of spontaneous recovery. The Wepman study reported the highest percentage of improvement, but it differs from the other studies both because of the population considered (young traumatized male patients) and because of the intensity and duration of treatment. Among the remaining three studies, recovery was poorest in the Aten et al. study, possibly because of the small number of therapy sessions (only 24 group sessions).

TREATED VERSUS UNTREATED PATIENTS

Another way of taking into consideration the effect of spontaneous recovery is to compare recovery in treated and untreated patients. It is supposed that, everything else being comparable, a difference in outcome between treated and untreated patients is to be ascribed to the specific effect of treatment. This experimental design has been frequently utilized in research on efficacy of aphasia therapy, and Table 4–4 reports the main studies.

Vignolo (1964) examined the records of 69 patients tested twice using a standard examination for aphasia (Basso et al., 1979); 42 patients were rehabilitated and 27 received no treatment. To be considered rehabilitated, a patient had to undergo a minimum of 20 therapy sessions over the course of at least 40 days. At the first examination the groups were not different for etiology (mainly vascular), age, time postonset, and type of aphasia. At the second examination, 14 of the 27 untreated patients were found to have improved, 12 were unchanged, and 1 deteriorated. Twenty-nine of the rehabilitated patients improved and 13 were unchanged on the second examination. Comparison between the percentages of improved treated

Table 4-4. Group Studies on Treatment Efficacy Comparing Treated and Untreated Patients

Authors	N of Patients Rehab. +	N of Patients Rehab. −	Duration of Therapy	N of Sessions	Pre/Post-evaluation	Results
Vignolo (1964)	42	27	min. 40 d	min. 20	SLE	No significant difference
Hagen (1973)	10	10	12 m	12 h/w	MTDDA	After 3 m, only rehabilitated patients continue to improve
Basso et al. (1975)	91	94	min. 6 m	3 h/w	SLE	(Oral production); higher percentage of rehabilitated patients improve
Gloning et al. (1976)	107		n.r.	n.r.	Gloning & Quatember (1967)	Significant effect
Levita (1978)	17	18 (hemiplegic)	8 w	5 h/w	FCP	No difference between groups at last exam (unknown severity at entrance)
Basso et al. (1979)	162	119	min. 5 m	3 h/w	SLE	Higher percentage of rehabilitated patients improve
Pickersgill & Lincoln (1983)	36	20	8 w	n.r.	PICA	No significant difference
Lincoln et al. (1984)	104*	87*	max 24 w	2 h/w	PICA	No significant difference
Shewan & Kertesz (1984)	52*	23*	up to 12 m	3 h/w	WAB ACTS	Significant difference
Poeck et al. (1989)	68	69	6–8 w	9 h/w	AAT	Significantly greater improvement in rehabilitated patients
Mazzoni et al. (1995)	13 (matched in pairs)	13	6 m	4–5 h/w	SLE	No difference at 4 m postonset; significant difference at 7 months postonset

* = high dropout rate. N = number; min. = minimum; d = days; w = weeks; m = months; h/w = hour/week; n.r. = not reported; SLE = Standard Language Examination (Basso et al., 1979); MTDDA = Minnesota Test for the Differential Diagnosis of Aphasia (Schuell, 1955); FCP = Functional Communication Profile (Sarno, 1969); PICA = Porch Index of Communicative Ability (Porch, 1967); WAB = Western Aphasia Battery (Kertesz, 1982); ACTS = Auditory Comprehension Test for Sentences (Shewan, 1979); AAT = Aachen Aphasie Test (Huber et al., 1984).

and untreated patients (71% vs. 52%) revealed no significant differences, although there was a trend toward greater frequency of improvement in the rehabilitated group. The study is important because it is one of the first to compare treated and untreated patients. It has, however, two shortcomings: the nonrandom allocation of patients to the treated and untreated groups and the small number of therapy sessions.

Twenty male patients with vascular disease were studied by Hagen (1973); 10 were rehabilitated for a year and 10 received no treatment due to a shortage of speech therapists. All patients were at least 3 months postonset when first evaluated, and the treatment trial began at 6 months postonset. Patients received 4 hours of individual therapy and 8 hours of group therapy per week. On pretherapy testing the groups were comparable on all language tasks except reading comprehension, which was better in the no-treatment group. After 3 months of treatment (9 months postonset) no difference was significant between the two groups, but only the rehabilitated patients continued to improve in the following months. This study shares with the Vignolo's study the shortcoming of the nonrandom allocation of patients, but it is otherwise methodologically sound; all patients were treated at least 6 months after onset and were rehabilitated for approximately the same amount of time. Moreover, the treatment time was sufficiently prolonged.

In a second study by the Milan group (Basso et al., 1975), recovery of oral expression was studied in 91 rehabilitated and 94 nonrehabilitated patients. Patients in the two groups were subdivided according to time postonset (less than 2 months, between 2 and 6 months, and more than 6 months); the minimum interval between the first and second evaluations was 6 months. Treated patients received 3 hours of rehabilitation per week. Improvement was defined as an increase of 2 points on a 5-point scale. The difference in the percentage of improved patients among the treated and untreated groups was significant in the three time groups, but the percentage of improved patients decreased as a function of the duration of aphasia before rehabilitation was initiated. The strengths of the study lie in the large number of patients studied and the inclusion of the variable time postonset in the statistical design.

Gloning and coworkers (1976) computed the prognosis for individual patients in a group of 107 aphasics by studying the effect of 19 variables, among which were sex, age, handedness, etiology, duration and severity of aphasia, and speech therapy, by means of a multiple linear regression analysis. The patients were tested at least three times: on entering the study, after 1 week, and approximately 18 months later. Speech therapy lasted for at least 6 months, but the authors do not specify its frequency or the number of treated patients. Older age (over 50 years), severe aphasia, and bilateral lesions were found to have a negative effect on recovery. Two variables were found to improve the prognosis: speech therapy and improvement of aphasia within 1 week. It is, however, difficult to understand what the second factor means because the time postonset at entry is not specified in the paper. All patients were recruited in hospitals, and it is likely that they were all acute patients, but it is not possible to locate along the time dimension the week interval with any certainty.

Levita (1978) compared 17 treated and 18 untreated hemiplegic, vascular aphasic patients first evaluated 3 months postonset. Traditional therapy was given daily (a half hour of individual therapy and an hour of group therapy) for 8 weeks, after which time the results of the two groups on the FCP were compared. No significant difference was found, but the FCP's scores before treatment were not available and it is not known whether the initial severity of aphasia was comparable in the two groups. This fact greatly limits the possible interpretations of the study's results.

Basso et al. (1979) studied the effect of therapy separately for oral production, written production, oral comprehension, and written comprehension in 162 treated and 119 untreated patients. The study design was the same as that in their previous study (Basso et al., 1975). Some of the patients were also included in the first study, and results for oral production were not totally independent of the previous results. In each modality the percentage of improved and unimproved patients was compared by means of a separate analysis. Improvement was defined as an increase of 2 points on a 5-point scale, which took into account processing of single words and sentences. Rehabilitation proved to have a significant effect in all four verbal behaviors, and time postonset had a significant negative effect on recovery. The effect of rehabilitation, however, was not significantly different in the three time groups. In other words, even if a smaller number of patients improved if they started rehabilitation more than 6 months postonset, the effect of rehabilitation was significant. The major drawback of this study is the nonrandom allocation of patients. The treated and untreated groups, however, did not differ significantly in age, educational level, etiology, and time postonset. In addition, untreated patients were not refused therapy; by far the most frequent reason for not being rehabilitated was geography: patients lived in places where no aphasia treatment was available.

Among other prognostic indicators of recovery in aphasic stroke patients, Pickersgill and Lincoln (1983) studied the effect of therapy. The patients were first evaluated with the PICA between 1 and 36 months postonset; the 36 treated patients underwent an 8-week therapy course, and 20 patients referred for occupational therapy to other hospitals made up the control group. No data are given on the intensity of therapy. Results indicate that the greatest recovery occurred in the first months poststroke, with no significant difference between the treated and untreated patients.

Lincoln et al. (1984) assessed patients at 10 weeks poststroke with the PICA and randomly allocated them to the treatment ($n = 104$) or no-treatment ($n = 87$) group; all patients were reevaluated at 22 and 34 weeks postonset. The treatment group was offered two sessions weekly for 24 weeks, after which time the no-treatment group was offered treatment. Most of the patients, from either the treated or the untreated group, dropped out of the study before completion of the treatment, and only 27 patients were given more than 37 therapy sessions. Treatment was delivered by speech therapists, who were left free to choose the type of therapy they considered the best. Comparison was done by the use of t-tests, and no significant difference was found between treated and untreated patients. The Lincoln et al. study appears to be well controlled, mainly because of the random allocation of patients to the treatment and no-treatment groups. This, however, does not ensure that results of the study are generalizable (see below). Aphasia therapy was delivered only twice a week for a short time; more intensive treatments could have produced different results.

Shewan and Kertesz (1984) compared recovery in four groups of aphasic patients. Three groups of patients were randomly assigned to three types of treatment: LOT (Shewan and Bandur, 1986), stimulation-facilitation therapy (Wepman, 1951, 1972; Schuell et al., 1955, 1964), and unstructured treatment. Speech pathologists provided therapy to patients in the first two groups, and nonprofessionals trained to stimulate communication in the patients (mainly nurses) provided therapy to the third group. The group of untrained patients was self-selected and was composed of patients who either did not wish to receive treatment or were unable to receive it. The reasons for their inability to receive treatment are not indicated in the study. The treated patients received 3-hour weekly treatment for up to 12 months, although many patients dropped out of the study. The reasons for the loss of patients to follow-up were constant across groups. The results of the study indicate that the two groups treated by speech pathologists improved significantly more than the no-treatment group, with no significant difference between the two rehabilitated groups.

Treatment provided by nonprofessionals did not result in significantly greater recovery than no treatment, although it approached statistical significance. Self-selection of the untreated group, however, limits possible interpretations of the study results.

Shewan and Kertesz also studied when treatment has its greatest effect. The patients were seen at entry (2 to 4 weeks postonset) and after 3, 6, and 12 months. Forty-nine patients who remained in the study for at least 6 months provided the database for this analysis. When recovery was compared for treated and untreated patients in the first 3 months, no difference was found; between 3 and 6 months, treated patients recovered significantly more than untreated patients. Between 6 and 12 months, the treated group more or less reached a plateau and the untreated group showed a slight decrement in performance.

The experimental design in the Poeck et al. (1989) study was not a direct comparison of treated and untreated patients. The amount of improvement of a group of 68 patients receiving intensive therapy (9 hours per week over 6–8 weeks) was corrected by the expected rate of spontaneous recovery, as determined by a previous study (Willmes & Poeck, 1984). About two-thirds of the patients showed greater improvement than expected by spontaneous recovery.

Finally, a carefully controlled study was conducted by Mazzoni and colleagues (1995), who compared recovery in 13 treated aphasic patients and 13 matched untreated controls. Patients were matched for sex, age, education, CT lesion, and type and severity of aphasia, and were all evaluated at 1 month postonset. The treated group received six therapy sessions per week for 3 months and 3–4 sessions per week for a further 3 months. The percentage of patients who met the criteria for recovery was not significantly different at 4 months postonset, that is, after 3 months of therapy, but it was significantly different 7 months postonset.

The results of the studies reviewed here do not allow firm conclusions to be drawn. This issue will be discussed later. The only point made here is that all these studies have been argued to have a common methodological weakness: the treated and untreated groups do not differ only in the presence/absence of therapy; they also differ in the amount of attention and conversational opportunities they were given. In other words, even if the treated groups were shown to recover significantly more than the untreated groups, a significant effect of therapy could not be unequivocally demonstrated. The difference could be due to an unspecified effect of attention and not to the specific techniques employed. Investigations that have taken this problem into account are reported below.

DIFFERENT THERAPEUTIC METHODS AND DIFFERENT "THERAPISTS" COMPARED

Probably the first study to compare different treatments was one by Sarno et al. (1970). Thirty-one vascular severely aphasic patients, at least 3 months postonset, were included in the study and subdivided into three groups: the first group received programmed instruction therapy, the second received traditional therapy, and the third received no therapy. Allocation was not random but due to uncontrollable reasons such as the limited availability of therapists or the location of the patients. All evaluations were performed with the FCP. The treatment's goal was the acquisition of six words—*one, two, red, blue, book, pen*—and ceased after 80 half-hour therapy sessions or when patients had acquired the six words. At the end of the treatment no significant difference was found among the groups, all showing small gains. It must be stressed, however, that the study had a very limited scope, perhaps because of the severity of the aphasia; the patients had to learn six words and use them in different combinations.

In another study, the progress of a group of patients ($n = 17$) receiving conventional therapy carried out by speech therapists was compared to the progress of a group of patients ($n = 14$) treated by nonprofessional volunteers, each instructed by speech therapists about the patients' disabilities (Meikle et al., 1979). Patients were assessed with the PICA at least 3 weeks after onset and were regularly reassessed at 6-week intervals. Twenty-one patients dropped out of the trial when they reached a plateau between two evaluations about 6 weeks apart. The mean duration of the therapy was 21 weeks for the nonprofessional group and 36 weeks for the speech pathologist group. Both groups showed some improvement, but no difference between the groups emerged.

The results of therapy delivered by volunteers and speech therapists were also compared in a study by David et al. (1982). Treatment lasted for 30 hours over a period of 15–20 weeks, and patients in the volunteers' and therapists' groups were followed for about the same length of time. Volunteers were given a detailed description of their patients' disorders but no instruction about therapy. Both groups showed a certain amount of improvement, but no difference was found between the two groups.

Three large, carefully designed collaborative Veterans Administration (VA) studies tackled the problem of the efficacy of aphasia therapy by comparing the effects of individual and group therapy (Wertz et al., 1981), of therapy delivered by speech pathologists and trained volunteers (Wertz et al., 1986), and of therapy delivered by speech therapists and home therapists (a spouse, friend, relative) (Marshall et al., 1989). In all studies the patients, all men, were assigned randomly to a treatment group. In the first VA study, the patients entered it at 4 weeks postonset and were then reassessed at 26, 37, and 48 weeks postonset. Thirty-two patients were assigned to group therapy and 35 to individual therapy. Therapy was delivered to all patients for 8 hours each week, and the study lasted for 44 weeks. Only 34 patients completed the 44-week course. Both groups made significant improvements, and the individually treated patients improved significantly more than those in the other group. Both groups continued to improve between 26 and 48 weeks postonset, although the recovery rate was lower than in the previous weeks. According to the authors, the late improvement can be assumed to result from the treatment because spontaneous recovery is generally considered complete by 6 months postonset.

The second VA cooperative study compared treatment administered by speech pathologists to treatment administered by trained volunteers. It also tackled the question of whether delaying therapy may have a negative effect on recovery. Three groups of patients were compared: the first group was rehabilitated by speech pathologists, the second group was rehabilitated by trained volunteers, and in the third group therapy started 12 weeks later, when the first two groups had completed their therapy course. The patients entered the study between 2 and 24 weeks postonset. Treatment was provided for 8 to 10 hours each week for 12 weeks. The results of the study indicate that all groups made significant improvements and that the group treated by speech pathologists improved more than the home-treated group. None of the differences, however, reached significance. Delaying therapy was not demonstrated to be harmful for the patients since the delayed-therapy group caught up with the others, after having received treatment, at the 24-week comparison.

In Marshall et al.'s (1989) study, 37 aphasic men received treatment for 12 weeks (8–10 hours of individual treatment per week) from a home therapist trained by a speech pathologist, and 31 aphasic patients were treated by speech pathologists. The patients entered the study between 2 and 24 weeks postonset. Both groups improved, but the differences between the groups were not statistically significant. A third group who started aphasia therapy after 12 weeks recovered significantly less than the first two groups during the same period, thus supporting the benefits of volunteer and speech therapist treatment over no treatment. The patients, however, caught up when therapy was delivered, confirming that deferring therapy by 12 weeks has no detrimental effect on recovery.

The three VA studies support the conclusion that therapy is effective. First, patients in the first study (Wertz et al., 1981) continued to improve after 6 months postonset, when spontaneous recovery should no longer have taken place. Second, in Wertz et al.'s study (1986) and in Marshall et al.'s study (1989), rehabilitated patients improved more than nonrehabilitated patients (who caught up when delivered therapy). By contrast, no difference was found according to whether therapy was delivered by a speech therapist or trained volunteers.

Finally, Hartman and Landau (1987) compared recovery in 60 stroke patients randomly assigned to two therapy groups: conventional therapy and supportive counseling, both delivered by professional speech therapists. Patients were first seen 1 month postonset and received therapy twice weekly for the following 6 months. The PICA test was administered at entry into the study and then monthly during therapy. Supportive counseling was conversationally based, and therapists were instructed not to provide suggestions for language practice but rather to discuss familiar topics with the patient. Both groups partially recovered, and no significant between-group difference was found.

Table 4–5 summarizes the studies discussed above.

In short, the studies comparing the effect of therapy carried out by speech therapists with the effect of therapy carried out by volunteers have not found greater efficacy of therapists. The only significant difference in this group of studies was found between two therapy regimens, individual therapy being more effective than group therapy (Wertz et al., 1981).

The question about the efficacy of aphasia therapy remains unresolved. Therapy has been claimed to be efficacious in all the clinical studies without a control group, but the studies failed to control for the effect of spontaneous recovery. More convincing evidence comes from studies with chronic aphasics and from some of the studies that compared treated and untreated patients, which found aphasia therapy to be efficacious. In addition, when compared with no treatment, treatments carried out by both speech therapists and volunteers were found to be more efficacious. However, papers that published results suggesting that aphasia therapy is effective have not aroused widespread interest. For the most part, they have been criticized for their limitations and rapidly dismissed. Prins and coworkers, for instance, argue that the statement by Wertz et al. (1981) that two groups of patients (one receiving individual therapy and the other group therapy) made a significant improvement "seems unwarranted, because the observed improvement can also be explained by test-retest effects" (Prins et al., 1989, p. 89). Moreover, Schoonen (1991), discussing the problem of the

Table 4–5. Efficacy of Different Methods or Different "Therapists" Compared

Authors	N of Patients	Treatments/ Therapists	Duration of Therapy	N of Sessions	Pre/Post- evaluation	Results
Sarno et al. (1970)	10–10–11	Programmed inst, classic, no treatment	3 m	80 1/2 h	FCP	No significant difference
Meikle et al. (1979)	17*–14*	th vs. vol	max 80 w (th: mean 36 w; vol: mean 21 w)	4 h/w	PICA	No significant difference
Wertz et al. (1981)	32*–35*	Group vs. individual therapy	44 w	8 h/w	PICA	Individual therapy significantly better
David et al. (1982)	48–48	th vs. vol	max 20 w	30 h	FCP	No significant difference
Wertz et al. (1986)	38*–43*	th vs. trained vol	12 w	8–10 h/w	PICA	No significant difference
Hartman & Landau (1987)	30–30	th vs. counseling	6 m	2 h/w	PICA	No significant difference
Marshall et al. (1989)	31–37	th vs. trained family member	12 w	8–10 h/w	PICA CADL	No significant difference

* = high drop-out rate; N = number; h = hours; w = week; m = months; h/w = hours/week; inst = instruction; th = therapists; vol = volunteers; FCP = Functional Communication Profile (Sarno, 1969); PICA = Porch Index of Communicative Ability (Porch, 1967); CADL = Communicative Abilities in Daily Living (Holland, 1980).

internal validity (see infra) of the studies on efficacy of aphasia therapy, concludes that there is a general lack of internal validity (only 3 of 35 efficacy studies reviewed, according to Schoonen, have an adequate design. But see Robey, 1994, for a critical review of this conclusion). He therefore accounts for the fact that so many studies have claimed to have demonstrated significant improvement as the result of luck, publication selectivity, invalid rating scales, and bias. Obviously, the same reasoning could be applied to all studies, but it is to be hoped that such blunders are not frequent in research. Furthermore, Schoonen's unsubstantiated claims should not be given serious consideration until he provides supportive evidence.

A further example of the skepticism with which positive studies on the efficacy of aphasia therapy are read is the response by Pederson and coworkers to a comment by Wertz on a previous paper by the same group. In that study, Pederson and coworkers asserted that in the majority of studies, aphasia treatment has not been found efficacious (Pederson et al., 1995). Wertz (1996) argued that most of the studies reported by Pederson et al. had in fact found a significant difference between treated and untreated patients. In their response to Wertz, Pederson and coworkers wrote, "No treatment is not a good control, because these patients may have their performances negatively affected by the decision not to treat them. ... It is only when no difference is found, that it is possible to draw a valid conclusion from a comparison with no treatment" (Pederson et al., 1996, p. 130). On the other hand, the message that therapy provided by speech therapists is no better than simple counseling or therapy delivered by volunteers has been immediately accepted by the scientific community, notwithstanding the fact that this group of studies displays obvious weaknesses and has been criticized on methodological grounds (Pring, 1983).

Leaving aside the question of the experimental soundness of the above studies, although the David et al. and Meikle et al. studies are commonly accepted as demonstrating the inefficacy of aphasia therapy, this is not the case. In these studies, the efficacy of aphasia therapy was not even their goal. The studies focused on insufficiency of particular therapy and not on therapy in general. David et al. (1983a) state, in response to Pring (1983), that "both our own study and that of Meikle et al., as well as many others of a similar nature, arose from the practical and organisational difficulties of the overpressed speech therapy service ... *our main concern was to evaluate the existing standard speech therapy provision in Britain*" (p. 74; emphasis added). In addition, in reply to Huber et al. (1983), they write, "Thus the most pressing need in clinical research in aphasia therapy is for investigation of the type of service which is currently available to post-stroke aphasic patients referred to our speech therapy departments" (David et al., 1983b, p. 692). The only conclusion one can draw from the Meikle et al. and David et al. studies is that the service currently provided in Great Britain is not sufficient and that we need to consider more appropriate therapy time.

DURATION AND FREQUENCY/INTENSITY OF THERAPY

A careful review of the studies that compared treated and untreated patients demonstrates that no significant difference was found in those studies where treatment was of short duration (Vignolo, 1964; Sarno et al., 1970; Levita, 1978; Pickersgill and Lincoln, 1983; Lincoln et al., 1984; Prins et al., 1989), whereas in all cases in which therapy lasted for longer periods of time, it was found to be effective (Hagen, 1973; Basso et al., 1975, 1979; Gloning et al., 1976; Mazzoni et al., 1995). As Howard and coworkers put it, "Intriguingly, the studies that report beneficial effects of treatment involved more intensive and prolonged reeducation programs than the studies that find no effect" (Howard et al., 1985, p. 818).

Some studies directly studied the effect of duration of therapy. Marshall, Tompkins, and Phillips (1982) investigated the effect of 11 factors that they felt might contribute to recovery, including the number of treatment sessions. The results of the stepwise regression analysis are important for the question of the duration of therapy because they indicate that the number of therapy sessions is the most powerful predictor of improvement.

In a retrospective study, the effect of length of treatment on improvement (3 months vs. 6 months) was investigated for oral production and comprehension. In both cases it was found to be significant (Basso, 1987).

Brindley et al. (1989) reported on a group of Broca aphasics. After a first period of therapy that lasted for 12 weeks, with two sessions per week, patients were given 12 weeks of intensive therapy with 25 hours per week. The group did not show any improvement in the first period but improved in the second, intensive period.

Finally, Denes et al. (1996b) compared the efficacy of intensive versus regular speech therapy in 17 acute global aphasics randomly allocated to intensive or regular therapy. Intensive therapy was delivered daily for 6 months and consisted of an average of 130 sessions; regular therapy was delivered three times per week for 6 months, with an average of 60 therapy sessions. Both groups showed improvement in all language modalities but the patients submitted to intensive treatment showed better results, which were statistically evident, however, only in the written language subtests.

In conclusion, intensive or protracted therapy has been found to have a significant effect on recovery, and when it was compared to shorter (Basso, 1987) or less intensive treatment (Denes et al., 1996b), its effect was found to be significantly greater.

META-ANALYSES

None of the above-reported studies taken singly, provide sufficient evidence for the efficacy of aphasia therapy. As already stated, they all have some methodological weaknesses, probably the most important being that allocation to the treated or untreated group was not random (with the exception of a few studies). Another important argument against these studies has been that other factors that are supposed to influence recovery (such as the patient's age, education, etiology, and so forth) might interact and pose particular problems for the experimental design.

The picture emerging from the literature is, however, convincing: if the therapy is sufficiently prolonged and/or intensive, it is generally effective. Clinical studies indicate that a higher proportion of rehabilitated patients improve and that the amount of improvement is larger in rehabilitated than in nonrehabilitated patients. It must also be stressed that a positive result showing the efficacy of treatment is more "powerful" than a negative result, which does not demonstrate that treatment has no effect but merely that a significant effect has not been found.

Yet, no general agreement has been reached. It has been stated with equal confidence that "Aphasia therapy works. It works so well that every neurologist, psychiatrist, and speech language pathologist responsible for patient management should refuse to accede to a plan that abandons the patient to neglect" (Darley, 1979, p. 629); or that "the effects of therapy in terms of recovery from aphasia are still uncertain" (Legh-Smith et al., 1987, p. 1488); or that "our conclusion as to the efficacy of language therapy can only be *doubt*" (Shoonen, 1991, p. 461; emphasis in the original).

In the field of social and medical sciences the use of meta-analyses is accepted. A *meta-analysis* is a quantitative procedure for assessing and synthesizing a collection of primary studies. It is the most frequently used quantitative procedure for calculating treatment efficacy on the basis of all treatment studies that report sufficient data to be reanalyzed. The results of a meta-analysis are the magnitude of the average effect size and its confidence interval, which allows one to estimate the degree to which a null hypothesis is false on the basis of all available evidence. The validity of a meta-analysis is determined in part by the completeness of the primary studies analyzed. In the case of aphasia therapy efficacy studies, the outcome of a meta-analysis determines the weight of the scientific evidence of the hypothesis that aphasia therapy is effective. In the past 10 years, the meta-analysis procedure has been repeatedly applied to aphasia therapy studies.

Whurr et al. (1992) reviewed 45 studies carried out from 1947 to 1988. They examined the influence of factors such as subject selection, test reliability and validity, and treatment characteristics on treatment outcomes. They concluded that the results of the meta-analysis demonstrate a significant effect of treatment, although the studies on the efficacy of aphasia therapy suffer from lack of internal and external validity. *Internal validity* is based on correct sampling and correct matching with normal controls with respect to putative interfering variables, such as, for instance, age and educational level. *External validity* refers to the generalizability of results; in other words, it is concerned with the stability of the results across other contexts or other experimental groups.

Robey (1994) reviewed 48 reports on the efficacy of aphasia therapy. He excluded the papers that did not meet the statistical requirements for inclusion, and in the 21 remaining studies he separately studied whether there was any recovery in untreated and treated patients and whether there was a difference in recovery between the two groups. In view of the fact that time elapsed since onset has a direct influence on the outcome, he analyzed separately the results for patients seen before and after 4 months postonset. Four conclusions emerged from the reanalysis of the eligible and published data:

1. The effect of treatment beginning in the acute stage of recovery is nearly twice as large as the effect of spontaneous recovery alone.
2. Treatment initiated after the acute period achieves a considerably smaller but appreciable effect.
3. The separation of treated and untreated populations exceeds the criterion value for a medium-sized effect and approaches the criterion for a large-sized effect when treatment is begun in the acute period.
4. The separation of treated and untreated populations in the chronic stage of recovery corresponds to a small-to-medium sized effect (Robey, 1994, p. 602)

In a second study, Robey (1998) examined a larger series of clinical trials to determine the replicability of his previous findings and to look for an answer to more focused questions about amount of treatment, types of treatment, severity of aphasia, and type of aphasia. Data for types of treatment and type of aphasia were too scant for a reliable answer. Amount of treatment was considered low when it did not exceed 1.5 hour per week, moderate when it consisted in 2–3 hours per week, and high when it consisted in 5 or more hours per week. Severity of aphasia was coded as moderate or severe; no data were available for mild aphasia. Furthermore, since time postonset is related to the amount of recovery, all the effects were studied at three different points in time: within 3 months postonset (acute), between 3 and 12 months postonset (postacute), and more than 12 months postonset (chronic). Robey considered as eligible 55 studies, all of which were coded for the variables considered. Results of the meta-analysis indicated that recovery in treated patients was superior to recovery in untreated patients and the difference was higher in acute patients; that intensive treatment was more effective than less intensive treatment, and that, when treated, acute severe aphasics recovered more than acute moderate aphasics. This last result is rather unexpected, but it is based on only one study of severe acute patients and two studies of moderate acute patients. A larger number of studies may well yield different results. From these results, Robey argues that aphasia therapy in general for aphasic patients in general is effective, and that it is now time to investigate more precise questions.

Finally, Greener et al. (1999) performed a thorough search of the literature from 1968 to 1998. The main aims of the study were to compare the outcome of treated and untreated vascular patients, and the outcome of patients treated by speech therapists and patients treated by volunteers. Studies had to be randomized, controlled trials. Only 12 studies were considered eligible; 45 were considered and rejected because they were not randomized, and 3 further studies were considered but rejected for various other reasons. Of the 12 eligible studies, only 2 compared treated and untreated patients (Lincoln et al., 1984; Wertz et al., 1986) and only 4 compared patients treated by professionals with patients treated by volunteers (Meikle et al., 1979; David et al., 1982; Wertz et al., 1986; Leal et al., 1993). Due to the paucity of data, a meta-analysis was not performed. The authors' conclusion is that aphasia therapy has not been demonstrated to be either clearly effective or clearly ineffective. However, they invite readers to be cautions about generalization of this result to the population of aphasic patients in general because of the quite stringent exclusion criteria.

The Brain Injury-Interdisciplinary Special Interest Group (BI-ISIG) of the American Congress of Rehabilitation Medicine has lately been developing recommendations for the practice of cognitive rehabilitation. The Cognitive Rehabilitation Committee developed clinical recommendations based on a thorough search and reading of the literature (Cicerone et al., 2000). The studies finally considered were classified according to the soundness of their experimental methodology in Class I, Class II, and Class III. Class I studies included prospective, randomized, controlled studies. Prospective cohort studies and clinical series with well-defined controls were defined as Class II studies. Clinical studies without controls and single case studies with appropriate methodology constituted Class III. Recommendations for clinical practice were organized into three types—practice standards, practice guidelines, and practice options. Practice standards are based on the highest level of evidence and practice options on the least.

Seven areas of intervention were considered: attention, visuospatial deficits, language and communication deficits, memory, executive functions and problem solving, multimodal interventions, and comprehensive-holistic cognitive rehabilitation. Forty-one studies concerned with language and communication deficits were reviewed and classified: 8 were classified as Class I studies, 7 as Class II, and 26 as Class III. An evaluation of the findings of the studies and of their level of evidence led the committee to conclude that there is enough evidence for recommending language and communication disorder rehabilitation as practice standards. In other words, the American Congress of Rehabilitation Medicine suggests that language rehabilitation should be always performed because there is sufficient evidence to demonstrate its usefulness.

One could argue that the recommendation of rehabilitation by the committee is self-serving, but the committee did not reach the same conclusions for other areas of possible intervention. Attention training for patients with traumatic brain injury, for example, is recommended only as a practice guideline, and the committee does not recommend rehabilitation of visuospatial disorders in patients without visual neglect because its benefits have not been clearly proven.

GROUP STUDIES AND SINGLE CASE STUDIES

Data from the group studies reviewed in this chapter are of several types, varying in scientific merit, reliability, and the provision of a basis for generalization. No single study has proved to be so comprehensive and rigorously designed and executed as to provide by itself an unequivocal answer to questions about the efficacy of aphasia therapy. Notwithstanding their methodological weaknesses, taken together and backed up by the results of the meta-analyses and by findings in chronic aphasic patients, they support the conclusion that language treatment leads to significant greater gains in a number of patients. There is, however, a more general and theoretical objection frequently raised against the group studies that have addressed the question of the effectiveness of aphasia rehabilitation.

Regardless of whether they have been well conducted or not, group studies (or randomized, controlled trials [RCTs]) have been criticized on theoretical grounds, and it has been argued that they cannot be used to evaluate the efficacy of aphasia therapy. An example is Howard's (1986) paper, which fueled an ongoing discussion about the advantages and disadvantages of group and single case studies for the evaluation of aphasia therapy effectiveness (cf. Fitz-Gibbon, 1986; Pring, 1986, 1987). It should be emphasized that we are not dealing here with the use of single case versus group studies in neuropsychology in general but specifically with the literature on their adequacy in the evaluation of the efficacy of aphasia rehabilitation.

Howard argued that "the effectiveness of aphasia therapy is not an issue that can be addressed by an RCT; in this case (and many others) it is an inappropriate scientific technique" (Howard, 1986, p. 91). He went on to illustrate the conditions necessary to justify the use of RCTs as a method of assessing treatment efficacy. He identified the features of the statistical design that allowed researchers to draw powerful conclusions from RCTs with the employment of streptomycin-TB in patients with tuberculosis and considered the extent to which these features apply to RCTs in aphasia therapy. He addressed three points: homogeneity of the populations studied, homogeneity of the treatments given, and sensitivity of the assessment techniques. The populations of the RCT with streptomycin were homogeneous with respect to the illness studied, as were the treatments given. In contrast, apart from a few studies that investigated relatively homogeneous groups of patients (only Broca or global aphasics, for instance), treated and untreated aphasics in the RCTs were unselected and all types of aphasic disorders were grouped together. The unavoidable problems in pooling heterogeneous patients together are that therapy may be effective for some but not all types of aphasic disorders and that the lack of homogeneity of the group can mask the effect of therapy for, say, Wernicke but not Broca aphasics. The second point referred to homogeneity of treatment. Even if it were demonstrated that the outcome of the intervention was favorable, the treatments adopted in the RCTs were not specified and probably varied from one study to another. It would therefore be impossible to use the same treatment with other patients and replicate the success. Finally, Howard argued that the techniques adopted to evaluate recovery are insensitive and therefore unsuitable to measure it.

These considerations led Howard to the conclusion that the question of the efficacy of aphasia therapy is too broad and not amenable to scientific discourse. More realistic questions would be, for instance, which treatments are effective and for what particular disorders. The solution of the problem, according to Howard, is to abandon clinical trials and to evaluate specific therapeutic interventions using single case studies (for an answer to Howard, see Fitz-Gibbon, 1986).

The researchers who have criticized the group studies generally have supported the use of single case studies for the evaluation of aphasia therapy efficacy (e.g., Coltheart, 1983; Howard, 1986; Howard & Hatfield, 1987; Byng, 1993).

Criticisms against the single case approach have not been as frequent as those against the group-study approach, but single case studies have not escaped criticism. Two general shortcomings of such an approach may be mentioned. One is the impossibility of controlled replication that would enable one to reject a previously reported result. The other is that the performance of individual patients may be idiosyncratic and too specific to permit meaningful generalization.

Two further objections are more directly related to the use of single case studies for the evaluation of aphasia therapy efficacy. First, in no single case is it possible to demonstrate beyond any reasonable doubt that recovery is due to the therapeutic intervention and not to some other undetected cause, such as spontaneous recovery or changes in lifestyle. One of the advantages of the group study approach is that it allows one to define the risk of concluding that aphasia therapy was effective when in fact it was not. Second, even if a certain method has been demonstrated to be effective for a specific patient, we still do not know whether it will be effective for another. This holds true because no two patients are alike, and it is not known whether the success of the intervention can be attenuated by individual differences.

Recently, several important developments in statistical research have concerned single-subject designs, and Robey et al. (1999) argue that the generality of treatment efficacy can be assessed through meta-analysis of several single case studies. They go on to say that "the capacity for single-subject studies to produce standard evidence regarding the effectiveness of a treatment for an individual is largely unrealized" (p. 468), and they offer some guidelines for the correct application of single-subject designs. It is to be hoped that Robey et al.'s suggestion will be taken up and that the question of the effectiveness of aphasia therapy will receive an important contribution from single case studies.

Without discussing the intricacy of the statistical evaluation of the advantages and disadvantages of group studies versus single case studies, I shall, nevertheless, try to place the problem of the group studies about aphasia therapy effectiveness into a historical perspective. Furthermore, in Appendix 1, two apologues are reported. They tackle a problem in the single case study and group study approaches—systematic sampling and casual observation—but are not concerned with the merits of either approach in general. The choice between single case and group studies mostly depends on the question asked. In Chapter 5 we will see that cognitive neuropsychologists have convincingly argued that to study the functional architecture of normal cognitive functions, group studies are inadequate and only single case studies are appropriate. By contrast, a well-conducted randomized, controlled trial gives reliable responses to such question as the efficacy of aphasia therapy that can be generalized to the population.

A HISTORICAL PERSPECTIVE

As aptly stated by Shallice, "it inevitably takes a long time to collect enough patients to form a series. . . . The slowness with which the series is assembled generally implies that it is necessary to set very wide criteria for the patients to be included" (Shallice, 1988, p. 209). In our 1979 study, for example, we (Basso et al., 1979) presented data from 281 patients that we had started to collect in 1965.

Unless patients are drawn from many centers, the collection of data always requires many years. Once the data are collected, one must analyze them and write the results, which means that the group studies have a very long gestation; when they are eventually published, the data are already rather old. Inspection of the years of publication of these studies reveals that most of them were published many years ago and that very few are relatively recent. They deal with patients rehabilitated many years ago, in the 1960s and 1970s, when theories about the nature of aphasia were not as detailed as they are today. In the 1960s, many authors assumed that there was only one form of aphasia that varied only in severity. Others acknowledged that there were different clinical types due to lesions of different brain regions. The analysis of the language disorder, however, was rather unrefined, and at best the deficits were described with reference to levels of language processing (phonemes, words, sentences). Given this theoretical background, "grouping" corresponded to theoretical positions of the time and it seemed reasonable to conduct group studies that, if well carried out, would allow generalization of the results to the aphasic population in general.

A criticism frequently raised against the group studies is that the treatment employed was not clearly specified, which made it impossible for another therapist to reproduce it. In this respect, it must be kept in mind that clinical studies were not concerned about the outcome of a specific treatment, such as learning to read 50 words or to name 50 pictures. They aimed to establish whether rehabilitation had a positive effect on the patients' language performance in their daily lives. An important difference between learning 50 words and becoming more proficient in language use is immediately perceivable. It is possible to describe in sufficient detail how a restricted treatment program has been carried out, but it is impossible to summarize in a paper how a number of aphasic patients with quantitatively and qualitatively different language disruptions have been rehabilitated. Manuals of aphasia therapy detail the therapeutic methods used by different researchers (e.g., Basso, 1977; Ducarne, 1986; Shewan & Bandur, 1986) and can be referred to for further information about the techniques used.

In brief, it is argued that the clinical studies have achieved their purpose. They have demonstrated that aphasia therapy can enhance recovery in some patients. However, although the question about the efficacy of aphasia therapy was once important, today it is obsolete because we know much more about the possible functional disruptions in aphasia and it no longer makes sense to address the issue in such general terms.

Many other questions remain unanswered. To list just a few: For which patients and damages is therapy efficacious? Which is the best therapeutic intervention? What intensity and duration of therapy are advisable?

CONCLUSIONS

This chapter reviewed studies on the efficacy of aphasia therapy regrouped according to how the problem was dealt with: clinical studies without a control group, treated chronic patients, treated and untreated patients, comparison of different methods, and meta-analyses of previous studies. Notwithstanding the greater evidence of the efficacy of aphasia therapy, the question is still unsettled. Many researchers argue that aphasia therapy efficacy can only be demonstrated by RCTs. However, the complexity of the behavioral and social sciences is such that random assignment of patients to either control or treatment conditions is frequently impossible but lack of randomization does not necessarily imply a lack of scientific power (Robey et al., 1999). Lack of precision in terminology can also add to the confusion. I have used the terms *efficacy* and *effectiveness* interchangeably, but they should not be confused.

Efficacy has been defined as "the probability of benefit to individuals in a defined population from a medical technology applied to a given medical problem under ideal conditions of use" (Office of Technology Assessment [OTA], 1978, p. 16). *Effectiveness* has been defined in the same terms except for conditions of use, which are not ideal but average (OTA, 1978). In other words, the difference between efficacy and effectiveness lies in the conditions of use, ideal in efficacy studies and average in effectiveness studies. In practice, it means that an efficacious treatment works under ideal conditions and *can* work under average conditions, whereas an effective treatment *does* work under normal average conditions. Researches about effectiveness should be carried out only once efficacy has been demonstrated.

It is not always easy to decide whether the outcome studies described in this chapter are efficacy or effectiveness studies. For most of them, the conditions were not average, although not ideal, and they can be considered efficacy studies. Lincoln et al.'s (1984) study, by contrast, was carried out under more average conditions. The treatment regimen was representative of clinical practice, and no specific type of speech therapy was advocated. The negative result of this study may simply signify that aphasia therapy is efficacious, as demonstrated by numerous studies, but it is not effective under average conditions in the United Kingdom. As suggested by the results of studies on intensity and duration of treatment, the reason for this difference may simply lie in the brevity of standard language treatments.

5

COGNITIVE NEUROPSYCHOLOGY

IT CAN BE ARGUED THAT the first cycle in the history of aphasia research comes to a close with the studies on efficacy of aphasia therapy reported in Chapter 4. The nature of the aphasic disorder was discussed in the second half of the nineteenth century and the first decades of the twentieth century, and two schools of thought—the associationist and the holistic—had faced each other. After relaunching of the associationist approach, objective methods of evaluating the disorder were devised. Therapy for aphasia became common practice, and its effectiveness was thoroughly investigated. Yet, the classic clinical approach had exhausted its propulsive spur, and a totally new approach was needed. This was to be the cognitive neuropsychological approach.

The 1950s saw the growth of a new scientific approach to cognition. Many of the various influences that were at the root of this new approach coalesced in 1956. The name given to this approach was *cognitive psychology*, which was also endowed with a birthday, September 11, 1956. A Symposium on Information Theory was in fact held at the Massachusetts Institute of Technology on that date, and many scientists from different disciplines, among whom were Noam Chomsky, George Miller, Allen Newell, and Herbert Simon, participated. The major goal of cognitive psychology was to learn more about how the mind works and to formulate descriptions of the processes that occur during the execution of a mental activity such as speaking, planning an action, recognizing a friend, or memorizing a fact.

The human processing system was likened to a computer with specialized subsystems, and flow chart diagrams were used to illustrate the various stages of processing. The growth of experimental psychology and the use of flow charts helped the development of explicit theories of the organization of the normal cognitive system. In addition, data obtained from the observation of brain-damaged patients began to be used, and inferences about the structure of normal, intact cognitive processes were drawn from impaired processing.

A name was needed for this new branch of cognitive psychology, and Coltheart wrote, "Since it is an approach to cognitive psychology, and since the data used come from patients with neuropsychological disorders, the term 'cognitive neuropsychology' would seem appropriate" (Coltheart, 1984, p. 2). However, at least in its early days, there was a sharp difference between clinical and cognitive neuropsychology, cognitive neuropsychology being a science about the mind and clinical neuropsychology about the brain. Yet, it must be noted that cognitive neuropsychology would not be possible if distinct cognitive components were not also spatially separated in the brain, and lately the brain has made its reappearance in cognitive neuropsychology. To cite just one example, McCloskey lists three objectives of cognitive neuropsychology, among which is "to explore the localization of cognitive functions in the brain" (McCloskey, 2000, p. 593).

The basic aims of cognitive neuropsychology are to provide a theory or model of normal cognitive processing and to explain performance in brain-damaged patients in terms of damage to one or more components of the normal cognitive function. The classic anatomo-clinical neuropsychological approach had provided knowledge about the relationships between lesion and function. Neuropsychologists found that brain damage does not always cause a general cognitive disorder, and they established the existence of many selective deficits suggesting that the brain is organized into distinctive areas of relative functional independence. However, in spite of the accumulation of knowledge derived from the study of neurologically impaired patients, the problem of inferring normal brain functions from behavioral dysfunctions was still a crucial issue in neuropsychology. Researchers were somewhat dissatisfied with the methodology of clinical neuropsychology. Shallice, for example, stated, "In the mid-1960s, then, neuropsychology did not appear to outsiders to be a very exciting field. The laborious group-study methods then standard seemed likely to produce a decreasing return for theory on empirical time and effort. The rococo splendors of the field's youth were generally forgotten" (Shallice, 1988, p. 14). Even more pessimistic were Caramazza and McCloskey, who wrote, "It is not an exaggeration to say that over one hundred years of research on cognitive disorders has shed little light on the nature of normal cognitive processes and the form of their dissolution in conditions of brain damage" (Caramazza & McCloskey, 1988, p. 519).

Researchers started to be more concerned about the nature of the cognitive mechanisms and the formulation of an explicit theory of cognitive functions and less interested in their localization in the brain. Major changes were introduced, which can be summarized as follows: cognitive neuropsychologists stressed the rigorous study of single patients and abandoned the group study approach; they argued for a functional approach to the study of the mind explicitly independent of the study of the brain, and they introduced the use of information-processing models, which provide a rational basis for the characterization of patterns of impaired performance in terms of damaged subcomponents.

This chapter is divided into two parts. The first part deals with some fundamental questions in cognitive neuropsychology. The assumptions that must be made for cognitive neuropsychology to be possible, the status of the single case study and the concept of syndromes in general, the use of association and dissociation of symptoms for studying the functional structure of a cognitive function, and the more recent analysis of error types for understanding the nature and processing of representations will be briefly considered. A final topic in the first part of the chapter is the possibility of differentiating disorders of access to unimpaired representations from damage of the representations.

The second part of the chapter describes the neoassociationist and cognitive syndromes of reading and writing disorders to illustrate the main differences between the two approaches.

ASSUMPTIONS

The use of pathological data for the study of the normal cognitive system is not straightforward; it requires some assumptions. The main assumptions of cognitive neuropsychology are the modularity assumption, the universality assumption, and the subtraction assumption. Cognitive neuropsychologists do not assert that these assumptions are true; they do, however, argue that they have to be true for cognitive neuropsychology to be possible.

The *modularity assumption* states that a complex cognitive function consists of a series of functionally independent subcomponents. Intuitively, it is easy to grasp the meaning of the word *module*. We can all imagine a machine (e.g., a computer) made up of subcomponents that perform different functions and interact with other parts of the machine. Even before the modularity assumption was explicitly asserted, functional independence of components within a cognitive system had already been demonstrated. Shallice and Warrington (1969), for example, described a patient with normal learning and impaired short-term memory. The converse pattern—normal short-term memory and impaired learning—found in amnesic patients provides evidence for the modular organization of the memory system.

Fodor (1983) characterized modules in a stringent way and listed a number of characteristics. Among other things, they are domain specific, computationally autonomous, and informationally encapsulated. *Domain specificity* refers to the fact that a module responds to only one particular sort of input; *computationally autonomous* means that it does not share general resources such as attention and memory with other modules; *informationally encapsulated* indicates that the module has access to a restricted and predetermined amount of information and carries out its own processing in complete isolation from the processes going on in other parts of the cognitive system.

According to Fodor, modules have a further property; they are *innate*, that is, they are part of our genetic endowment. This statement, however, is no longer accepted because of the existence of systems that are modular in many important aspects but are not innate. The best examples are the reading and writing systems (see below), which apparently behave like other modular cognitive systems but which are culturally transmitted, have been only recently acquired in phylogeny, and must be acquired through learning by every child.

Fodor's criteria for the characterization of modules are highly specific and very strict, but most cognitive neuropsychologists admit that cognitive systems can have different degrees of modularity. Modular systems are generally illustrated by diagrams, in which boxes correspond to modules or components and arrows correspond to the flow of information.

The *universality assumption* states that the structure of a cognitive function is universal, that is, there are no significant individual variations in the functional structure of cognitive systems; if the functional structure varied within individuals, it would not be possible to make inferences from one patient to another. This assumption is not peculiar to cognitive neuropsychology, but cognitive neuropsychologists have stated it explicitly.

Finally, the *subtraction assumption* states that no new cognitive structure is created as a consequence of the lesion and that an impaired cognitive system is basically the same as a normal system except that some of its operations are impaired. In other words, pathological transformations of the normal cognitive function obey constraints determined by the normal structure of the system and can be inferred from the analysis of the normal structure. If this were not so, studying impaired systems would not foster our knowledge about normal systems.

As stated earlier, cognitive neuropsychologists do not assert that these assumptions are true. They must be considered such for cognitive neuropsychology to work. However, it is possible to bring some evidence that cognitive neuropsychology works and therefore that its assumptions are substantially correct. In the past 20 years, much coherent evidence about the structure of cognitive systems has accumulated and data from cognitive neuropsychology have also been used to explain data from normal subjects. If any of the assumptions were wrong, this result would not have been possible. Consider, for example, the universality assumption. If the cognitive system were not very similar (if not exactly the same) in every one of us, data from different patients would point to two or more different cognitive structures. If, on the contrary, as has happened, results from various patients suggest the same cognitive structure, the assumption of universality is reinforced. The same line of reasoning holds for the other two assumptions. If they were wrong, it would not have been possible for cognitive neuropsychology to accumulate coherent and reliable data. The degree to which patients' performances converge and are interpretable by making similar assumptions is an indication of the extent to which the proposed theory of the normal cognitive structure is confirmed by patients' data.

SYNDROMES AND SINGLE CASE STUDIES

Syndromes are a collection of symptoms that co-occur. They may co-occur because they have an underlying common cause or because of damage to adjacent areas of the brain—in other words, because they are functionally correlated or because of anatomical proximity. Regrouping of the patients in syndromes was undertaken primarily for medical purposes and proved to be very useful. During the neoassociationist period of neuropsychology it was the only systematic basis for patient classification, and much information was gathered by comparing groups of patients. Groups were formed on the basis of either similar lesions (left or right hemisphere, frontal, parietal, and so forth) or similar impairments, such as Broca aphasia, Wernicke aphasia, and acalculia. Little by little, syndromes tended to be elevated to the status of theoretical entities and to be transformed into evidence of the necessary co-occurrence of their symptoms. The main objection made by cognitive neuropsychologists to the use of syndromes for the constitution of experimental groups was that the classic aphasia categories were not based on the presence of any necessary and sufficient symptom.

Poeck, considering the problem of aphasic syndromes from a neurologist's point of view, agreed that they are "to a large extent, artifacts produced by the vascularization of the language area" (Poeck, 1983, p. 84) and not natural combinations of symptoms that necessarily co-occur. However, he defended their usefulness since about 80% of vascular aphasic patients cluster very strongly in well-defined subgroups because of the little interindividual variation in the distribution of the branches of the middle cerebral artery. "Therefore it is justified and indispensable to base group research on aphasia ... on vascular patients and to divide these patients in well-defined subgroups" (Poeck, 1983, p. 85). On the other hand, according to Schwartz (1984), the evolution of the classic taxonomy has become increasingly empirical and unfounded on a theoretical basis, and it has reached a "polytypic" structure. Members of the same category, she argued, do not share any single attribute but only have a family resemblance. Broca aphasics, for instance, do not share any single necessary feature, and generalizations from the performance of one group of Broca aphasics to other groups of Broca aphasics is unjustified. Schwartz argued that aphasia syndromes are not "real entities" because "one cannot delineate for each category an 'essence' or idealized pattern which is invariant and hence shared by all members of the group" (Schwartz, 1984, p. 5). Accordingly, the use of intensive single case studies was advocated by cognitive neuropsychologists.

In neuropsychological research the single case was of central importance in the early years of development of the field; neuropsychology owes much to the careful description of rare patients with remarkable disorders. After World War II the privileged status of the single case came to an end, and single case studies were substituted for by group studies. Patients were selected for the presence of a syndrome (or symptom) or for the site of the lesion and were studied with standardized batteries. Within the past 20–30 years the role of single cases for the theoretical interpretation of data has been increasingly recognized, and single case studies have been argued to be the best or even the only methodology for making inferences about the normal cognitive system.

Caramazza and McCloskey (1988), for example, wrote: "valid inferences about the structure of normal cognitive systems from patterns of impaired performance are only possible for single-patient studies" (p. 519). Their argument is that the performance of a patient on a given task is the output of the normal system affected by the functional lesion; however, a patient's functional lesion is unknown, and study of the patient includes the identification of the components that are damaged. Averaging results from two or more patients is not feasible because the functional lesions are different and interfere differently with the execution of the experimental task. It is not possible to guarantee that any two patients are functionally homogeneous.

Shallice (1988) argued that this is an extreme position and labeled it *ultra-cognitive neuropsychology*. A lively debate between supporters of the single-case-only approach for the study of normal cognitive processes and supporters of a less rigid position took place. A whole issue of *Cognitive Neuropsychology* (1988, vol. 5, n. 5) was dedicated to the first round of discussion about the single-case-only approach.

One of the criticisms raised against the single case study is that it is impossible to replicate since no two brain lesions are exactly the same and it is impossible to find two patients who show exactly the same functional damages. This is not an insurmountable obstacle. Replicability can be within the patient if crucial findings can be replicated within the same patient on more than one occasion. Replicability across patients is made possible by the use of the multiple single case studies method. When results from several nonidentical patients can be accounted for by the same theory about the normal cognitive mechanisms, the theory is reinforced rather than weakened by the diversity of results.

ASSOCIATIONS AND DISSOCIATIONS

For the study of functional structure, one type of neuropsychological finding—dissociations—has been considered to have a special status. A dissociation occurs when a group of patients (or a single patient) perform poorly on one task and at a normal level (or significantly better) on another task. We talk in this case of a *simple dissociation*. One interpretation of the dissociation is that the two tasks are subserved by two different functions, which explains why they are separately impaired. Yet, it remains possible that the two tasks are subserved by the same function but have different levels of difficulty, and the more difficult task shows greater impairment than the easier one when the single subserving mechanism is impaired.

A much stronger basis for hypothesizing independent functions is the *double dissociation*. According to Shallice (1988), the major successes of the use of single case studies have been the demonstration of the independence of specific subsystems with the double dissociation paradigm. A double dissociation occurs when patient A is impaired in task X and (nearly) unimpaired in task Y, and patient B presents with the reverse pattern of performance: disruption of performance in task Y and (near) normal performance on task X. This is generally considered sufficient experimental evidence to argue that tasks X and Y are dependent on different cognitive processes. A double dissociation can also be present in a single patient. Rapp and Caramazza (2002), for example, described a patient who could write nouns better than verbs but showed the opposite pattern—verbs better than nouns—in speaking.

Association of symptoms is more difficult to interpret, as symptoms can co-occur simply because of the vicinity of the neural areas on which they depend and not because they reflect a functionally necessary association (see Shallice, 1988, for discussion). Caramazza (1986), however, argued that whenever a model predicts that a given functional lesion will cause the co-occurrence of a certain number of symptoms, the finding of such an association of symptoms is theoretically relevant. If dissociation of the symptoms expected to follow from damage to a single component should be observed, it would provide counterevidence for the proposed model. A case of a theoretically important association of disorders is patient IGR (Caramazza et al., 1986). This patient showed impairment in reading, writing, and repetition of nonwords, and the errors consisted primarily in single-letter and phoneme substitutions. This pattern of impairments was interpreted by the authors as necessarily coexisting. The functional architecture for reading, writing, and repetition assumed by the investigators predicted in fact that a single functional damage to the phonological output buffer (see Chapter 6) would result in precisely this pattern of impairment.

ERROR ANALYSIS

The study of brain-damaged patients for gaining insights into the structure and functioning of normal systems is fraught with problems. Yet, the study of a malfunctioning machine can be more informative than the study of a perfectly working one.

In the realm of language processing, for example, much has been learned based on the study of normal speech errors, which show a variety of regularities and distributional properties that have been used to make some hypotheses about the underlying structure of language. Among the most informative speech errors are word and segment exchanges. Exchanges are subject to excursion constraints; word exchanges, for example, involve words from the same grammatical class that exchange across different phrases ("Well you can cut *rain* in the *trees*," from Garrett, 1982). Sound exchanges generally involve sounds from words from different grammatical classes but within the same phrase ("And this is the *l*arietal *p*obe" (parietal lobe), from Garrett, 1982). This observation can be explained if one presupposes a multiphrasal level in language processing where lexical items have already been retrieved (and can be exchanged) but have not been phonologically specified and a single-phrasal language processing level where the phonological forms of the words are specified and segments of words can be exchanged.

As noted earlier, one of the most important and early tools of cognitive neuropsychology was the study of dissociations, which permitted the identification of the components of the system, how the components relate to each other, and a proposed model of the system's functional architecture. The second step in cognitive neuropsychology research consisted in studying the representations and internal mechanisms of each component. To do so, the study of the types of errors that arise from damage to each component is necessary. The impaired performance of patients can be richly structured, and in-depth analyses of their performance can help us to understand how components are internally organized. In Chapter 6, data from patients LB (Caramazza & Miceli, 1990) and HE (McCloskey et al., 1994) with damage to the orthographic output buffer are reported. It will be seen that a careful analysis of their errors has enabled the investigators to propose a highly structured internal organization of orthographic structure at the level of the graphemic buffer.

ACCESS AND STORAGE DISORDERS

A frequently drawn distinction is that between deficits of access to unimpaired stored representations and damage to stored representations. The distinction is considered important not only on theoretical grounds but also because of its bearing upon therapy. Warrington and Shallice (1979) attempted to account for certain differences among patients with deficits to the semantic system and suggested four variables to distinguish access and storage disorders. A fifth criterion was added subsequently by Warrington and McCarthy (1983). According to these criteria, patients with damage to stored representations should be consistent in their responses, show a frequency effect, be better at making decisions about superordinate than subordinate information, present no effects of priming, and be insensitive to the rate of presentation. On the other hand, patients with an access disorder should be inconsistent in their responses, have a small frequency effect, be equally damaged in their knowledge of superordinate and subordinate information, show a priming effect, and be better at lower rates of presentation.

Intuitively, consistency of responses appears to be a convincing argument for differentiating between access and storage disorders. If a representation is lost, it will never be possible to retrieve it; if, on the other hand, it is not lost but difficult to access, it is conceivable that under some facilitatory circumstances it can be accessed. In addition, Warrington and Shallice (1979) maintained that a storage disorder will be characterized by a frequency effect since frequent items are argued to have a lower threshold or a higher resting state, and it is presumable that they are more resistant to damage; on the other hand, the characteristic variability of an access disorder should reduce the frequency effect. As for the third variable— differences in accessing superordinate and subordinate information— Shallice (1988) argues that for both types of disorders it will be easier to identify the superordinate category than the specific item. Attribute information is then easier to obtain in the case of an access disorder because the superordinate information should facilitate access to the specific attributes. As for priming, the line of reasoning is similar to that of consistency of responses. If an item is lost, it should not be possible to prime it, whereas in case of a retrieval deficit, priming may be possible. Finally, Warrington and McCarthy (1983) suggest that damaged access procedures become refractory and are unable to operate immediately after having operated. They necessitate large intervals to operate again. Accessibility of an item at lower but not at higher rates of presentation is a further characteristic of an access disorder.

Rapp and Caramazza (1993) take issue with this characterization of the access–storage dichotomy. They claim that the empirical findings on which it is based are not very robust, and that the five criteria are independent of one another and represent an arbitrary list. They argue that theories about the internal organization of the semantic system are underspecified and do not allow one to draw reliable conclusions. For each of these criteria they propose a theory that would predict the opposite results, such as inconsistency of responses with a storage disorder and consistency with an access disorder. However, notwithstanding the critics, these criteria for distinguishing between access and storage disorders have generally been accepted by clinical aphasiologists. The question of the relevance of the access–storage dichotomy for aphasia therapy will be treated in Chapter 8.

In the second part of this chapter, disorders of reading and writing will be reviewed and the classical and early "cognitive" syndromes will be illustrated. Today the multicomponent nature of most cognitive syndromes is recognized, and although labels such as *deep dyslexia* or *surface dysgraphia* are still used, they are not meant to point to a unitary functional damage.

THE DYSLEXIA AND DYSGRAPHIA SYNDROMES

When discussing the neoassociationist syndromes in Chapter 2, I reported whether or not reading and writing were concurrently impaired with oral language but did not discuss them in detail. In the rest of this chapter, the classic and early cognitive syndromes of reading and writing disorders are briefly described. This will permit a direct comparison of the two approaches and serve as an introduction to the cognitive neuropsychological approach that will be the topic of the next two chapters. For an understanding of the cognitive reading and writing syndromes, reference to a simple model of the structure of the normal function will suffice; the model will be better described in Chapter 6.

The Classic Alexia Syndromes

A recent neuroanatomical classification of reading disorders is that of Benson and Ardila (1996). In keeping with the objectives of classical neuropsychology and the analysis of aphasia, Benson and Ardila describe three main forms of alexia: parietal-temporal alexia, occipital alexia, and frontal or third alexia.

Parietal-temporal alexia. Reading disorders in parietal-temporal alexia are generally associated with writing disorders. The alexia and the agraphia may be total, and both the ability to read aloud and the ability to comprehend written language are disturbed. Generally, patients cannot read numbers or music. In addition to the alexia and agraphia, patients have oral language disorders that are, however, mild. Recovery of reading, although not complete, is not infrequent.

Occipital alexia. Described by Dejerine (1892), this form of alexia is frequently called *pure* alexia because of the absence of other language disorders. Patients with pure alexia are generally unable to identify even single letters, and they cannot read aloud. A few can identify single letters, but the process is slow. They cannot read words in a global way, except for some very short and common words. When they do succeed in identifying a word, they understand it, in contrast to patients with parietal-temporal alexia. Pure alexic patients can write but are unable to read what they have written. Due to the lesion's location, right hemianopia is present in most cases.

Frontal alexia. As indicated by the name, the lesion that causes this form of alexia is localized in the frontal lobe and is generally accompanied by Broca aphasia. Classic neuropsychology did not assign to Broca's area any role in reading and writing competence, which was ascribed to the angular gyrus region. Lictheim (1885), having observed reading disorders in some Broca aphasics, argued that this symptom complex resulted from two different lesions, one in Broca's area (giving rise to disorders of oral output) and one in the angular gyrus (giving rise to the reading disorder). Benson stated that "just how a frontal alexia could be explained, using the prevalent theories of language, was never settled" (Benson, 1979, p. 114). However, he observed that frontal alexia is qualitatively different from the other alexias. According to Benson, frontal alexic patients fail when asked to name individual letters, but they understand at least isolated written words; reading aloud and comprehension are better for nouns than for other classes of words.

Besides these main forms of alexia, Benson and Ardila acknowledge the existence of other forms of reading disturbances, such as aphasic alexia (reading disorders that occur as a feature of many aphasic syndromes), which they argue are not reading disorders per se.

The Classic Agraphia Syndromes

Researchers have long assumed that writing requires phonological mediation, that is, that it is not possible to activate written word forms directly from semantics but that in order to write a word the phonological form of the word must be activated first. One of the most accurate analyses of writing in line with the phonological mediation hypothesis is that of Luria (1970), who identified a series of necessary steps. To write a word, one must first activate its phonological form, analyze it acoustically, identify the sequence of phonemes that compose the word, and, finally, translate each phoneme into a grapheme.

The supposed subordination of writing to oral language and the rarity of isolated agraphia may in part explain the lack of interest in writing disorders aphasiologists have manifested for a long time. In 1979, Benson wrote that "while there have been attempts to utilize graphic evaluation for clinical purposes, using both anatomical and psychological correlations, none have proved consistently useful to date" (Benson, 1979, p. 122). He recognized only dominant frontal agraphia (due to a lesion of the left frontal lobe), dominant parietal-temporal agraphia (with a lesion in the left parietal-temporal region), and nondominant agraphia (due to damage to the posterior right hemisphere). Years later, with Ardila (Benson & Ardila, 1996), he described four different forms of agraphia.

Aphasic agraphia. These writing disturbances are present in most aphasics and show little difference from their oral language counterparts. For example, Broca aphasics have agrammatic writing, conduction aphasics make grapheme substitutions, and so on.

Pure agraphia. Some patients have been described with relatively isolated agraphia without other marked language disorders (e.g., Basso et al., 1978). The lesion was either left frontal (Penfield & Roberts, 1959; Dubois et al., 1969) or left parietal (Russell & Espir, 1961; Kinsbourne & Rosenfield, 1974; Rosati & De Bastiani, 1979; Auerbach & Alexander, 1981).

Apraxic agraphia. Constructional skills are necessary to produce well-formed letters, and constructional apraxia or limb apraxia may cause writing disorders unrelated to aphasia. Rare cases of a selective deficit of the graphic motor program, however, have been described in patients who do not show other apraxic disturbances and whose oral spelling is relatively preserved (Roeltgen & Heilman, 1983; Baxter & Warrington, 1986; Costlett et al., 1986; Anderson et al., 1990).

Visuospatial agraphia. Visuospatial analysis is necessary to write. Posterior lesions of the right hemisphere can cause a visuospatial impairment and a purely mechanical, nonaphasic variety of writing disorder.

The Cognitive Dyslexia Syndromes

Figure 5–1 presents a schematic model of the structure of the dual-route reading model assumed here. The model assumes a semantic-lexical route passing through the orthographic input lexicon, the semantic system, and the phonological output lexicon and a nonlexical route that utilizes the grapheme-phoneme conversion rules. Reading and spelling of familiar words can be carried out by the semantic-lexical route. Reading of the word *chair*, for instance, can be explained by hypothesizing that the sequence of letters (*C H A I R*) is held in the abstract letter identification system for its successive identification; the word is then recognized in the orthographic input lexicon. The output of the lexicon accesses the

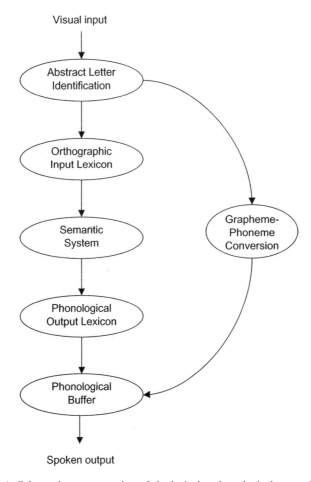

Figure 5–1. Schematic representation of the lexical and nonlexical routes for reading.

semantic representation of *chair* in the semantic system, which in turn accesses the phonological representation of the word *chair* for output. This is then held in the phonological output buffer for successive articulation. Reading of orthography-to-phonology irregular words must follow this lexical-semantic route. Correct reading of a word such as *pint* that does not rhyme with *mint* must be lexically driven.

Normal literate subjects can read irregular words and are also able to give a phonologically plausible rendition of new words or legal nonwords, which cannot be achieved through the lexical route. Reading of novel or unfamiliar words involves converting the sequence of constituent graphemes into corresponding phonological sequences, and this is what the grapheme-to-phoneme conversion mechanisms do. The model is described in more detail in Chapter 6.

Deep dyslexia. The most important defining symptoms of deep dyslexia are the impairment of nonword reading and the presence of semantic paraphasias. Deep dyslexia has been the first type of dyslexia described within the framework of cognitive neuropsychology. Marshall and Newcombe (1966, 1973) described patient GR, who made frequent semantic errors in word reading (*ill* was read as *sick*, *bush* as *tree*). A second interesting phenomenon of GR's reading was that it was affected by word class: nouns, for instance, were read better than verbs.

Deep dyslexia is not a functionally homogeneous syndrome, being a multicomponent deficit due to the lesion of two components of the reading system: the nonlexical route and the semantic route. The locus of damage to the semantic route can vary, although the semantic system itself is frequently damaged. The number of semantic paraphasias varies widely from patient to patient (56% of GR's errors were semantic compared to only 10% of those made by Shallice and Coughlan's [1980] patient GS), and it is not clear how many semantic paraphasias there must be in order to classify a patient as having deep dyslexia. Moreover, orthographies vary in the degree of correspondence between graphemes and phonemes. Alphabetic orthographies can be classified according to their orthographic depth, namely, the transparency of their grapheme-to-phoneme and phoneme-to-grapheme correspondence. An orthography is said to be *transparent* or *shallow* when letters are isomorphic to phonemes, and it is said to be *opaque* or *deep* when some letters have more than one sound and some phonemes can be written in more than one way. It has been argued that in transparent orthographies, such as Spanish, semantic paraphasias are absent or at least less frequent than in opaque orthographies, such as English (Ardila, 1991).

The other characteristics of deep dyslexia are visual errors (GR read *wife* for *life*, for instance), derivational errors (reading *entertain as entertainment*), concreteness effect (concrete words are read better than abstract words), and the grammatical class effect (nouns, for instance, are generally read better than verbs).

Impairment of the conversion rules easily explains why patients with deep dyslexia have difficulty reading nonwords, and impairment of the semantic system easily explains why they make semantic errors. The relationship between the other symptoms and the functional damage is not nearly as obvious (for a discussion, see Shallice, 1988).

Surface dyslexia. Surface dyslexia was first described by Marshall and Newcombe in 1973. In surface dyslexia the nonword reading route is relatively preserved and the lexical-semantic route is impaired. The patient can read nonwords and words with regular spelling; errors in reading irregular words generally consist in regularization errors. If a printed word fails to activate the corresponding representation in the phonological output lexicon because of damage somewhere along the lexical route, the application of sublexical conversion rules will allow a plausible phonological pronunciation. Finally, patients will have difficulty comprehending homophone words such as *nun* and *none, route* and *root*. The only basis patients have for comprehension is the phonological form they have produced through the conversion mechanisms, and they have no clue as to which one of the two meanings of the phonological form was written.

In transparent orthographies, like Spanish, surface dyslexia is difficult to demonstrate. If all words can be read by applying conversion rules, all words will be read correctly, regularization errors will not be present, homophones will also be homographs, and all the possible meanings will be correct. Regularization errors can, however, occur when reading unknown foreign words that have come to be regularly used in oral language, such as *jeans*.

Similarly to deep dyslexia, surface dyslexia is not a homogeneous syndrome; damage to the lexical route can be at the level of (or access to) the orthographic input lexicon, the semantic system, or the phonological output lexicon (see Fig. 5–1). In the first case the surface dyslexic patient will also have understanding disorders of written words; in the case of damage to the semantic system there will be difficulties in the comprehension and production of spoken and written words, and errors will frequently be semantic. Finally, damage to the output phonological lexicon will cause naming disorders (see Chapter 6).

Phonological dyslexia. This form of dyslexia was first described by Dérouesné and Beauvois (1979). It follows damage to the nonlexical route. Reading of nonwords is impaired and reading of known words preserved. The dissociation between preserved and impaired processes must be striking and statistically significant, but in no published case was the dissociation complete—that is, 100% correct in reading one type of material and 0% correct in another type—in this or any of the other forms of dyslexia.

Researchers do not agree on the units of analysis of the conversion rules, which can be the grapheme, the syllable, or a still larger unit; moreover, the processes underlying the conversion rules are only partially understood. Mitchum and Berndt (1991) identify three different processes: segmentation of the sequence of graphemes, grapheme-to-phoneme conversion, and assembly of phonemes. Depending on which of these stages is/are impaired, the phonological dyslexic patient presents different disorders.

The Cognitive Dysgraphia Syndromes

Figure 5–2 is a schematic representation of the writing model assumed here with a lexical-semantic route and a conversion route. The lexical-semantic route passes through the phonological input lexicon, the semantic system, and the orthographic output lexicon. As for writing of novel words, the same reasoning carried out for reading applies to the spelling of unfamiliar words. The sequence of heard phonemes must be converted into the corresponding sequence of graphemes by applying the phoneme-to-grapheme conversion rules of the language.

Deep dysgraphia. First described by Bub and Kertesz (1982a), deep dysgraphia is the analogue in writing of deep dyslexia. Damage to the nonlexical route causes difficulty in nonword writing; damage to the semantic system causes errors in word writing, the most characteristic being the semantic paragraphias. Bub and Kertesz's patient also had a concreteness effect (concrete words were written better than abstract words) and a grammatical class effect (nouns were written better than verbs and closed-class words). A few cases of deep dysgraphia are on record (Assal et al., 1981; Nolan & Caramazza, 1983; Patterson & Shewell, 1987), although it remains a relatively rare syndrome.

Surface (or lexical) dysgraphia. Surface dysgraphia, first described by Beauvois and Dérouesné (1981), is interpreted as a consequence of damage to the lexical route. Writing of nonwords is preserved (or

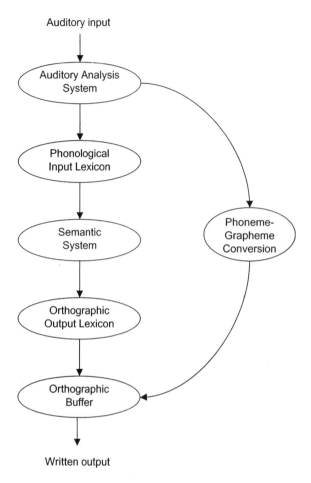

Auditory input

Auditory Analysis System

Phonological Input Lexicon

Semantic System

Phoneme-Grapheme Conversion

Orthographic Output Lexicon

Orthographic Buffer

Written output

Figure 5–2. Schematic representation of the lexical and nonlexical routes for writing.

significantly better than writing of words); writing of regular words is similar to writing of nonwords; the most frequent errors in writing of irregular words are phonologically plausible errors. This is explained by the fact that patients with surface dysgraphia can only use the phoneme-to-grapheme conversion rules to write words; regular words can be rendered correctly because they honor the conversion rules, but irregular words can only be rendered phonologically. A number of English-speaking patients with lexical agraphia have been described (Hatfield & Patterson, 1983; Roeltgen & Heilman, 1984; Goodman & Caramazza, 1986; Baxter & Warrington, 1987). In a totally transparent orthography, surface dysgraphic patients would make no errors since all words, known and unknown, could be spelled correctly using the conversion rules.

Phonological dysgraphia. Described by Shallice (1981), phonological dysgraphia follows damage to the nonlexical writing procedure. Nonword writing is impaired or impossible but writing of known words, whether regular or irregular, is still possible, provided that the words are understood. Lexical writing is based on the operation of the lexical-semantic route; if a word is not understood, activation of the word in the orthographic output lexicon by the semantic system cannot take place and the patient is unable to write the word. A few patients with phonological dysgraphia have been described (Bub & Kertesz, 1982b; Roeltgen et al., 1983; Baxter & Warrington, 1985)

CONCLUSIONS

Description of the reading and writing disorders well exemplifies the differences between clinical and cognitive neuropsychology. Clinical neuropsychology studies brain–behavior relationships and uses groups of patients with similar lesions to identify specific patterns of cognitively damaged behavior. Cognitive neuropsychology focuses on the mind. It starts from models of normal processing, supposedly modular, and uses pathological data with the double aim of verifying normal data and better specifying the functional models. Its main tool was initially the study of dissociation, subsequently supported by analysis of errors. Group studies have been more or less abandoned in favor of single case studies. The assumption of universality supported the generalization of hypotheses based on results of a single patient to the cognitive structure in general, and the subtraction assumption allowed researchers to use data from patients to make inferences about the normal structure.

The next two chapters are concerned with cognitive neuropsychology. Cognitive neuropsychologists have devoted much time and effort to the study of the lexicon, and our knowledge of words has probably been the most thoroughly investigated topic in cognitive neuropsychology. Models of the lexical system are fairly detailed and well illustrate the cognitive neuropsychological approach. Moreover, they have been frequently used to motivate treatments of lexical disorders. Chapter 6 illustrates a widely accepted dual-route model of the structure of the lexicon based on data from brain-damaged patients, and Chapter 7 reviews cognitive studies on rehabilitation of language disorders.

THE LEXICON

THE STRUCTURE OF THE LEXICON and how lexical representations interact is one of the most thoroughly investigated topics in cognitive neuropsychology. The interest in our knowledge of words can be easily understood if we consider that besides production and comprehension of words, reading and writing also involve lexical processing. Moreover, models of word processing are easier to elaborate than models of sentence processing (which are in fact less detailed and more controversial), and it is understandable that they have attracted the interest of researchers.

This chapter describes a model of the functional structure of the system underlying the use of single words in such tasks as comprehension, naming, reading, and spelling. Its aims are to illustrate how brain-damaged patients with lexical disorders have been investigated and how the results of these studies have been used to constrain the model and to present a sufficiently clear and detailed description of the structure and processing of the lexicon to guide both diagnosis and targeted rehabilitation.

Most of the models currently popular in cognitive neuropsychology are articulated as information processing models and share certain common features. This chapter illustrates the functional structure of a widely accepted lexical system. Not all the assumptions made by this model are universally accepted, and slightly different interpretations and models have been proposed. The intention here is to outline a current model that can explain most patterns of performance in single-word processing, not to provide a thorough review of the whole literature on word processing. This entails the risk of some rigidity and oversimplification, but I argue that the model is sufficiently detailed for guiding rehabilitation.

The chapter is organized in two parts. The first part deals with the various components and their connections. The core functional structure of the lexicon includes a single amodal semantic system, phonological and orthographic input and output lexical components, working memory systems (or buffers), and mechanisms for the conversion of sublexical units from orthography to phonology and from phonology to orthography. I will also argue that lexical and sublexical mechanisms interact. The second part of the chapter deals with the internal organization of each part of the lexical-semantic system and uses data from brain-damaged patients with selective functional disorders.

STRUCTURE OF THE LEXICAL-SEMANTIC SYSTEM

The first distinction must be drawn between the meaning of a lexical item and its form (phonological and orthographic). The performance of brain-damaged patients with selective lexical disorders demonstrates both the preservation of the meaning of words with disorders of word forms and the preservation of word forms with disorders of their meaning. Figure 6–1 presents the structure of a lexical-semantic system with a single amodal semantic system interrelated with the distributed lexical components. The arrows indicate the flow of information between the boxes, and the boxes represent repositories and processors of information.

The distributed nature of our knowledge of word forms is widely recognized, but it is still disputed whether there is a single amodal semantic component or multiple modality-specific semantic systems (for a discussion see Caramazza et al., 1990; Shallice, 1993).

Semantic System

Selective impairment of semantics in lexical processing has been demonstrated by Hillis et al. (1990) in patient KE. This patient made semantically related errors in reading, writing, naming, and comprehension. The word *arm*, for instance, was read as *finger* and written *hand* to

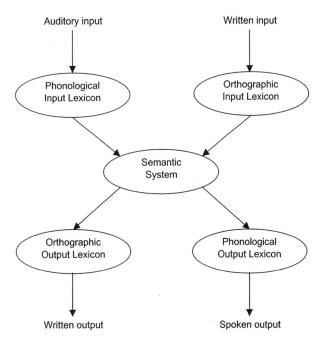

Figure 6–1. Schematic representation of a model of the lexical-semantic system representing the lexical and semantic components.

dictation; when he was presented with the picture of an arm, he said *finger* and wrote *leg*. In auditory- and written-word–picture matching tasks, he also made frequent semantic errors. These were the most frequent errors across all modalities of input and output and occurred with essentially the same frequency. The pervasiveness of the semantic errors and the similarity of their frequency make it difficult to attribute them to independent and separate damage to the input and output lexicons. They speak for relatively restricted damage to a common semantic mechanism.

Input and Output Lexicons

As Figure 6–1 shows, the lexical component consists of a distributed set of sub-components interconnected through the semantic system. A major distinction is drawn between input and output components, that is, components involved in the comprehension as opposed to the production of words.

The distinction between input and output components is quite reasonable. In auditory word comprehension the input lexicon must compute phonemic information, whereas for output, what must be computed by the phonological lexicon is semantic information. The same reasoning applies to the input and output orthographic lexicons. The input lexicon must compute orthographic information and the output lexicon must compute semantic information.

Allport and Funnell (1981), however, argued that there is no compelling evidence in favor of the separation between input and output components and that a single phonological lexicon can handle both the recognition and the production of spoken words. A single orthographic lexicon, they believe, can do the same with written words, and only the accessing processes differ for input and output. They maintained that "on grounds of parsimony" the single phonological (and orthographic) lexicon view is preferable.

Ellis and Young (1988) pointed out that a single (phonological) lexicon involved in the comprehension and production of words cannot explain results from patients (so-called deep dysphasics) who produce semantic paraphasias in repetition (Michel & Andreewsky, 1983; Howard & Franklin, 1988; Katz & Goodglass, 1990; Martin & Saffran, 1992). In a one-lexicon model, the same representations in the phonological lexicon are used for both recognition and production of spoken words, and semantic paraphasias in repetition are not easily explained. Only mediation from the input to the output lexicon through the semantic system can account for semantic paraphasias in word repetition.

A further argument in favor of the existence of separate input and output lexicons comes from the observation of patients with damage restricted to the comprehension or the production of single words. Heilman et al. (1976) described a patient who was able to name pictures but unable to comprehend spoken language. The failure in comprehension could not be attributed to impairment in auditory perception because the patient had good repetition, and integrity of the semantic system was inferred from the patient's naming capacity, although it was not specifically examined. The comprehension disorder, the authors argued, must be located between an intact auditory analysis system and an intact semantic system, probably at the level of the phonological input lexicon.

Patients with the opposite pattern—intact comprehension of single words and word-finding difficulties—are common and have been considered to provide evidence of independent damage to the output lexicon (Gainotti et al., 1986; Kay & Ellis, 1987; Miceli et al., 1991a, 1996). Gainotti and coworkers (1986), for instance, studied a group of 13 aphasic patients with clear-cut word-finding difficulties in spontaneous speech and in a confrontation naming task. Eight patients showed clear impairment on tasks evaluating lexical-semantic comprehension, but the remaining five patients had "purely expressive anomia" with preserved semantic knowledge and damage at the stage where the selected semantic representation is specified into the appropriate phonological form.

Phonological and Orthographic Lexicons

A further distinction is drawn between modality-specific components, namely, phonological and orthographic components. The mechanisms involved in phonological and orthographic processing are computationally independent. In reading, for instance, visual information must be converted into orthographic information, which, in turn, must be processed lexically; in comprehending oral language, lexical information must be extracted from phonemic input, which is processed from acoustic input. In production, initial information is semantic for both oral and written output. In oral production it must then be transformed into a phonological abstract representation of the word that must finally be articulated, whereas in written production it must be transformed into an abstract orthographic representation and then into graphic movements.

Not much research has been carried out on the mechanisms of written word production, and it has long been maintained that orthographic knowledge is fundamentally parasitic upon phonological knowledge. The phonological mediation hypothesis states that in reading for comprehension, it is necessary to generate the internal phonological representation of the word's written form before accessing its meaning. In spelling, it is argued, the orthographic form of the word cannot be directly accessed from the semantic system; access to the orthographic representation is gained through the phonological lexicon.

Goodglass and Hunter (1970) compared oral and written production in two patients, one with Broca aphasia and the other with Wernicke aphasia. They found that the oral and written productions of each patient were similar but that they differed between the two patients. The qualitative similarity between the oral and written productions in either of the two patients and the opposite pattern they showed between the patients were considered evidence that "written language is, at least in part, the formulation of spoken language converted to graphic form" (p. 34).

However, a few patients have been described with better-preserved written naming than oral naming. Lhermitte and Dérouesné (1974) described the first two cases of this kind. One patient with a left-hemisphere vascular lesion produced many phonemic errors in oral production, whereas her writing was correct. The second patient, who had suffered head trauma, correctly named only 3 of 50 pictures in the spoken modality; most of his errors were neologisms. In the written modality he correctly named 44 of the same 50 pictures. For *bicyclette* (bicycle), for instance, he said "fogran" and wrote [bicyclette]; for *peigne* (comb) he said "bradin" and wrote [peigne]. It is interesting to note that the authors did not consider that their results demonstrate the independence of the orthographic representations from phonological mediation. On the contrary, they argued that it is not possible to write without previously formulating orally what one wants to express. In their words, "Il n'est pas possible d'écrire sans qu'au préalable la pensée ait engendré une suite d'activités neuronales qui s'attachent à la formulation linguistique orale" (p. 32). To explain the observed dissociation between better written than oral naming and production in these patients, they hypothesized a disconnection between (unimpaired) abstract language capacity and its (unimpaired) articulatory implementation.

Two further patients have been described with Wernicke aphasia, phonemic errors in oral production, and better-preserved written over oral naming (Ellis et al., 1983; Patterson & Shewell, 1987). Finally, Hier and Mohr (1977) and Bub and Kertesz (1982b) described two patients who frequently made no responses in the oral modality and correctly named a few stimuli in the written modality. The difference between oral and written naming was particularly striking in patient MH (Bub & Kertesz, 1982), who named 3 of 40 pictures orally and 34 in writing. Four further responses were recognizable but misspelled.

Other results have also been taken as evidence that phonological mediation is not necessary in orthographic lexical access. Miceli and colleagues (1997), for example, reported on a patient whose responses in a picture-naming task were inconsistent when he had to respond in different modalities (oral then written or written then oral) but not when he had to give two responses in the same modality. To the picture of pliers, for example, he responded "pincers" and wrote [saw] and to the picture of peppers he wrote [tomato] and said "artichoke." This never happened when the two responses were in the same modality. (For a review of dissociations in reading and spelling see *Cognitive Neuropsychology*, vol. 14, n. 1, 1997.)

The opposite dissociation, better-preserved oral than written naming, has long been considered normal and not worth reporting. It is only recently, in the wake of evidence that orthographic representations are not necessarily phonologically mediated, that these patients have attracted attention. Hillis et al. (1999) reported the performance of a patient, RCM, with left frontal damage who presented a striking dissociation between oral and written picture naming. Oral and written comprehension and oral naming were within normal limits, whereas her written naming was markedly impaired. The writing impairment in word spelling (RCM could not spell nonwords because of damage to the nonlexical route) could not be ascribed to postlexical damage because most of her errors were semantic, writing [airplane] when shown the picture of a bus or [owl] for eagle. Moreover, the impairment could not be due to damage to the semantic system itself or to the phonological output lexicon because she could correctly name the pictures, indicating correct semantic processing and preserved phonological representations.

To sum up, thus far we have assumed three main distinctions in lexical knowledge types: semantic, phonological, and orthographic. In addition, we have assumed that phonological and orthographic knowledge is modality specific and that the lexical subcomponents are interrelated through a single semantic system.

Phonological and Orthographic Buffers

Besides the lexical and semantic components, Figure 6–2 depicts a mechanism for the recognition of heard phonemes and one for the recognition of graphemes, as well as a phonological and an orthographic output buffer. The motivation for proposing the existence of a working memory component, or buffer, in an information processing system such as the lexical model is straightforward. The working memory component temporarily stores representations in preparation for subsequent processes, keeping information available while it is being processed.

On the input side, processes in the auditory/phonological analysis system abstract from the detail of the acoustic stimulus and compute an auditory representation that serves as input to the phonological lexicon. Damage at this level has been considered to be the cause of word deafness, a deficit that interferes with the patient's auditory comprehension (see infra).

A task performed with ease by normal readers is the identification of a letter regardless of its particular form. Skilled readers can easily read unfamiliar typefaces, which means that the reading system must include a component for the identification of letters. The abstract letter identity system is a working memory system that recognizes letters independently of their font and letter case and holds them for subsequent processing. Damage to the abstract letter identification system impairs the patient's

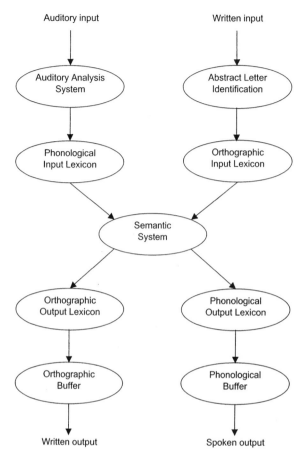

Figure 6–2. Schematic representation of a model of the lexical-semantic system representing the lexical and semantic components and the buffers.

ability to recognize letters and prevents him or her from reading normally. The letter-by-letter reading strategy present in some patients has been interpreted as caused by damage to the abstract letter identity system. As for the output buffers, the phonological output buffer holds the lexical phonological representation while it is converted into phonemes for oral production, and the orthographic output buffer holds the lexical orthographic representations activated in the lexicon while they are processed sequentially for conversion into graphic patterns for written spelling.

Damage to the phonological or the graphemic output buffer should result in a pattern of performance characterized by the presence of errors in all tasks, independent of the modality of input or output, qualitatively and quantitatively similar for known and novel words. It should not be affected by lexical factors and should be interpretable by phonological and orthographic properties, respectively. Finally, since the buffer is a working memory system, there should be a length effect, with longer words and nonwords being more difficult to process than shorter ones.

Patients with selective deficits in each of these systems are described below.

Sublexical or Conversion Procedures

As stated in Chapter 5, normal literate subjects can read and spell novel words by converting the unforeseen sequence of graphemes into the corresponding sequence of phonemes and the new sequence of phonemes into the corresponding sequence of graphemes. Figure 6–3 depicts the nonlexical routes for reading and writing.

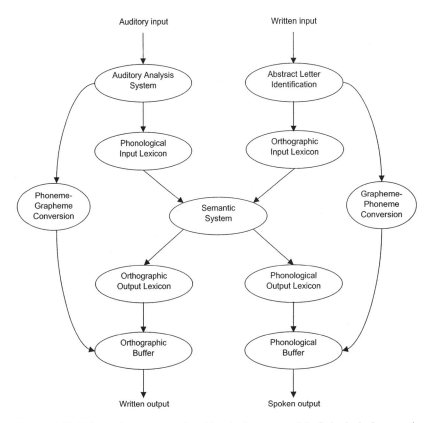

Figure 6–3. Schematic representation of a dual-route model of the lexical-semantic system.

Patients with selective damage of nonword reading (so-called phonological dyslexics) have been described, among others, by Beauvois and Dérouesné (1979), Cuetos et al., (1996), and Dérouesneé and Beauvois (1985). Patients with selective damage of nonword writing have been described by Assal et al. (1981), Bub and Kertesz (1982b), Baxter and Warrington (1983, 1985), Kremin (1987), Roeltgen et al. (1983), and Shallice (1981).

Although not represented in Figure 6–3, there is a third transmission route, which translates heard phonemes into spoken phonemes. Between a heard phoneme and a spoken phoneme there is a one-to-one correspondence, and very few patients have been described who can repeat known words better than novel words (McCarthy & Warrington, 1984; Howard & Franklin, 1988).

Interaction Between Lexical and Nonlexical Processes

Some models of the lexicon assume the existence of a third reading route, which directly connects the input orthographic lexicon to the output phonological lexicon. This nonsemantic lexical route has been proposed to explain the performance of patients with severely impaired comprehension who can read some orthophonologically irregular words (Schwartz et al., 1980a; Funnell, 1983; Bub et al., 1985). It has been argued that in these patients, reading of irregular words cannot have been accomplished by the semantic route, because of the damaged semantic system, or by the nonlexical conversion mechanisms that by definition do not allow reading of irregular words. Hence, a direct route that bypasses the semantic system must exist. Other, rarer patterns of performance have also been regarded as evidence for the existence of a third direct lexical route (see Hillis & Caramazza, 1995, for review).

An alternative explanation to the lexical nonsemantic direct route is an interaction between lexical and nonlexical mechanisms (Hillis and Caramazza, 1991, 1995; Patterson & Hodges, 1992). According to this account, information from the nonlexical routes interacts with representations in the phonological (or orthographic) output lexicon. Figure 6–4 illustrates this further connection.

Interaction between semantic and nonlexical mechanisms is not incompatible with the third direct route for reading. Hillis and Caramazza (1991), however, analyzed the performance of all the published cases reported as evidence of the existence of a third direct lexical nonsemantic route for reading and argued that, in all cases, interaction between lexical and

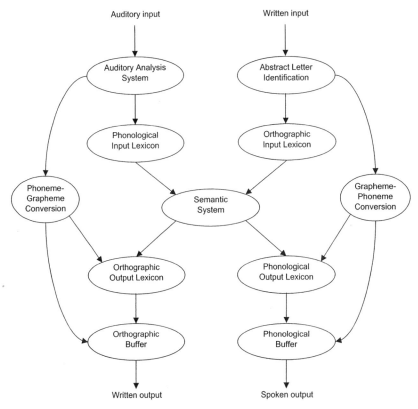

Figure 6–4. Schematic representation of a dual-route model of the lexical-semantic system representing interaction between lexical and nonlexical processing.

nonlexical mechanisms could also explain the results. In a later paper, Hillis and Caramazza (1995) presented further evidence in support of the interaction hypothesis. They described three patients with different functional lesion loci, all of whom were able to read aloud some irregular words that they did not produce correctly in naming tasks. GLT was held to have partial damage to the semantic system and partial damage to the grapheme-to-phoneme conversion procedures; JSR had damage to the output phonological lexicon and additional damage to the grapheme-to-phoneme conversion procedures; RBI had only partial damage to the semantic system. Their performance across a variety of reading tasks is best explained, according to the authors, "by assuming that partial semantic information and at least partial sublexical information contributes to the activation of lexico-phonological representations in reading by these patients" (p. 190).

Further support for interaction between sublexical and lexical-semantic procedures comes from a different task. A few patients with semantic disorders were asked to perform double naming tasks, that is, say-then-write and write-then-say. The errors were semantic and the responses were inconsistent when, in addition to the semantic disorder, the patients had severe damage to both phoneme-to-grapheme and grapheme-to-phoneme conversions (Beaton et al., 1997; Miceli et al, 1997; Rapp et al., 1997). Responses, however, were the same when the sublexical procedures were undamaged (Miceli & Capasso, 1997). Miceli et al. (1999) considered this pattern of results as consistent with interaction between lexical and nonlexical mechanisms. The first response given by the patient can in fact constrain the second response if the sublexical procedures are at least partially efficient because the patient can read what he or she has just written or write what he or she has just said. In cases of severe damage to the sublexical conversion procedures this cannot be done. If this interpretation is correct, a patient with damage to only one of the two conversion procedures should give inconsistent responses only when the first response is given in the modality (orthography, for instance) in which the conversion procedures (orthography-to-phonology) are damaged, but not when the first response is given in the other modality with unimpaired conversion procedures. Miceli et al. (1999) presented evidence from such a patient.

ECA had damage to the semantic system and to phoneme-to-grapheme conversion. In double naming tasks requiring the production of a written and then an oral response, he was always consistent. He gave, however, inconsistent responses in the say-then-write condition because the oral response could not constrain the written response due to damage to the phoneme-to-grapheme conversion mechanisms. The difference between the number of inconsistent responses in the say-then-write condition and the write-then-say condition was statistically significant.

INTERNAL ORGANIZATION AND PROCESSING

Thus far we have considered only the architecture of the lexical system. The second part of the chapter illustrates how the phonological, orthographic, and semantic representations are organized and how information is processed in each component. The most peripheral input components will be described first, and the information flow will be followed downstream up to the most peripheral output components.

Auditory Analysis System

The first stage of auditory word recognition is performed by an auditory analysis system that identifies phonemes in the speech wave and holds them in a working memory system until the sequence of phonemes is complete. The sequence is then transmitted to the phonological input lexicon, where a match is sought with a stored representation. If no match is found, the word is not recognized as a known word. Depending on whether the sequence of phonemes is or is not recognized as a stored representation in the phonological input lexicon, it is further processed by the lexical or the nonlexical system. Damage to the auditory analysis system should result in impaired phoneme identification, thus providing an altered input to the phonological input lexicon and the phoneme-to-grapheme and input-to-output phoneme conversion procedures, impairing word comprehension and the processing of lexical and nonlexical stimuli in writing to dictation and repetition.

Luria (1970) argued that impaired phonemic identification is the primary underlying deficit in comprehension disorders but reported no confirmatory experimental data.

Blumstein and coworkers (1977a, 1977b) investigated the ability of groups of aphasic patients to make a same–different discrimination when presented with pairs of stimuli. Stimuli consisted of real words, novel words, or synthetically generated stop consonants. Aphasic patients were variously impaired in phoneme identification and discrimination but, all in all, the authors did not find a relationship between impaired phonemic perception and impaired auditory comprehension, thus lending no support to Luria's hypothesis about the origin of comprehension disorders in aphasia. Impaired phoneme perception, however, has frequently been considered the cause of pure word-sound deafness, a circumscribed disorder limited to auditory stimuli. Patients can no longer repeat, understand, or write to dictation auditorily presented stimuli. In its purest form, perception of nonspeech sounds is normal, but it is frequently the case that recognition of nonverbal sounds is also impaired.

Patients with pure word-sound deafness have been described by Albert and Bear (1974), Auerbach and coworkers (1982), and Miceli (1982), among others. The precise nature of the deficit underlying pure word deafness has been debated and a prephonemic locus of impairment has been sometimes suggested. Albert and Baer and Auerbach and coworkers, for instance, showed that their word-deaf patients had deficits in the processing of rapidly changing nonspeech stimuli. They therefore argued that word deafness is not limited to language processing but rather extends to processing of rapid acoustic stimuli of any kind, including phonemes.

In conclusion, there is evidence that unselected groups of aphasic patients have damage to the auditory analysis system but that impaired identification of phonemes has no relationship with the auditory comprehension disorder (Blumstein et al., 1977a, 1977b). Word-sound deaf patients with severe auditory comprehension disorders have impaired phoneme perception, but the deficit has sometimes been considered prephonemic (Albert & Baer, 1974; Auerbach et al., 1982).

Abstract Letter Identification System

Just as phoneme identification is a necessary step for further processing of phonemes, letter identification is the first step in the processing of written words and nonwords. Damage to the abstract letter identification system should therefore equally impair the reading of known and new words. In pure alexia, or letter-by-letter reading, patients read single words by identifying one letter at a time, with the obvious consequence that the more letters there are in a word, the longer it takes the patient to read it. The hallmark of pure alexia is in fact a length effect.

Arguin and Bub (1993, 1994), Kay and Hanley (1991), and Reuter-Lorenz and Brunn (1990) have argued that letter-by-letter reading depends on impaired single-letter processing or a deficit in abstract letter identification, and Behrmann and Shallice (1995) have asserted that there is no convincing evidence of normal letter processing in any patient with letter-by-letter reading. In accordance with this interpretation of letter-by-letter reading is a recently described case involving patient GV (Miozzo & Caramazza, 1998). The authors argued that GV had preserved visual processing abilities and normal knowledge of letter shapes but that she could not access knowledge about their graphemic identity, thus preventing her from accessing the orthographic input lexicon and the semantic system.

Not everyone, however, agrees on interpreting letter-by-letter reading as a disorder of the abstract letter identification system, and it has frequently been maintained that the deficit is not specific to reading. As in word-sound deafness, it has been argued that more general visual perceptual disorders underlie the reading impairment (for a review see Behrmann et al., 1998).

More challenging for the letter identification damage interpretation is a relatively recent finding. It has been shown that some pure alexic patients are able to access lexical information after an exposure duration that is too brief to allow correct reporting of words. A degree of implicit or covert reading has been demonstrated by some letter-by-letter readers who performed well above chance in lexical decision and semantic categorization tasks, suggesting that the deficit occurs only after an adequate orthographic representation is activated (see *Cognitive Neuropsychology*, vol. 15, n. 1–2, 1998).

Phonological and Orthographic Lexicons

Evidence from brain-damaged patients and the theoretical principle of economy invite us to assume that the internal organization of the lexical subcomponents is similar in the input and output lexicons as well as in the phonological and orthographic lexicons, except for the obvious differences due to the specificity of the modality or the code—at least unless there is evidence to the contrary. Three important organizing parameters of the lexicon have been shown to be grammatical class, morphological structure, and frequency of use.

Grammatical class. An interesting observation in aphasia is that words in different grammatical classes appear to be independently disrupted. The two word classes that have been shown to dissociate most frequently are nouns and verbs (cf. Shapiro et al. 2000, and references therein).

Selective sparing of nouns relative to verbs has been reported many times, usually in clinically agrammatic patients (Miceli et al., 1984, 1988b; Williams & Canter, 1987; Kohn et al., 1989; Zingeser & Berndt, 1990; Kremin & Basso, 1993; Berndt et al., 1997; Silveri & di Betta, 1997; Breedin et al., 1998; Rapp & Caramazza, 1998). Caramazza and Hillis (1991) describe the performance of two patients who had good comprehension of spoken and written words but who showed selective deficits in production of verbs in only one modality of output: SJD produced semantic errors in naming verbs only in the written modality, while HW produced semantic errors with verbs in oral but not written naming, even when identical words were used as nouns and verbs ("there is a *crack* in the mirror" vs. "don't *crack* the nuts in here"). The authors conclude that grammatical class distinction is redundantly represented in the phonological and orthographic output lexicon components.

The opposite dissociation, namely, verbs reliably better preserved than nouns, has been less frequently documented but is not rare and is generally found in anomic patients (Miceli et al., 1984, 1988b; Zingeser & Berndt, 1990; Rapp & Caramazza, 1997; Silveri & di Betta, 1997). Zingeser and

Berndt (1988) described a severely anomic patient whose verb production was superior to his noun production. This pattern of performance precludes any explanation that relies on the argument of a difference in processing difficulty between nouns and verbs, since both nouns and verbs can be selectively impaired or spared.

Doubts about the appropriateness of an interpretation based on grammatical classes were raised by Allport and Funnell (1981), who pointed out that nouns tend to be higher in imageability than verbs. This difference may introduce a potentially confounding effect, resulting in the interpretation of phenomena that may be semantic in nature as a grammatical class effect. However, factors such as imageability or the inherently greater complexity of verbs compared to nouns (they are acquired later and have a greater range of meanings, for instance) cannot account for all the grammatical-class dissociations reported in the literature.

Morphology. A second important organizing parameter of the lexical forms is morphology. Words like *under, cat,* and *eat* are monomorphemic, but the majority of words can be broken down into morphemes. A word such as *added* is composed of the verb *add* and the inflectional affix *ed,* which indicates past tense; the word *madness* is composed of the adjective *mad* and the derivational affix *ness,* which transforms it into a noun. When we hear a previously unfamiliar word formed by a known root and a known suffix, such as *devilishly* ("He looked at her devilishly"), we can easily understand it (in a devilish manner) because of our knowledge of the rules that govern production of morphologically complex word forms. We are also able to produce a new morphologically complex word such as *chicly* or *fetchingly* by unconsciously applying the correct rule.

An important question is whether and how morphological structure is represented in the lexicon. Two contrasting views were initially developed: that words are represented in the lexicon either as nondecomposed wholes (Butterworth, 1983) or as morphologically decomposed forms.

Miceli and Caramazza (1988) have described an Italian patient, FS, who made morphological errors in spontaneous speech and in single-word processing. They asked the patient to repeat lists of words in order to investigate the locus of his damage. The majority of FS's errors were morphological substitution errors. In single-word repetition tasks he frequently substituted the inflectional specifications for gender and number in repeating nouns and adjectives, and for person, tense, and aspect in repeating verbs, all of which are obligatory in Italian. However, his derivational morphology was almost intact. Badecker and Caramazza (1991) presented data from patient SJD's reading of single words. Her reading showed a significant effect of parts of speech (nouns and adjectives were read better than verbs and function words) and a length effect. More pertinent to the present question is that SJD's reading was affected by the morphological structure of the words; morphologically less complex words were read better than morphologically complex words. When reading, for instance, a list of homophones, one affixed and one unaffixed (such as *links* and *lynx*), she made significantly more errors in reading the affixed members of the list. At odds with the whole-word hypothesis is another result. SJD produced morphological errors that did not result in real words. She read *newing* for *newer* or *discussionly* for *discussing*, producing illegal combinations of a root and an affix. Badecker and Caramazza convincingly argued that these are compositional errors and not whole-word substitutions.

Illegal combinations of a root and an affix were also present in the spontaneous production of an Italian jargonaphasic (Panzeri et al., 1990). Panzeri and coworkers maintained that this result speaks against a whole-word model, according to which morphologically simple and complex words are retrieved as a whole from the speaker's store of words. They claimed that morphologically complex words are put together at the moment of production.

A compromise solution between the full-listing and full-parsing theories is now popular: high-frequency complex words are thought to be stored as wholes, while less frequent forms are thought to be stored as decomposed forms. An alternative view is that whole-word retrieval and on-line composition may occur in parallel.

Frequency. A final aspect of the internal structure of the phonological and orthographic lexical components is frequency of word use, as measured by objective counts of written and spoken language. In a lexical decision task, normal subjects respond faster to high-frequency than to low-frequency words, and this holds true independently of the modality of input—auditory or written. In other words, the activation threshold of a word is related to its frequency of use in the language. In aphasic patients, word frequency is an important determinant of success or failure in word retrieval, suggesting that high-frequency words have lexical representations that are more easily available than those of low-frequency words. Recently, it has been argued that subjective familiarity rather than frequency is the relevant variable (Gernsbacher, 1984), but the two variables are strictly interrelated—a familiar word being also a frequently used word—and it is difficult to tease their effect apart.

To conclude, it appears that the lexical components have an internal organization. No evidence has been reported of a different internal organization of the lexicons, and the hypothesis that it is the same for the input and output lexicons and for the phonological and orthographic lexicons has been upheld. The internal representations are organized according to frequency/familiarity and grammatical class and there is some evidence that (at least high-frequency words) are morphologically decomposed.

Semantic System

A lexical item is generally thought to be represented by a bundle of semantic features that, taken together, describe the concept. The concept *lion*, for instance, can be represented by the features animal, wild, carnivorous, four-legged, and so forth. The compositionality of the semantic representations allows us to define the categorical relationships among lexical items. Items that belong to the same semantic category have more semantic features in common than items belonging to different semantic categories, so that *lion* and *leopard* will have more common semantic features than, say, *lion* and *table*.

An important characteristic of the internal structure of the semantic system has been inferred from observations of patients with selective deficits of specific semantic categories. Warrington and McCarthy (1983) published the case of a globally aphasic patient, VER, whose comprehension of words referring to animals, flowers, and food was relatively preserved compared to her comprehension of words referring to artifacts. The following year, Warrington and Shallice (1984) reported four patients with herpes simplex encephalitis who were much more impaired in producing and understanding the names of living than nonliving things. Since their first seminal paper, many further reports of patients with selective damage to knowledge of living things have been published. A few cases of selective damage to knowledge of nonliving things have also been published (for a review see Caramazza & Shelton, 1998; Gainotti, 2000). This double dissociation has generally been taken to suggest that the semantic system is categorically organized.

The simple observation of patients with selective semantic disorders, however, does not warrant the conclusion that semantic categories represent an organizational principle of the semantic system. In other words, the observed dissociations do not unequivocally demonstrate that animate and inanimate concepts are functionally independent. Other explanations are possible.

Warrington and Shallice (1984) argued that the observed dissociation was a by-product of a more basic dichotomy concerning the different distribution of the visual and functional information associated with the meaning of words pertaining to the animate or the inanimate category. The meaning of animate concepts is mainly based on visual characteristics, whereas the meaning of inanimate object is based on functional characteristics. An important difference, for instance, between a horse and a zebra is visual: the zebra has stripes. The main difference between a fork and a spoon, which are visually similar, lies in the different purpose for which they have been manufactured that determine their use: the spoon is used for eating liquid food, the fork for holding solid food and carrying it to the mouth. The visual–functional hypothesis predicts that selective damage to visual semantic information will mostly impair knowledge of animate concepts, whereas damage to the functional attributes will particularly impair inanimate concepts. Some authors have attempted to verify Warrington and Shallice's hypothesis by testing patients' knowledge about visual and functional attributes of living and nonliving things. If Warrington and Shallice's hypothesis were true, patients with apparently selective sparing of knowledge of artifacts should have better knowledge about the functional than the visual attributes of both categories, and patients with selective sparing of knowledge of living things should have better knowledge of the visual attributes, independent of the category. However, this prediction has not been supported in many patients with selective impairment of living categories or in those with impairment of nonliving categories (for a review, see Laiacona & Capitani, 2001).

To make things worse, the pattern of spared and damaged categories varies greatly from patient to patient and cannot be easily explained. JBR, one of the patients described by Warrington and Shallice (1984), for instance, had impaired knowledge of animals, vegetables, and food but also of musical instruments, which do not belong to the animate category. On the other hand, CW (Sacchett & Humphreys, 1992) had better-preserved knowledge of animals and plants and was more impaired for artifacts and also for body parts, a category that is generally impaired together with the animate categories.

Two recently published papers that present an overview of this issue came to different conclusions. Caramazza and Shelton (1998), considering the published cases, argue for a categorical organization of knowledge in the brain that, they maintain, is the result of evolutionary pressure. To survive in ancient times, people had to learn to respond quickly to predatory animals and to recognize edible and medicinal plants. This could have resulted in dedicated neural mechanisms for the domains of animals and plant life. In this view, knowledge is categorically organized only for animals and plant life. Artifacts do not form a category but are identified, by contrast, as not being animals or plant life. Gainotti (2000), on the other hand, after reviewing the existing evidence, reached a completely different conclusion. He argued that the outcome of his survey was consistent with "the first of these models [which] assumes that a differential weighting of visual-perceptual and associative-functional attributes underpins the dissociations between living and non-living beings" (p. 555).

Borgo and Shallice (2001) have recently published a new case of a patient, MU, who had suffered from herpes simplex encephalitis, with a marked category-specific deficit for living things. The investigators tackled the question of whether such a dissociation can be explained by category-specific organization of the semantic system or whether an explanation based on sensory versus functional attributes is more consistent with results from brain-damaged patients. They explored novel categories—edible substances, materials, and liquids—chosen because they do not pertain to the category of living things but are highly dependent upon their sensory quality. MU was better with man-made artifacts and equally poor with living things and the three experimental categories. This finding was taken by the authors to support a sensory/functional organization of the semantic system.

A third model has been proposed to explain cases of categorical dissociation. It has been suggested that the basic difference between living and nonliving categories is the degree of correlation among different properties of concepts. Living items are characterized by correlated properties ("having legs," for example, correlates with "can run"), whereas artifacts have a higher proportion of distinctive properties (Devlin et al., 1998). According to this hypothesis, the dissociation between living and nonliving categories depends on the severity of the disorder, living things have densely interconnected properties and are more resistant to brain language than nonliving things that have more distinctive properties.

Devlin et al.'s model, however, cannot explain cases of selective deficit for living things because, according to their hypothesis, nonliving categories should selectively fail when damage to the semantic system is moderate; when damage is severe, both living and nonliving categories should fail.

Nor can the sensory-functional theory be considered a valid general explanation. The sensory-functional theory implies that a disproportionate deficit for living categories should be associated with a prevailing deficit for visuoperceptual information. Although some early case reports apparently supported this prediction, more recent and better-controlled studies have demonstrated that in a substantial number of cases, living categories impairment was balanced between visuoperceptual and functional-associative knowledge (for review and discussion, see Caramazza, 1998).

The domain-specific account (Caramazza & Shelton, 1998) seems to offer a more plausible explanation of the results. It does not specify the fine-grained mechanisms according to which category-specific knowledge is represented in the brain, but it can account for the cases of balanced impairment of perceptual and associative knowledge of natural categories, and it is compatible with the few reported cases of dissociation within the realm of natural categories, such as that of patient EW (Caramazza & Shelton, 1998).

Phonological Output Buffer

The buffer, as noted earlier, is a working memory system where word and nonword stimuli are temporarily held for further processing. Damage to the buffer should have the following consequences: errors should be present in all spoken tasks independently of the modality of input or output and should be present for all types of stimuli, words and nonwords. Errors should be explicable by phonological principles, and lexical factors (word frequency, grammatical class) should not affect performance since the buffer is located postlexically. Finally, and perhaps most importantly, there should be an effect of stimulus length. Many investigators have described patients with a reportedly phonological output buffer deficit. Patients IGR (Caramazza et al., 1986), MV (Bub et al., 1987), RR (Bisiacchi et al., 1989), and LT (Shallice et al., 2000) presented similar pictures, albeit with some important differences. Caramazza and coworkers (1986) argued that damage to the phonological buffer should result in a common pattern of errors in reading and repeating, as well as in writing, because they assume the existence of a phoneme-to-grapheme conversion between the phonological output buffer and the orthographic output buffer. A length effect and phonologically related errors, which should consist of substitutions, insertions, deletions, and transpositions, should also be present. IGR (Caramazza et al., 1986) had this pattern of errors but, contrary to what one would expect from damage to the buffer, he made no word errors. To explain this result, the authors argued for the existence of a direct route from the phonological output lexicon to the articulatory system, bypassing the buffer. LT (Shallice et al. 2000) presented a picture very similar to that of IGR but was more severely damaged and, most importantly, his reading, repeating, and writing of words were also impaired. According to Shallice and coworkers, there is no direct route between the phonological output lexicon and the articulatory system; processing of nonwords, they argued, necessitates a greater amount of resources than processing of words. IGR, with a less severe disorder, could still process words but was impaired in nonword processing. LT, with a more severe disorder, was more impaired than IGR in nonword processing and was also impaired in word processing.

In sum, although theoretically the function of the phonological buffer appears clear—to hold a stimulus in working memory for its successive elaboration—there is no complete agreement about the consequences of damage at this level.

Orthographic Output Buffer

There have been reports of patients whose writing deficit could be interpreted as a selective disturbance within the orthographic output buffer (Miceli et al., 1985; Caramazza et al., 1987; Posteraro et al., 1998). As predicted, a length effect was present in all patients (longer words were more difficult than shorter ones), and errors were equally present in the writing of novel and known words. The most frequent errors were deletions and substitutions of letters.

A detailed analysis of the spelling errors of LB (Caramazza et al., 1987), an Italian patient with damage to the orthographic output buffer, led Caramazza and Miceli (1990) to argue that graphemic representations do not consist simply of linearly ordered sets of graphemes but are highly organized. If the linear order of letters were the only information available at this level, substitutions of graphemes should be random. Caramazza and Miceli, however, found that this was not the case. LB made 741 letter substitutions. In 736 cases (99.3%), vowels were substituted for by vowels and consonants by consonants, thus supporting the hypothesis that substitutions are not random. In addition, almost all the single-letter deletions (311/313) involved a consonant in a consonant cluster or a vowel in a vowel cluster. Finally, regular consonant-vowel words were written better than complex words with consonant clusters, the only exception being words with consonant geminates. Based on these and other results not detailed here, Caramazza and Miceli argued that graphemic representations have a multidimensional structure, each dimension representing distinct information. The information about the nature (consonant or vowel) of a letter, for instance, is represented independently of the identity of the letters; at a higher level, the syllabic structure of the word is represented. Finally, the information about the presence of a geminate is independent of any of the preceding levels of information.

These conclusions were largely confirmed by the study of another patient, HE, who had damage to the orthographic output buffer (McCloskey et al., 1994). On the basis of the patient's spelling errors, McCloskey and coworkers maintained that spelling representations are not linear sequences of letters; they have a multidimensional structure that encodes separately letter identity, consonant/vowel status, and the presence of geminates.

Conversion Rules

Input to output phonology. Damage to transmission from input to output phonology should cause difficulty in the repetition of novel words, with spared repetition of known words that can be normally processed by the lexical-semantic route. We have just seen that IGR (Caramazza et al., 1986) presented with such a dissociation, but his impairment was argued to depend on damage to the phonological output buffer rather than transmission from input to output phonology. Two further patients have been described with better-preserved word than nonword repetition: ORF (McCarthy & Warrington, 1984) and MK (Howard & Franklin, 1988). ORF's repetition was better for words than nonwords and was significantly influenced by stimulus length. McCarthy and Warrington (1984) argued for "an impaired auditory/phonological transcoding process" (p. 482) to explain ORF's repetition impairment but the reported data are not sufficient to discriminate between a transcoding and a buffer damage. MK's (Howard & Franklin, 1988) results speak more clearly in favor of damage to the transcoding process. MK could repeat 58 of 200 words but none of 19 monosyllabic nonwords. What is more important, however, is the fact that there was a significant effect of word length, but the advantage was for longer rather than shorter words, speaking against damage at the buffer level.

All in all, patients with better preserved word than nonword repetition are rare. One reason could be that conversion between input and output phonemes is easy and resilient to brain damage, being a simple one-to-one correspondence.

Grapheme-to-phoneme conversion. Reading of novel words cannot be carried out via the lexical route because novel words cannot be recognized as words; it can only be carried out by applying the specific rules that permit the conversion of graphemes into phonemes. Data from neuropsychology have been used to construct a model of nonlexical reading, and three functionally independent processing components have been proposed (Dérouesné & Beauvois, 1985).

The first operation required is the segmentation or parsing of the input letter sequence into graphemes. Defined in terms of phonemes, a grapheme consists of the letter or letters that correspond to a phoneme. Thus the word *baker* has five letters but only four phonemes and hence four graphemes. The second operation, grapheme-to-phoneme conversion, involves the assignment of a phonological representation to each grapheme. Orthographic rules must also be stored at this stage. In French or Italian, for instance, the letter [C] must always be converted into /k/ except when it is followed by the letters [I] or [E], in which case it must be converted into /s/ in French and /tʃ/ in Italian. Moreover, in French, when [C] is followed by [H] it changes to /ʃ/. The Italian words *cena* (dinner) and *cane* (dog) are both formed by four graphemes, each corresponding to a phoneme, but to be able to convert the first grapheme into the correct phoneme, one must know beforehand which letter it is followed by. Finally, the nonlexical segments that are the output of the grapheme-to-phoneme conversion must be blended and produced as a single unit to be stored in the phonemic buffer for subsequent articulation. Patients with nonlexical reading impairments and with disorders at one or more of these processing stages are on record. LB's (Dérouesné & Beauvois, 1985) performance in reading nonwords aloud was better when there was a one-to-one letter–sound correspondence then when two letters corresponded to a single phoneme. LB's performance was also better when he was told whether a four-letter nonword corresponded to three or four phonemes than when he did not know whether or not each letter corresponded to a phoneme. Dérouesné and Beauvois took this as evidence of damage to the parsing procedure. Phoneme blending was also impaired in LB.

Patients who are able to identify letters but unable to sound them out are considered to have a deficit in the grapheme-phoneme association. LR (Mitchum & Berndt, 1991; Berndt & Mitchum, 1994) is a case in point, although his impairment was not restricted to grapheme–phoneme association. LR was a deep dyslexic patient with poor nonword reading. Careful examination of his nonword reading demonstrated that all three components of the grapheme-to-phoneme conversion mechanisms—grapheme parsing, grapheme–phoneme association, and phoneme blending—were impaired.

Phoneme-to-grapheme conversion. Damage to phoneme-to-grapheme conversion procedures causes difficulty in nonword writing. By analogy to reading, this form of writing disorder has been called phonological agraphia by Shallice (1981).

Roeltgen et al. (1983) described four patients with phonological agraphia and agrammatic spontaneous writing. The authors argued that their patients' nonword writing was impaired at two different levels. In order to write a nonsense word, one must first perform an acoustic analysis, then segment the nonsense word into phonemes, and finally convert the phonemes into graphemes. Impaired acoustic analysis, currently carried out by the auditory analysis system, could not be the cause of the patients' writing disorders because the patients had relatively intact nonword repetition and better writing of words. In order to test the second stage of the phoneme-to-grapheme conversion process, patients were asked to write the corresponding grapheme when a phoneme was spoken. Patients 2 and 3 performed this task perfectly, patient 4 did not understand the task and could not be examined, and patient 1 correctly wrote only 3 of 16 graphemes. Patients 2 and 3, however, despite correct writing of single graphemes, could not write three-phoneme nonwords. Roeltgen and coworkers interpreted these results as proof of their interpretation that nonword writing is not a single process but one that requires at least a segmentation process and phoneme–grapheme association. Patients 2 and 3 were impaired at the segmentation level, and patient 1 had impaired phoneme–grapheme association (and possible also segmentation).

As can be seen, the hypothesized processes in nonword writing closely correspond to those hypothesized for nonword reading, with the exception of the third process, blending or assembling, which apparently is not required for nonword writing because individual graphemes can be written in succession without having to be assembled beforehand. Cases of phoneme-to-grapheme conversion deficits are rather rare, and no in-depth analysis of the writing disorder analogous to the analysis of the phonological reading disorder has been performed.

LOCATING THE FUNCTIONAL LOCUS OF DAMAGE

Cognitive neuropsychology is based on the assumption that the language system is organized in separate components that can be impaired selectively by brain damage, although it is exceptional for a patient to have a selective deficit that honors the functional structure of the cognitive system.

A cognitively based assessment aims to provide information about which components and/or processes are impaired and which are still functioning, but locating the functional damage is not an easy task. Hypotheses have to be formulated and investigated. Correct performance of nearly every task requires the integrity of more than a single component, and each component is used in the performance of many tasks. Decisions about the nonfunctionality of a specific component can be reached only through the converging evidence of many different tasks. In general, the integrity of a component can be confidently deduced from a correct response in a task that involves that component in its execution. By contrast, it is more difficult to interpret an error because it can be caused by malfunctioning of any of the components involved in the execution of the task.

In the following discussion, for each component, a task specifically directed at evaluating its integrity will be illustrated. However, a given component can operate normally only if it receives normal inputs, that is, if all the connected upstream components are undamaged. It is not possible, for example, to investigate the integrity of the phonological input lexicon if the auditory/phonemic input system is damaged because the input to the lexicon is distorted. Before discussing specific tasks, the importance of controlling the materials employed should be mentioned. Words, for instance, must be controlled for all the variables that can affect responses. Frequency of use and familiarity, for example, must be controlled in comprehension and production tasks, and word length when assessing the integrity of the buffers. The compilation of the test materials requires a lot of time and effort. Today a few screening battery are available, such as PALPA (Kay et al., 1992) for English-speaking aphasic patients and the Batteria per l'Analisi dei Deficit Afasici (Miceli et al., 1991b) for Italian-speaking patients.

In indicating the best-suited task for the evaluation of each component, the input components will be considered first and the more peripheral output components will be considered last.

Discrimination of auditory minimal-pair nonwords (same/different) can be correctly performed only if the auditory/phonemic input system is undamaged. Poor performance in the discrimination task may be due to impaired hearing or impaired phonemic perception. The abstract letter recognition system discriminates written minimal pairs of nonwords regardless of their particular font and letter case. To assess its integrity, the patient can be asked to perform a same/different task with written minimal-pair nonwords or to match letters in different cases.

Auditory and written lexical decision tasks tap the integrity of the phonological and orthographic input lexicons, respectively. Failure to recognize that a novel phoneme or letter string is not a word, as well as failure to recognize that an auditory or written word is a word, implies an impaired phonological or orthographic input lexicon. As already stated, however, damage to the input auditory analysis or the abstract letter identification system must first be excluded.

Intact naming can be taken as good evidence that the semantic system is undamaged because confrontation naming requires prior activation in the semantic system, unless one assumes the existence of a direct route from the visual recognition of objects to the phonological output lexicon, bypassing the semantic system. Yet, no convincing evidence of this kind exists (but see Kremin et al., 2001, for a possible case). In the case of impaired naming, damage to the semantic system can be inferred by the coexistence of comparable comprehension and production disorders in oral and written tasks. In the case of damage to the semantic system, moreover, the expected errors are semantic.

Oral and written confrontation naming is also the task of choice to evaluate the output lexicons. Reading aloud and writing to dictation are also frequently used, but reading (and writing) can be performed via the nonlexical route. Only reading (and writing) of irregular words necessitates the activation of the corresponding representations in the output lexicons, although interaction between lexical and nonlexical processing predicts that a partially damaged output lexicon and an undamaged (or mildly damaged) conversion procedure can be sufficient to allow reading (or writing) of irregular words. Damage to the output phonological buffer is indicated by (equally) poor repetition of words and nonwords with a length effect. As for the orthographic output buffer, (equally) poor writing of words and nonwords and a length effect are expected in the presence of damage.

The conversion procedures are tackled by repetition, reading aloud, and writing to dictation of nonwords. Reading, repetition, and writing of words should be correctly performed.

Also of great importance to the diagnosis is the analysis of error types. The type of error is suggestive of its functional origin, although there is no one-to-one correspondence between the type of error and the functional damage. Semantic errors, for instance, generally follow damage to the semantic system but have also been described in patients with damage to the phonological output lexicon (e.g., Caramazza & Hillis, 1990). Phonological errors can be traced back to damage to the phonological output buffer or the phonological output lexicon; if they are found only in repetition tasks, they can be due to damage to the input-to-output phoneme conversion mechanisms or to the grapheme-to-phoneme conversion mechanisms when found only in reading tasks. Morphological errors are less frequent than semantic and phonemic errors and are suggestive of damage to the phonological (or orthographic) output lexicon.

CONCLUSIONS

In this chapter a theory of the structural components of the lexical system and of their processing has been sketched. As already stated, the model of lexical processing has been extensively illustrated because it is one of the most thoroughly investigated topics in cognitive neuropsychology and because it has frequently been referred to to motivate treatments for lexical disorders.

First, the meaning and the form of words were distinguished, and separate representations for the modality (input and output) and the code (phonological and orthographic) of word forms were assumed. Working memory systems were also considered necessary, as were specialized mechanisms for grapheme-to-phoneme and phoneme-to-grapheme conversions. This or a similar model of the lexical-semantic system is generally accepted, and most recent therapeutic interventions have taken the model as a basis for a detailed diagnosis of the patient's functional damage. In the next chapter, reportedly cognitive interventions will be reported and the real impact of the model in constraining therapy will be evaluated.

7

COGNITIVE
REHABILITATION

AS STATED IN CHAPTER 5, COGNITIVE neuropsychology
fostered an approach to the study of aphasia that was radically different from the classic clinical approach that related verbal behaviors, such as
comprehension and reading, to specific cerebral areas. Cognitive
neuropsychologists assumed that cognitive tasks are not unitary but rather
are the result of a series of cognitive processes, which they endeavored to
clarify. Chapter 6 illustrated how a behavior such as naming a picture or
reading a word is accomplished. The aim of this chapter is to establish
whether and how such cognitive models of language processing have
affected implementation of rehabilitation. Selected case studies of patients
reportedly rehabilitated following the cognitive neuropsychological
approach are considered, and the intervention procedures are compared to
the more traditional clinical approaches described in Chapter 3.

Hopefully, the selection is sufficiently representative of the literature
on the subject. It includes two books (*Cognitive approaches in neuropsychological
rehabilitation*, edited by Seron and Deloche [1989], and *Cognitive neuropsychology and cognitive rehabilitation*, edited by Riddoch and Humphreys [1994])
and three special issues of three journals (*Aphasiology*, vol. 7, n. 1, 1993;
Neuropsychological Rehabilitation, vol. 5, n. 1–2, 1995; and *Brain and Language*,
vol. 52, n. 1, 1996). The reviewed studies are grouped according to the

targeted disability: naming disorders, sentence production, reading, and writing.

NAMING DISORDERS

Raymer, Thompson, Jacobs, and Le Grand (1993)

Raymer et al. (1993) devised a phonologically based treatment to train four patients with severe anomia. All were chronic patients with a clinical diagnosis of Broca aphasia. To localize their functional damage, the four subjects (CG, RJ, MR, and RE) were administered a battery of six lexical tasks: oral and written picture naming, auditory and written word/picture matching, word reading, and word repetition. Based on the patients' performance, the authors concluded that they differed in some aspects of lexical processing, but common to all was a severe written naming disorder and failure of lexical-semantic information to access phonological representations. In addition, a semantic impairment was present in all patients except CG. The experimental stimuli included two sets of 30 monosyllabic picturable nouns; each set included 10 target words, 10 rhyming words, and 10 semantically related words. To evaluate the effects of treatment, a single-subject multiple baseline design across behaviors and subjects was used. Each treatment session was initiated with probe tasks that included oral naming, reading, and written naming of the 20 control items. During treatment, patients were asked to name the 10 target pictures; in case of failure, phonological cueing was offered, first a rhyming word, then the initial phoneme of the target word, and finally the whole word. At whatever level the patient produced the correct name, he or she was asked to repeat it five times and then naming was reattempted. Each target word was presented two or three times per session, and training was continued until 80% of the target words were correctly produced or for a maximum of 15 sessions. Treatment was then applied to the second set of 30 words. At the end of the treatment, all subjects showed improved oral naming of target pictures but none reached criterion (80% correct) within 15 treatment sessions. Generalization to untreated (rhyming and semantically related) words and untreated tasks (reading and written naming) varied across subjects. CG, who showed improved naming of untreated words as well as improved reading of all words and writing of some treated words, attained the largest degree of generalization. MR, by contrast, did not show any generalization.

The authors concluded that the results of the experiment indicated that a phonologically based treatment can be effective for patients with different naming disorders. They argued that access to the phonological form of the treated words could have been reached in two ways. The phonological information provided by the examiner and the structural representation of the object could have reached the phonological output form directly, bypassing the semantic system. If this were the case, the treatment would not be helpful for patients with semantic disorders. Alternatively, the representation of the object together with the phonological information provided by the examiner could have activated the lexical-semantic information and the corresponding phonological form. Repeated activation of the target concept in the semantic system and the phonological form in the lexicon may have caused some change in the retrieval mechanisms. In this case, patients with either a lexical-semantic or a phonological deficit could benefit from the phonological treatment. This second interpretation seemed preferable to the authors, who concluded that the research demonstrated the importance of cognitive neuropsychological models in guiding the development of appropriate treatments.

This conclusion, however, seems unwarranted for a number of reasons. The experimental investigation carried out to identify the locus of damage failed to pinpoint the locus of the deficit. Patient CG's most frequent errors, for instance, were "unintelligible attempts to utter target words" in naming, reading, and repetition, suggesting to the authors "a primary locus of verbal impairment at the level of the phonological output lexicon" (p. 32). The errors, however, are also suggestive of an articulatory deficit and are not incompatible with output buffer damage. No pre- or postlexical processes are taken into consideration in the paper, and it is not possible to adjudicate between a lexical and a postlexical disorder. Furthermore, the results are used post hoc to infer the functional locus of damage. An access deficit was credited to those patients who showed generalization to untrained stimuli and a degradation deficit to those who did not show any generalization to untrained items.

Finally, two patients showed generalization to written naming, which improved during treatment. To explain this result, Raymer and coworkers argued for a direct influence of the output phonological lexicon on the output orthographic lexicon. In other words, they argued for a direct route from output phonology to output orthography, not included in the lexical model that was used to evaluate the patients' naming abilities. In addition, if this were the case, the errors in written naming should be phonologically based, but no analysis of errors was provided. Finally, the implemented treatment is not new, and the relationship between it and the model that guided the initial evaluation is not obvious.

Greenwald, Raymer, Richardson, and Rothi (1995)

Greenwald and coworkers (1995) evaluated the outcome of two experimental programs and a control program of naming treatment for two patients with multiple loci of deficits in the cognitive processes underlying confrontation naming.

SS, a 66-year-old right-handed retired truck driver, suffered a left-hemisphere cerebral infarction 6 months prior to treatment. Two weeks after onset he had anomic aphasia, severe alexia and agraphia, memory disorders, and impaired visual object processing. MR, a 71-year-old right-handed retired clerical worker, suffered a left-hemisphere hemorrhagic lesion. At 2 weeks postonset she had anomic aphasia, severe alexia and agraphia, and oral and limb apraxia. She was 8 months postonset when treatment was started.

Extensive testing of naming processing was carried out with reference to a model of normal lexical processing. In the context of this model, impairment in activation of lexical phonology from semantics was disclosed in both patients. In addition, MR had a mild semantic disorder. Both patients were better at naming to auditory definition than at confrontation naming, and impairment in activation of semantics from viewed objects was diagnosed.

The phonological impairment—impaired activation of lexical phonology from semantics—was treated first, and a phonological cueing hierarchy was used. Forty picturable nouns (20 to be treated and 20 to be used as controls) were selected, and the patients were asked to name each picture to an auditory definition because it was held that successful oral naming under such a condition requires semantic access and lexical retrieval. When the patients failed, a phonological cueing hierarchy was used (first sound, first two sounds, name of the picture) for the treated items. The 20 experimental pictures were subdivided into two sets. The two patients were first trained to name 10 experimental pictures (set 1 for SS and set 2 for MR) for 20 therapy sessions and then the other 10 experimental pictures (set 2 for SS and set 1 for MR). At the end of the treatment, SS demonstrated better naming of the 20 experimental pictures and some generalization to the control pictures. MR showed improvement in naming the experimental pictures but no generalization.

The 20 control pictures of treatment one were then used for treatment program two, which targeted the semantic impairment—impaired activation of semantics from viewed objects. This time, a visual-semantic cueing hierarchy was prepared for each stimulus word and was offered to the patients whenever they failed naming. They were first requested to say the semantic category of the stimulus; the examiner then pointed to a characteristic visual feature of the target and asked the patient to describe and name it. Two or three visual features were considered for each picture. After each question, the examiner summarized what had been said and asked the patient to name the picture. If the patient still failed after all the visual characteristics had been described, the examiner provided the name and asked the patient to repeat it three times. For both patients, treatment two resulted in improved naming and no generalization to untrained items. To control whether improvement in oral naming in the two treatment programs was due to simple rehearsal, an oral repetition treatment for picture naming was administered (treatment three), which resulted in a statistically nonsignificant improvement for SS and a statistically significant improvement for MR. The patients' performance immediately returned to baseline after treatment three, but degradation was more gradual after treatments one and two.

Greenwald and coworkers argued that two treatment programs targeted at two presumed impairments—phonological cueing for lexical retrieval damage and visual-semantic cueing for visual-semantic processing—were more successful than an aspecific control treatment—repetition—providing evidence for the usefulness of a cognitive diagnosis to guide treatment. However, the theoretical relationship between the functional damage—impaired activation of lexical phonology from semantics—and the treatment—phonemic cueing—is not clear since access to phonology is supposed to be semantically and not phonologically coded. Moreover, MR also showed a statistically significant improvement in the nonspecific control treatment, although decline was more rapid than in the two experimental conditions. Finally, whereas the visual-semantic treatment is innovative, the implemented phonological therapy is not new and has frequently been used.

Le Dorze and Pitts (1995)

Le Dorze and Pitts (1995) reported a treatment study involving a 67-year-old severely anomic woman, RT. As in the previously reviewed studies, the working hypothesis was that techniques designed to target the patient's specific disorder(s) should be more efficacious than more general and aspecific interventions.

Six months postonset, RT was found to have well-articulated but reduced speech. Repetition and reading aloud of words and sentences were preserved, but comprehension was impaired; anomia was severe, with better written than oral confrontation naming. A clinical diagnosis of mixed transcortical aphasia was reached. Further testing suggested problems in accessing semantic information and word-form information in naming tasks. Four different therapeutic techniques were devised, and their relative effect on the patient's severe word-finding difficulties was compared. The first treatment simultaneously targeted RT's two basic disorders, namely, the semantic disorder and the word-form disorder; in the second treatment only word-form retrieval was treated, and in the third only the semantic disorder. Finally, the fourth treatment did not specifically tackle any disorder. In addition, there were two control conditions that consisted in repeated opportunities to name without help. The semantic technique consisted in word–picture matching tasks with semantically related distractors. In word-form training RT was asked to read the target word and try to remember it; she was then given the first letter of the word and asked to name the picture. Both the semantic and the word-form training were implemented in treatment one. The fourth treatment consisted in word–picture matching tasks with unrelated distractors. In each condition the patient was asked to name a set of five different stimuli that were taken from consistently failed items. In each session, the four treatments and the two control tasks were implemented.

After six sessions RT reached criterion, namely, 80% correct in two consecutive sessions, for the semantic-phonological technique and the experiment was terminated. Recovery was also present with treatments two and three but did not reach criterion. No improvement was demonstrated following the fourth treatment and the two control conditions. Posttesting two days after treatment was terminated revealed some maintenance of the effects of therapy. According to the authors, the experiment demonstrated that "substantial improvement occurred when therapy was oriented towards the patient's disorders" (p. 63).

It must be stressed, however, that each treatment was based on the acquisition of only five words and that the criterion was 80%. This means that after six therapy sessions the patient was able to name four of five pictures on two consecutive days in treatment one. She named three of five pictures in treatments two and three, and two days later she only named some of them. It is difficult to evaluate the real importance of a treatment based on such a small number of stimuli. Moreover, Weidner and Jinks (1983) had already shown in a group of nonfluent patients that two cues (different combinations of the written word, a phonemic cue, and a sentence-completion cue) were more effective than any of the same cues given in isolation.

To conclude, the implemented techniques are not new, and comparison with more clinically guided interventions is difficult because of the small number of stimuli used in each treatment.

Miceli, Amitrano, Capasso, and Caramazza (1996)

Miceli and colleagues (1996) presented the results of the naming rehabilitation of two chronic anomic patients, RBO and GMA, with unimpaired comprehension and damage to phonological lexical forms. For both patients, damage was localized at the level of the output lexicon, and therapies requiring the patients to retrieve the phonological forms of the target words were devised. For each patient, a pool of consistently comprehended but incorrectly produced words was selected (90 pictures for RBO and 80 for GMA). RBO was asked to name a set of 30 written words and to repeat a second set of 30 words. Thirty words served as controls. Sets 1 and 2 were treated for 5 consecutive days each, and in each session the 30 words were presented 10 times in random order. Errors were immediately corrected. After each session RBO was asked to name the 30 experimental pictures. Treatments for GMA were slightly different. During treatment one, the stimulus picture and the corresponding written word were presented simultaneously and GMA was asked to read them. In treatment two only the written word was presented and he was again asked to read it, and in treatment three only the picture was presented and he was asked to name it and offered the first phoneme in case of failure. The three treatments were delivered separately, for 7 consecutive days each, and the stimuli were presented 10 times per session.

Changes were observed in both patients after each treatment program. All remediation programs required the oral production of the words under treatment, and it is the authors' conviction that training on any task that requires the oral production of the to-be-treated word should result in improvement in patients with output lexical damage and spared semantic production. In addition, no generalization to untreated words was noted and this too was a predictable result because, according to the model, there is a one-to-one relationship between a lexical-semantic representation and its corresponding phonological form.

Once again, the implemented techniques are not new, but the strict relationship between the predictions from the model (improvement with all treatment, and no generalization to untreated items) and the results allows the authors to conclude that "the model of lexical processing described in the Introduction has been useful in guiding hypotheses for treatment of naming disorders in RBO and GMA" (p. 179).

Table 7–1 summarizes data from the above described studies on naming disorders.

SENTENCE-LEVEL DISORDERS

Garrett's Model of Sentence Production

Classic rehabilitation has relatively underestimated sentence production and comprehension, and only a handful of suggestions may be found in the literature. Recently, the model of normal sentence production developed by Garrett (1975, 1980) has provided a useful framework for the interpretation of sentence production impairments in aphasia. Based on the study of speech errors in normal subjects, Garrett postulated five levels of functionally independent components of normal sentence production. The model claims that the levels of representation are serial and that the flow of information is top-down, without any feedback.

First, there is the message level. The representations at this level are nonlinguistic conceptual ideas of what one wants to say. At the message level, information about the content of the message the speaker wants to communicate is not the only information available. As illustrated in Figure 7–1, memory demands, discourse constraints, and the speaker's motivations are also included.

Next is the functional level, where abstract lexical entities represent concepts of things, actions, and attributes extracted from the message level. The logical relationships among these abstract entities are also established at the functional level, thus making explicit the conceptual interpretation of "who is doing what to whom." At the functional level items are semantically and syntactically specified, but they are not yet phonologically specified.

At the positional level, the phonological forms of the specific lexical items chosen to express the functional-level relationships are made available, as well as the grammatical elements of the syntactic frame into which the lexical items will be inserted. Two distinct levels—functional and posi-

Table 7–1. Treatment Studies of Naming Disorders

Patients (Authors)	Aphasia Type	Time Postonset	Functional Damage	Treatment	Stimuli	Implementation	Results	Follow-up
CG, RJ, MR, RE (Raymer et al., 1993)	Broca	Chronic (>1 year)	Damaged access to lexical-semantic and phonol representations	Phonol cueing	10 target 10 rhyming 10 semant related	2–3 times per d/15 sessions	Some improvement for all subjects. No one reached criterion. Variable generalization	(2 m) maintenance
SS MR (Greenwald et al., 1995)	Optic aphasia Anomic	6 months 8 months	Impaired activation of semantics from visual input and of phonology from semantic input	(1) Phonol cueing (2) Visual/semantic cueing	20 target 20 control	2–3 times per d/20 sessions	Improved. No generalization	(10 d) decline
RT (Le Dorze & Pitts, 1995)	Mixed transcortical	6 months	Semantic disorders; word-form disorders	(1) Semantic and phonol (2) Semantic (3) Phonol	5 words per treatment	6 sessions	Treatment one: 80% Treatments two and three: 60% No generalization	(2 d) some maintenance

(continued)

Table 7–1. Treatment Studies of Naming Disorders—*(continued)*

Patients (Authors)	Aphasia Type	Time Postonset	Functional Damage	Treatment	Stimuli	Implementation	Results	Follow-up
RBO	Anomic	18 months	Damage to phonol output representations	(1) Reading (2) Repetition	30 words for each treatment, 20 controls	10 times per d/5 days	Significant improvement for all treatments. No generalization to untreated items	(25 d) maintenance
GMA (Miceli et al., 1996)	Anomic	1 year		(1) Written w + picture (2) Written w (3) Picture	20 words for each treatment, 20 controls	10 times per d/7 days		(17 m) maintenance

d = day; m = month; phonol = phonological; semant = semantically; w = word.

tional—that mediate between the message level and the spoken sentence are necessary to explain the distributional properties of speech errors in normal subjects. As stated in Chapter 5, word exchanges take place across phrases and generally involve words of the same grammatical class. These exchanges indicate a level where grammatical class is specified but not the phonological form of the words. Segment exchange errors occur within the same phrase and can involve words of different grammatical classes. They indicate a level where the phonological form of words within a phrase is specified.

At the phonetic level, the output of the positional level is converted into a phonetically coded representation for successive translation into an articulatory program. Motor execution of the sentence takes place at the final articulatory level.

Figure 7–1 illustrates Garret's model as depicted by Mitchum (1992).

These same representational levels are sometimes used to describe the process of sentence comprehension, notwithstanding some obvious differences between the two processes. Production starts from a concept to be expressed and ends as a string of articulated morphemes. Comprehension starts from an auditory message and ends as a concept. There is, however, a widespread assumption that the information required at the functional and positional levels is similar for production and comprehension, although addressed in the reverse order.

Garrett's model is lacking in detail, but for want of a more detailed one, it has often guided the diagnosis of sentence production disorders in aphasic individuals.

Mitchum, Haendiges, and Berndt (1993) and Mitchum and Berndt (1994)

These two investigations addressed the rehabilitation of two clinically very different patients who were, however, treated in a very similar way. The main difference was the modality used, written for EA and oral for ML.

EA (Mitchum et al., 1993), an engineer with 18 years of education, was a nonfluent aphasic with poor oral naming and naming of verbs more impaired than naming of nouns; he also had difficulty producing and understanding sentences. ML (Mitchum & Berndt, 1994) was a fluent aphasic with frequent phonemic paraphasias, impaired word retrieval, and poorly structured sentences.

Mitchum and colleagues (1993) and Mitchum and Berndt (1994) used Garrett's model to identify the functional locus of impairment of EA and

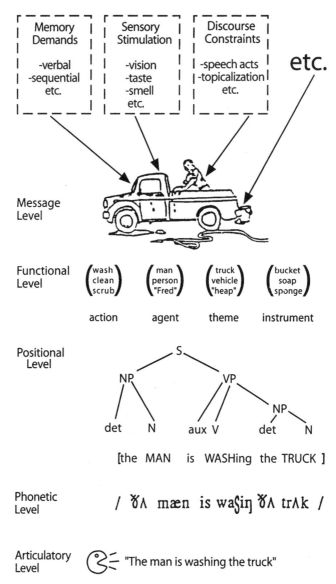

Figure 7–1. Garrett's model of sentence production (from Mitchum, 1992).

ML and to plan therapy. Despite their different clinical pictures, detailed analysis of their sentence production showed the presence of similar deficits: poor verb retrieval and difficulty in the application of the grammatical elements related to verbs. The investigators argued that failure to extract a correct verb concept from the message-level representation can impair retrieval of the correct abstract representation of verbs at the functional level. Alternatively, verb selection at the functional level can be correctly performed, but the phonological form cannot be retrieved at the positional level. In either case, impaired verb retrieval can, in turn, be a primary deficit that can explain subsequent failure in the execution of related processes.

An intervention aimed at facilitating verb retrieval was instantiated in EA (written verb retrieval) and ML (oral verb retrieval). The patients were repeatedly presented with 16 (EA) or 8 (ML) action pictures and asked to write (EA) or say (ML) the action name. The intervention method was successful in both patients, but only EA demonstrated improved retrieval of verbs in sentence production. EA also showed improved sentence construction with the same verbs, but only when he was asked to describe a picture. Mitchum and colleagues (1993) argued that the underlying cause of EA's sentence construction deficit was the lack of availability of verbs, as demonstrated by his enhanced ability to use a lexical verb in his written sentences, whereas it was not in ML's case.

The second treatment tackled the patients' poor ability to access the grammatical elements that form a verb phrase. The patients were shown sequential pictures of an ongoing action and were required to retrieve the target verb in its correct form in sentences that described the target activity before it happened, while it was happening, and after it had happened. Fourteen actions were treated. The stimuli used to elicit the correct tense were "about to happen," "right now," and "already done." For both patients the treatment was efficacious. The ability to construct a grammatical frame enhanced their capacity in sentence construction.

The success of the same intervention with two different aphasics (EA was a nonfluent aphasic and ML was a fluent aphasic) was considered by the authors as evidence that to be efficacious, therapy must not aim at the level of the overt symptoms, disregarding the underlying causes. Rather, it must focus on specific processing impairments identified by comparing the patients' performance to a model of the normal system.

As stated in Chapter 6, cognitive models of sentence processing are far less detailed than models of words processing and do not constrain therapy in the same way. They have, however, determined a major change in therapy. Classic interventions for sentence disorders were based on the (tacit) assumption that sentences are processed linearly. It was assumed that new sentences are created by filling in the slots of a basic sentence type (e.g., Naeser, 1975). Facilitation of verb retrieval as the first step in sentence construction acknowledges the hierarchical structure of sentences.

Haendiges, Berndt, and Mitchum (1996)

EA's production of written sentences improved substantially following the above-described treatment, but his understanding of semantically reversible sentences continued to be fairly impaired relative to his good comprehension of nonreversible sentences. Haendiges and colleagues (1996) devised a targeted intervention that was not overtly instructive. The intervention employed orally presented sentences using sentence–picture-matching tasks and avoided the use of *wh*-questions since EA had great difficulty understanding them. There were three conditions. In condition one, EA had to verify whether a sentence spoken by the examiner matched a single picture. There were 20 pictures, and the stimuli were the correct passive and active sentences and the reversed passive and active sentences (e.g., "The woman is splashing the man," "The man is splashed by the woman," "The man is splashing the woman," and "The woman is splashed by the man"). In condition two, the forced-choice condition, two pictures were presented and the patient had to point to the picture that matched the sentence spoken by the examiner. The 20 pictures were the same as in condition one, and sentences were active and passive reversible sentences. Finally, in condition three, the patient was presented with 1 of the 20 pictures, and the examiner spoke both the active- and passive-voice sentences corresponding to the picture and indicated to the patient that both sentences correctly described the picture. EA was seen twice a week for 17 sessions. Marked improvement was evident only after the differences between active and passive sentences were explicitly demonstrated in condition three. Comprehension of untreated sentences also improved, but the difference between pre- and posttreatment conditions was not significant and improvement was not maintained 7 weeks posttreatment. Comprehension of untreated written sentences did not improve.

The authors argue that they used "the relatively new methodology of targeted treatment study" (p. 298) and that the study's results indicate that even in a severely aphasic chronic patient a targeted intervention can have a positive outcome. However, the relationship between a model of sentence processing and the implemented therapy is not clear. The simple observation of the patient's difficulty in processing passive sentences could have persuaded the therapist to treat by having the patient listen to the difference between a passive and an active sentence.

Thompson, Shapiro, and Roberts (1993) and Thompson, Shapiro, Tait, Jacobs, and Schneider (1996)

These two investigations will be reported together because the treated patients, the linguistic framework within which they were evaluated, and the treatments were similar. Two patients participated in the first study (Thompson et al., 1993) and seven in the second study (Thompson et al., 1996). The investigators examined the effects of a linguistic-specific treatment on acquisition and generalization of *wh*-interrogative structures in agrammatic patients. Linguistic theories, they argued, should be used to understand normal sentence processing and identify what has gone awry in the aphasic patient under study. The therapy is based on Chomsky's (1982) government-and-binding theory—specifically, the *move-alpha* rule, a single general movement rule that allows one to derive from the underlying d-structure the s-structure of sentences with moved elements. According to the theory, there is a deep structure representation of a sentence in which the arguments of a verb are in their canonical position. Verbs have in fact an argument structure that specifies the number of entities that are necessarily part of the meaning of the verb. The arguments specified by the verb are obligatory, and the mental representation of the verb includes information about the argument structure. The verb *eat*, for example has a two-argument structure, and its thematic roles specify an agent (the doer of the action, who does the eating) and a patient (the undergoer of the action, what is eaten).

According to the move-alpha rule, sentences can be generated from the d-structure by moving some of the arguments to other positions. For instance, in a passive sentence like "The boy is being kissed by the girl," the grammatical subject ("boy") of the verb ("is kissed") has been moved out of its d-structure position of object ("the girl is kissing the boy"), leaving behind a trace. The trace links the moved argument to its position in the d-structure.

The *wh*-word of *wh*-interrogatives originates at the d-structure and is moved to its initial sentence position in the s-structure. The s-structure sentence "What is Bill eating?" can derive from the d-structure "Bill is eating the cheese." The object noun phrase—"the cheese"—is replaced by a *wh*-word, which is moved to the initial sentence position (COMP, for complementizer). A trace of the movement is left behind and coindexed with the *wh*-word. Figure 7–2 is a diagram illustrating the move-alpha rule for formation of a *wh*-interrogative sentence.

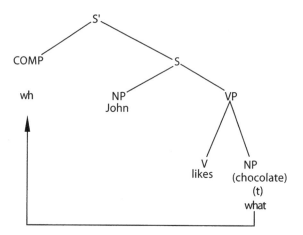

Figure 7–2. Diagram illustrating the "move-alpha" rule for formation of a *wh*-interrogative sentence.

The two patients, JM and PH, of the first study and the seven of the second study were all clinically agrammatic; they produced primarily simple, active, frequently incomplete sentences and had difficulty producing sentences with moved constituents, such as passive and *wh*-interrogatives. A single-subject experimental paradigm was used with the nine agrammatic patients. Patients were first shown a written sentence ("The girl is kicking the man" or "The man is sending flowers," for instance) and taught to identify the verb and the thematic roles—agent and patient—of the noun phrases. They were then presented with "What" and "Who" cards, with the sentence constituents on individual cards, and asked to replace the sentence constituent corresponding to a given question with the correct *wh*-morpheme. When told, for example, "You want to know the person the girl is kicking," they had to select the "Who" card. When told "You want to know the thing the man is sending," they had to select the "What" card. Finally, the patients were asked to move the *wh*-morpheme to its correct initial position and produce the surface form of the *wh*-question ("Who is the girl kicking?" or "What is the man sending?"). In the first study, only "Who" and "What" questions derived from the movement of the direct object, directly governed by the verb, were included. In the second study, "When" and "Where" questions were also dealt with.

"When" and "Where" questions are formed by moving an adjunct not governed by the verb that can be absent without the sentences becoming unacceptable. In the sentence "John is eating an apple in the park," for example, the direct object "an apple" depends directly on the verb "is eating," whereas "in the park" is optional and does not depend on the verb.

A total of 90 sentences were constructed for the first study and 80 for the second study. Treatment was provided twice a week for a total of 48 sessions for JM and 34 sessions for PH. In the second study, treatment was provided twice a week and lasted for 10 to 18 weeks.

After treatment all patients improved in *wh*-question production. Generalization varied across patients. Generalization to untreated but less complex exemplars of a treated structure was noted in all subjects. Four subjects in the second study showed the widest generalization, which was evident across all *wh*-interrogative structures. According to the authors, these data indicate that when the linguistic underpinnings of the language deficits are considered and the treatment strategy is based on these findings, the treatment is efficacious.

The study is an example of explicit teaching of a linguistic rule—the move-alpha rule. This type of therapy moves away from the classic clinical approach and moves a step forward in the attempt to treat the underlying functional deficit instead of the presenting clinical symptoms.

Table 7–2 reports for each patient the functional damage, the type of sentence-level treatment, and its results.

READING DISORDERS

Four patients with reading disorders are described in this section; one patient, EE, (Coltheart & Byng, 1989) had surface dyslexia, two patients, SP (Bachy-Langedock & De Partz, 1989) and LR (Berndt & Mitchum, 1994), had deep dyslexia, and a fourth patient, SI (Berhmann & McLeod, 1995), had letter-by-letter reading. The lexical route was treated in EE, the nonlexical route in SP and LR, and the abstract letter identification system in SI.

The reading disorder, type of stimuli, implementation of therapy, and treatment results are briefly reported in Table 7–3.

Coltheart and Byng (1989)

EE was a 40-year-old left-handed man who had fallen from a ladder and suffered an extensive hemorrhagic contusion of the right temporal lobe and a large hematoma extending over the left temporal and parietal lobes. Evacuation of the right hematoma was performed the same day, and 2

Table 7–2. Treatment Studies of the Sentence Level

Patient (Authors)	Aphasia Type	Time Postonset	Functional Damage	Treatment	Stimuli	Results
EA (Mitchum et al., 1993)	Agrammatic	5 years	Impaired verb retrieval Impaired S production	(1) Repeated written verb naming (2) Written verb-tense production	(1) 16 transitive verbs (2) 14 three-sequence action pictures	(1) Improved verb retrieval (2) Improved S production
EA (Haendiges et al., 1996)	Agrammatic	5 years	Impaired comprehension of reversible S	(1) Verification of reversible S (2) Forced choice (3) Listening to active and passive S	20 active and 20 passive S	Marked improvement
JM, PH (Thompson et al., 1993)	Agrammatic	13 and 40 months	Impaired *wh-*interrogative construction	Trained to move S constituents to form interrogatives	90 S to elicit *what* and *who* interrogatives	Improved
ML (Mitchum & Berndt, 1994)	Fluent para-grammatic	7 years	Impaired verb retrieval Impaired S production	(1) Repeated oral verb naming (2) Oral verb-tense production	(1) 8 transitive verbs (2) 14 three-sequence action pictures	(1) Improved verb retrieval (2) Improved S production
7 patients (Thompson et al., 1996)	Agrammatic	19 to 198 months	Impaired *wh-*interrogative construction	Trained to move S constituents to form interrogatives	80 S to elicit *what, who, when,* and *where* interrogatives	Improved

S = sentence.

Table 7–3. Treatment Studies of Acquired Reading Disorders

Patient (Authors)	Time Postonset	Reading Disorder	Treatment Target	Stimuli	Implementation	Results and Follow-up
EE (Coltheart & Byng, 1989)	4 months	Surface dyslexia with damage to the orthographic input lexicon	(1) Direct learning of irregular words (2) Reading of frequent words	(1) 12 treated words and 12 controls (2) 27 treated words and 27 controls	(1) Reading words with a visual cue (2) Same	Learning of all treated words
SP (Bachy-Langedock & DePartz, 1989)	3 months	Deep dyslexia	Grapheme-phoneme conversion with the use of code words	(1) Simple graphemes (2) complex graphemes (3) 3 grapheme-conversion rules	(1) Association of letters with code word (2) Isolation of the first ph of the code word (3) complex g reading	Improved (correct but slow reading)
LR (Berndt & Mitchum, 1994)	10 years	Deep dyslexia	Grapheme-phoneme conversion	(1) 18 predictable graphemes	(1) Phonological awareness (2) Grapheme-phoneme conversion for 18 predictable ph using word code (3) Phoneme blending	Phonological awareness not improved Conversion improved Blending not improved
SI (Behrmann & McLeod, 1995)	11 months	Letter-by-letter reading	Parallel processing of letters	Lists of 20 words	Manipulation of length of words and time of exposure on a computer	Improved identification of final letters; no change in reading time

ph = phoneme; g = grapheme.

weeks later the left hematoma was evacuated. The patient was tested for his reading capacity 4 months later. Testing revealed that EE had surface dyslexia: better reading of regular than irregular words, with regularization errors and relatively spared reading of nonwords. Coltheart and Byng argued that a diagnosis of surface dyslexia cannot determine a sufficiently focused treatment because disruption of the lexical procedure can arise at different stages of reading: written word recognition, word comprehension, and retrieval of the output phonological representations. It was therefore necessary to identify the specific locus of impairment in EE. A thorough evaluation of EE's reading enabled the investigators to conclude that the major source of his reading impairment was not at the level of the output lexicon because when he misread a word he generally failed to understand it, demonstrating that the damage was at a higher level. Nor was it at the level of the semantic system since auditory comprehension was fair and far less affected than reading comprehension. The major source of EE's dyslexia must have been at the level of written word recognition. This conclusion was supported by the pattern of EE's comprehension when reading homophones. When reading *I*, for instance, he said "got two" and pointed to his eyes, suggesting that comprehension took place only after the written word had been phonologically recoded.

Coltheart and Byng chose a whole-word training strategy. They decided to rehabilitate such words as *south, rough*, and *though*, whose spelling pattern is one of the most inconsistent in English. They selected 24 words, 12 to be treated and 12 to serve as controls. They paired the experimental words with a picture representing the meaning of the word to help EE associate the written word with its meaning. EE was instructed to read aloud the words with the help of the picture for 15 minutes every day. Successively, the second group of 12 words was treated in the same manner and group one words were not treated. At the end of the first period, which lasted for 2 weeks, EE demonstrated recovery in both the treated and untreated words, with superiority for the treated words. At the end of therapy, which lasted for 5 weeks, he had learned to read all 24 words.

In a second therapy study, EE's reading of the 458 most frequent words in Kucera and Francis' norms (Kucera & Francis, 1967) was assessed. He misread 54 words that were then subdivided into two groups: 27 to be treated and 27 to serve as controls. Some kind of mnemonic symbol was drawn on the to-be-treated words (for the word *society*, for instance, faces were drawn inside some letters) and EE had to practice them at home. At the end of the treatment, performance was better for both the treated and untreated words and was superior for the treated words. A third therapy study followed the same lines as the second, using other words, with similar results.

Coltheart and Byng ascribed the learning of the treated word to the effects of therapy. The nonspecific effect (recovery of untreated words) was argued to be due to the fact that EE had learned to use a mnemonic technique.

Use of a cognitive model allowed the authors to localize precisely the functional damage at the level of the orthographic input lexicon and to constrain the choice of words to be rehabilitated (homophones and irregular words), but pairing of written words with pictures is certainly not a new approach for treatment of written word comprehension. More innovative appears to be the use of mnemonic symbols.

Bachy-Langedock and De Partz (1989)

SP (Bachy-Langedock & De Partz, 1989) was a left-handed man who at the age of 31 suffered a sudden left cerebral hemorrhage that was surgically evacuated. Three months later, the patient had fluent aphasia with word-finding difficulties and phonemic paraphasias. Reading and writing were severely impaired. An extensive reading examination disclosed deep dyslexia. SP could not read nonwords, and his word reading, though superior, was also impaired. Errors consisted mainly of no responses, semantic paraphasias, derivational paralexias, and function word substitutions. The reading therapy aimed at the reorganization of the grapheme-to-phoneme conversion mechanisms and used SP's better-preserved word reading. In the first stage, a word code starting with a given letter was selected and the patient was taught to say the word when he saw the letter. When this association had been firmly established for all the letters, SP was required to fade the production of the word and to say only the first phoneme. He then practiced reading simple nonwords in which each letter corresponded to a phoneme. In stage two, SP was taught to identify complex graphemes, that is, graphemes that correspond to more than one letter. The most frequent graphemes were chosen, and again a lexical relay strategy was used based on the patients ability to read some content words. To learn to produce the phoneme /o/ to the corresponding grapheme [AU], the homophone word *eau* (water) was used. After 9 months of intensive therapy, SP showed marked recovery in the reading battery and stage three was started. It was devoted to the learning of three graphemic conversion rules that had caused most of SP's errors in the reading battery. One of these was the conversion rules for the letters [C] and [G] that in French are always read /k/ and /g/, except when they are followed by [E] and [I], in which case they change to /s/ and /dʒ/. In addition, when [C] is followed by [H] it changes to /ʃ/, but this rule was not drilled. At the end of therapy, the patient could read slowly but correctly; in reading texts, he simultaneously used the conversion rules mainly for verbs and function words and the lexical route for some frequent nouns.

This is an example of a creative and well-conducted therapy, but it is not clear in what sense it should be considered cognitive. SP was first taught a word code, which allowed him to produce the first phoneme of the to-be-read word, and then the conversion rules for two frequently used letters—[C] and [G]. The same therapy could have been implemented without having reached a diagnosis of deep dyslexia but merely by observing SP's superficial symptoms.

Berndt and Mitchum (1994)

LR (Berndt & Mitchum, 1994), a severely nonfluent aphasic with better object than action naming, was almost 10 years postonset when the reading treatment was implemented. Her reading pattern was quite similar to that of SP. Both were deep dyslexic with impaired nonword reading, better reading of high- than low-imageability words, and semantic errors. In LR's case, the author's decided that grapheme-to-phoneme conversion rules would be treated in the hope that some knowledge of the conversion rules would reduce the number of her semantic errors. Knowing, for instance, that the word *effort* starts with the letter [E] would prevent her from reading it as *difficult*, as she had done at pretherapy testing.

Testing before starting therapy indicated that LR had problems with all three components of nonlexical reading: grapheme parsing, grapheme–phoneme association, and phoneme blending. Grapheme–phoneme association could be carried out for a few isolated letters only, and she had great difficulty blending phonemes into words. She did not appear to have any concept of phonemes since she could neither appreciate that spoken language can be analyzed into component sounds nor divide printed words into syllables.

Studies of developmental reading disorders have shown that phonological awareness is generally impaired in patients with developmental phonological dyslexia, and it is generally supposed that the acquisition of reading occurs in parallel with the development of phonological awareness (e.g., Masterson et al., 1995). In consideration of the widespread damage to all components of the model, some preliminary work was done on phonological awareness, such as phonological segmentation. Berndt and Mitchum decided to treat phonological segmentation before treating grapheme–phoneme associations because they argued that phonological processes "are presumably required to generate the sublexical segments to which graphemes must be mapped, and … govern the combination of sublexical segments at the blending stage" (p. 513).

Color-coded tokens were used to represent different phonemes. LR was given, for instance, three tokens (two green and one red) and was asked to arrange them to represent the sequence /p/, /p/, /I/, and then to rearrange them to represent the sequence /p/, /I/, /p/.

This attempt to have the patient acquire phonological segmentation separately from the processes involved in grapheme–phoneme association failed, and LR was taught grapheme-to-phoneme correspondences for 18 predictable graphemes. This was done, as with SP, by linking each grapheme to a cue word, segmenting the initial phoneme, and producing it in isolation. LR learned the grapheme–phoneme associations fairly easily, but she was then unable to blend the phonemes she had produced one by one.

The last phase of therapy consisted in the treatment of the blending component, starting with simple consonant + vowel or vowel + consonant associations. After extensive treatment, her ability to blend three-phoneme words was unchanged. When reassessed at the end of treatment, the number of errors in reading a list of 72 words was practically unchanged (47 errors pretherapy and 39 errors posttherapy) but the pattern of errors was different. Semantic errors had diminished and visual errors were more frequent.

Berndt and Mitchum interpreted the change in her error pattern as the consequence of her partial acquisition of grapheme–phoneme associations that allowed her to reject a semantic error that did not bear any phonological relationship to the target. Her partial recovery, however, did not allow her to read the entire target word using the nonlexical procedures.

LR, like SP, had a multiple reading impairment—damage to both the lexical and the nonlexical routes—and the decision to treat grapheme–phoneme association was made for both patients. The analysis of the cognitive processes underlying grapheme-to-phoneme conversion mechanisms is more accurate in Berndt and Mitchum's paper and the therapy is more constrained but unsuccessful. Publication of an unsuccessful treatment is one of Berndt and Mitchum's merits because such treatments are rarely reported, although they can be as informative as successful ones.

Berhmann and McLeod (1995)

SI, a 46-year-old woman with letter-by-letter reading following a posterior cerebral artery infarction, underwent a 9-week intensive therapy program. Pretherapy assessment demonstrated relatively good letter identification even under rather brief exposure and increasing reading reaction times with increasing word length, which is the hallmark of letter-by-letter dyslexia. Words were read somewhat better than nonwords, and the first letter was identified better than the last. The therapy program aimed at encouraging parallel processing of the first and last letters of words, with the hope that this would reduce the sequential left-to-right processing of letters and the reading time. SI was presented with a list of words on a computer screen and was asked to report the first and last letter. Length of words and exposure duration were manipulated. SI was first presented with words of increasing length (from three to seven letters) at a given duration; when she reached criterion with seven-letter words the duration of exposure was decreased by 100 milliseconds and the procedure was repeated. At the end of treatment SI was better at reporting the final letter of words and nonwords, but this did not translate into better reading of words. From this lack of direct transfer from improved letter identification to word recognition, the investigators conclude that the link between the two processes is not as transparent as was foreseen and that a more efficacious therapy for letter-by-letter readers could be a compensatory procedure rather than directly tackling the deficit.

WRITING DISORDERS

This section reports the therapy for three patients. Therapy was aimed at nonlexical writing in the first patient and at the orthographic output buffer in the other two patients. In one case, the orthographic output lexicon was also retrained.

Table 7–4 reports the main data from these studies.

Carlomagno and Parlato (1989)

Carlomagno and Parlato (1989) presented the case of a patient with severe reading and writing disorders and described a therapeutic intervention for his writing deficit. The patient was a 60-year-old right-handed man with a high school education. He was 1 year post onset of a cerebrovascular acci-

Table 7-4. Treatment Studies of Acquired Writing Disorders

Patients (Authors)	Time Postonset	Writing Disorder	Treatment Targets	Stimuli	Implementation	Results and Follow-up
1 patient (Carlomagno & Parlato, 1989)	2½ years	Severely agraphic; both routes impaired	Ph → G conversion by the use of a lexical relay strategy	30 CV syllables 40 CV syllables Consonant clusters	Syllabic segmentation → code name → initial syllables	Considerable improvement; maintenance 2 months later
JES (Aliminosa et al., 1993)	3 years	Impaired OOL and OOB Impaired Ph → G conversion	OOL and OOB	18 target words 18 controls	(1) Delayed copying (2) Writing to dictation	Significant improvement (no generalization; no follow-up)
AM (De Partz, 1995)	2 years	Impaired OOB Slightly impaired OOL Impaired Ph → G conversion	OOB	30 decomposable words 30 nondecomposable words	Delayed copying (suggested strategy: decompose words)	Word-specific improvement, higher for decomposable words

OOL = orthographic output lexicon; OOB = orthographic output buffer; Ph → G = phoneme-to-grapheme; CV = consonant-verb.

dent when first seen by the authors and $2\frac{1}{2}$ years postonset when the writing training began. In the $1\frac{1}{2}$ years that preceded treatment, the writing disorder was stable. Careful examination disclosed normal comprehension on the token test (De Renzi & Faglioni, 1978), a sensible test for the evaluation of auditory comprehension, and no spoken language impairment except for rare and frequently self-corrected phonemic paraphasias in spontaneous speech and repetition. The writing disorder was severe and no particular pattern of impairment was evident, although his nonword writing was usually worse than his word writing. The most frequent errors were insertions, deletions, and substitutions that, however, did not violate Italian orthographic rules. The absence of a clear pattern of writing impairment suggested severe damage to both the lexical and nonlexical writing routes. In reading, the patient was better at reading regular than irregular words and was moderately impaired in reading nonwords. His better reading of regular words than nonwords was considered evidence of his using of a lexical strategy in reading, although this, according to the authors, was accomplished by the grapheme-to-phoneme conversion mechanisms. Further proof came from an experiment in which he was requested to match a spoken nonsense syllable to one of eight written syllables or to one of eight written words (names of Italian towns) whose first syllable corresponded to the spoken ones. He was only 30% correct in the first task but 96% correct when he had to match a spoken syllable to the name of a town (the syllable /ca/, for instance, with the written word *Catania*). These results were interpreted as being consistent with damage to the lexical reading route, relatively preserved nonlexical reading, and use of a lexical strategy in reading by grapheme-to-phoneme conversion.

Carlomagno and Parlato argued that three conditions must exist to reorganize the damaged processes underlying a behavioral deficit. First, one must have a sufficiently detailed model of the normal function. Second, one must be able to identify the defective processes of the patient. Finally, some processes must be sufficiently spared to permit their use for the reorganization of the damaged function. Regarding implementation of therapy for this patient, the authors suggested that the two-route model of writing fulfilled the first condition; identification of the patient's disorder as damage to both writing routes fulfilled the second condition; and his relatively preserved orthographic competence fulfilled the third. Since he demonstrated a lexical strategy in reading by the grapheme-to-phoneme route, the authors decided to treat his nonlexical writing by suggesting the use of a lexical relay, similar to the strategy he used in reading.

The rehabilitation program consisted in using code names—names of Italian towns or proper names—whose first syllables represented as many Italian syllables as possible. The patient was then taught to identify the syllables in the to-be-written word and for each syllable find the corresponding code name. Only consonant-vowel (CV) words were used in this phase. Finally, he was asked to write the word using the first syllable of the code names in the correct order. When asked to write *vero* (true), for instance, he first had to decompose the word into the two syllables /ve/ and /ro/, then find the code names (Venice and Rome), and finally write down the first syllables of the code words, [VE] and [RO]. Subsequently, only nonwords were used and the patient was trained on consonant clusters and diphthong decomposition; the nonword *canca*, for instance, had to be segmented into ca + n + ca. He was instructed to use only the first letter of the code word instead of its first syllable when appropriate. In this example he had to find the code word *Catania*, write [CA], find the code word *Napoli*, write the first letter [N], and find again the code word *Catania* and write [CA].

After 5 months of rehabilitation, the patient had greatly improved and his errors could be explained by the use of phoneme-to-grapheme conversion, being therefore consistent with the rehabilitation strategy adopted.

Nothing in this study, however, seems to be dictated by cognitive neuropsychological models. The patient had a severe multiple writing disorder and, due to its severity, no attempt was made to qualify it in a more detailed way. Treatment consisted in the use of a word code—names of towns—which is not a new technique and is not specifically tailored to the patient's disorder.

Aliminosa, McCloskey, Goodman-Schulman, and Sokol (1993)

A further example of remediation of an acquired dysgraphia was described by Aliminosa and coworkers (1993). The patient, JES, a right-handed man who had suffered a cerbrovascular accident 3 years previously, had nonfluent aphasia with severe writing disorders. Assessment of his spelling suggested damage to the orthographic output lexicon, the orthographic output buffer, and the conversion mechanisms. Damage to the orthographic output lexicon was inferred from the finding of a word frequency effect. Damage to the orthographic output buffer was based on the finding that short words were written better than long words, that errors were a function of letter position (JES was more likely to make errors in the middle of the word than at its beginning or end), and that the errors consisted mainly of substitutions, deletions, insertions, and transpositions. Finally, damage to phoneme-to-grapheme conversion was inferred from JES's failure to write any nonwords. A remediation program was designed for the orthographic output lexicon and the buffer. The conversion mechanisms were not taken into consideration.

Aliminosa and coworkers assumed that training could have different effects, depending on the functional locus of the lesion. With damage at the level of the output orthographic lexicon, effective training should cause item-specific recovery; with damage at the level of the buffer, recovery should generalize to untrained items. If, as predicted by test results, both the lexicon and the buffer were damaged, there should be some generalization to the untrained items and better recovery of the trained items.

Two sets of 18 words matched for frequency, length, word class, and number of syllables were constructed. Set A words were used for rehabilitation and set B as controls. At baseline, JES was 14% correct for set A and 11% for set B. The first training phase consisted in delayed copying of set A words. Whenever JES misspelled a word, it was shown again and the patient was asked to copy it after a delay. In the second phase, JES had to write the words to dictation. When misspelling occurred, he looked at the correctly written word and wrote it again after the card was removed. Training was terminated when all the words were written with 100% accuracy over five consecutive trials. Each training phase lasted for 2 weeks and consisted of two training sessions and four independent practice sessions per week. At posttesting a week later, set A and set B words were dictated in random order. JES was 100% correct for set A and 17% correct for set B.

Aliminosa et al. argued that these results are difficult to reconcile with partial recovery from a buffer deficit because no generalization to untreated words was found. They suggested three possible explanations. First, JES could have learned a strategy to subdivide words into smaller units and load these, one by one, in the buffer, thus explaining how he could write the target words correctly, notwithstanding his still existing buffer deficit, but this strategy was not generalized to untreated items. The second interpretation is that their diagnosis was wrong and that JES did not have a buffer deficit at all. According to the authors, the length effect, the types of errors, and all the symptoms generally considered as evidence of a buffer deficit could just as well be explained by damage to the orthographic output lexicon. The length effect, for instance, is simply the consequence of the fact that "the longer the word the greater the potential for degradation of the graphemic representation" (p. 67). However, if all the effects attributed to damage to the output buffer can be explained by damage to the output lexicon, it follows that a third interpretation of JES's results is possible, namely, that one might question the very existence of the buffer. This was the interpretation the authors favored.

Aliminosa and colleagues argued that the importance of the study is twofold: demonstration of the effectiveness of a therapeutic method for the rehabilitation of writing disorders and illustration of how therapeutic procedures can be used to test the functional diagnosis. However, they do not give any independent reason for questioning the existence of the buffer except the patient's results. Yet, for any pattern of results, it is possible to devise a model that explains it.

De Partz (1995)

AM (De Partz, 1995) was a 64-year-old right-handed man who suffered a cerebrovascular accident with a left parietal-occipital lesion 2 years before testing. At the time of testing, AM showed an acoustico-phonological deficit, phonemic paraphasias in all production tasks, and unimpaired written comprehension of words, sentences, and paragraphs. Writing was severely impaired for words and nonwords and presented a curious phenomenon: in writing words, AM wrote letters in a nonlinear order. He generally started writing the word from the first letter and then went on in an apparently random order, leaving a space when he skipped a letter and coming back to it later. A detailed analysis of his writing abilities led De Partz to conclude that he had a deficit involving the orthographic output buffer. Specifically, there was a length effect; errors consisted of substitutions, deletions, and insertions; and his error rate was higher in the middle of words. A mild deficit of the orthographic output lexicon was also hypothesized based on the presence of a word frequency effect. Writing of nonwords was impossible, and the deficit was ascribed to his acoustico-phonological damage.

De Partz argued that her patient was similar to JES (Aliminosa et al., 1993) and that Aliminosa and coworkers were too hasty when they discounted a segmentation strategy at the base of JES's improvement. She therefore decided to teach her patient, with a buffer deficit like that of JES, a segmentation strategy in order to verify whether or not such a strategy could be ruled out as a possible explanation for JES's results.

AM was taught to divide long words into segments and to dictate them to himself separately. Two sets of 30 words matched for frequency and letter length were prepared. Half of the words in each set—part A—consisted of words that contained a lexical segment (cravache [crop]), for instance, where <u>vache</u> is a word [cow]). The other half—part B—consisted of similar words that, however, did not include a lexical segment (cramique [a Belgian pastry], where <u>mique</u> is a nonword). The lexical part of the words with a lexical segment (<u>vache</u>) and the corresponding nonlexical part of the other words (<u>mique</u>) were underlined, and the patient was instructed to pay attention to the decomposition of the word.

At baseline the patient correctly wrote two words in part A and three in part B of the first set of 30 words, which was then presented for delayed copying. AM's attention was drawn to the underlined letters, and training was carried out in five sessions. After training, AM demonstrated word-specific improvement: treated words were 76.6% correct and untreated words were 6.6% correct. Words comprising a lexical segment were written better than nondecomposable words, but the difference was not statistically significant.

The remaining 30 words in the second set were then treated in five sessions, and AM demonstrated improvement on both types of words; she was also found to have acquired a lexical segmentation strategy since words that comprised another word were significantly better written than non-decomposable words. A follow-up a month later still showed the effects of training.

De Partz argued that the word-specific improvement supports the initial diagnosis of damage to the orthographic output lexicon, and the use of a lexical segmentation strategy that of damage to the buffer. The word-specific improvement can in fact be traced back to an improvement of representations in the lexicon; the use of a lexical segmentation strategy allows better functioning of the buffer and better recovery of decomposable words.

According to De Partz, the importance of the study lies in the fact that it illustrates how a therapy program can be used to demonstrate whether the initial cognitive analysis of the deficit (deficit of the orthographic output buffer in the present case) was correct. At the same time, it demonstrated how Aliminosa et al.'s (1993) patient's results do not clearly indicate that he did not have a buffer deficit. JES, as well as AM, could have applied a segmentation strategy even if this had not been deliberately taught.

This case illustrates a clear example of a therapeutic intervention rationally linked to the identified functional damage and to hypotheses about the processing of the damaged component.

CONCLUSIONS

What all these treatments have in common is the identification of the functional damage in relation to a model of normal processing, a clear description of the therapeutic program and of its expected effect, careful implementation of the program, and a detailed description of the outcome. All these are obvious advantages and permit replication of the therapeutic intervention with similar patients.

However, apart from the first—identification of the functional damage—these characteristics are not new in aphasia therapy and had already been recommended by the modification behavior approach. The behavior modification approach was based on a rigorous methodology, which required that a baseline be established and a treatment planned in detail and implemented in a standardized way. The obvious difference between these two approaches lies in the different emphasis on initial diagnosis. The programmed instruction approach was not based on a theoretical analysis of the language disorder. By contrast, the cognitive approach starts from a detailed model of the structure of the normal function and seeks to locate the patient's deficit within this model. A more precise diagnosis is important for aphasia therapy because it allows more specifically focused treatments. The starting point is therefore totally different.

Yet, the initial evaluation is not always as detailed as the model allows it to be, and conclusions about the patient's functional damage are frequently based on insufficient data.

In regard to the implementation of the treatment, many of the treatments so far described can hardly be considered cognitive. In fact, there is nothing new in the treatment carried out for anomia. An important difference does exist, but it does not refer to the type of intervention but rather to its range. In the clinical studies reported in Chapter 4, rehabilitation aimed at a general improvement of the patients' language capacity. In most of the cognitive studies reported here, few experimental stimuli were used (from a minimum of 5 to a maximum of 90), and patients were asked to learn them. It is not known whether the same technique would be successful with a large number of words, but only such a result would be of any impact on the patient's daily living. These studies illustrate the methods therapy might use rather than therapy itself.

Other intervention strategies, particularly for sentence-level disorders, are more innovative and more specifically directed to the deficit.

IN SEARCH OF
A THEORY OF
APHASIA THERAPY

THE PURPOSE OF THIS CHAPTER IS to propose a working model of a theory of aphasia therapy. However, I will argue that, for the time being, a theory of aphasia rehabilitation that can explain known facts and predict new ones is beyond our reach, and a conscious effort to collect meaningful and organized data is a necessary prerequisite.

To define the word *theory* is not easy. A theory comprises the general principles of a science, a system of ideas explaining something; it should account for the existing data and predict outcomes that have not yet been tested. A theory gains support as the predictions made are confirmed and it loses support when its predictions are not confirmed, making it necessary to revise the theory or develop a new one. Aphasia therapy has not progressed sufficiently to support the development of a fully articulated theory of aphasia rehabilitation. Mitchum et al. (2000), for instance, write, "In our view, it is premature to attempt to propose a theory of therapy, especially in light of the limited detail presented in the models of language processing that are available" (p. 312). However, merely collecting data and refining models of language processing will not lead to the foundation of a theory. Empirical data and detailed models are of assistance in formulating a theory, but an important body of empirical data and sufficiently detailed models (at least for single-word processing) are already available.

Moreover, future empirical data will not be more useful in constraining a theory if we do not make a conscious effort to provide a *rationalized* organization of facts about therapy. It is unrealistic to think that we can wake up one morning and find out that we have enough empirical data and detailed models to construct an elaborate and lasting theory. Collection of data must be systematic and based on predefined hypotheses if we want to use them to lay the foundation of a theory of aphasia therapy. We have to start from a few straightforward statements because we currently ignore the answers to most questions to which a theory of aphasia therapy should respond. The first and most important step in the construction of a theory of rehabilitation is to agree on some basic principles and accumulate knowledge as it becomes available. A cooperative effort is necessary for building a common framework to which to add all new knowledge coming from different sources and disciplines. This could help to avoid scattering what we know in various loose ends that are never tied up.

To speak of a theory of aphasia therapy is in any case a gross simplification. Just as we cannot talk about aphasia because there is no such thing as a single aphasia, we cannot talk about a theory of rehabilitation, although it is possible that some general rules are valid for many if not all aphasic disorders.

A theory of aphasia therapy should at least incorporate (*1*) a model of the cognitive processes to be treated and specific hypotheses about the functional damage(s) present in any given patient; (*2*) knowledge of which types of functional damage are amenable to amelioration, and which are not; (*3*) specific hypotheses about how neural mechanisms relate to recovery; (*4*) whether and which other factors, besides the damage itself, have an effect on recovery; (*5*) a theory of learning in brain-damaged patients; (*6*) and, last but not least, how to remediate each functional damage, namely, which tasks are to be utilized and how to implement them.

Caramazza and Hillis (1993) discussed the framework for a remediation theory and argued that the development of such a theory requires a model of the cognitive system to be treated, a detailed hypothesis about the damage(s) in the patients to be treated, and a motivated hypothesis about how therapy modifies the damaged processes. The third of Caramazza and Hillis' points will be the main focus of this chapter since the model of the cognitive system and hypotheses about how it can be damaged have been treated in previous chapters.

In this chapter, the current experimental evidence about some of the topics that must be included in a theory of aphasia therapy will be considered. How to remediate functional damages will be treated in more detail in the next two chapters.

FUNCTIONAL DAMAGE AND
THE NORMAL COGNITIVE STRUCTURE

Many researchers have asserted that cognitive neuropsychology has provided the grounds for a more rational intervention (e.g., Howard & Hatfield, 1987; Behrmann & Byng, 1992). They probably meant that cognitive neuropsychology allows one to identify more precisely than in the past the patient's functional damage, which should be the focus of the therapeutic intervention. Cognitive neuropsychological models of word and sentence processing do in fact allow us to reach a detailed diagnosis of many patients' functional damages, particularly with regard to single-word processing. Models of production and comprehension of sentences are not as detailed as those of single-word processing, but they suggest new and interesting ideas about intervention. In short, although still perfectible, our current knowledge about the location of functional damages is sufficient to constrain therapy in a meaningful way.

FOR WHICH FUNCTIONAL DAMAGES IS
IMPROVEMENT POSSIBLE?

The second important question concerns whether or not the damaged components to be treated are amenable to improvement. As noted in Chapter 4, previous group studies have reliably demonstrated that aphasia therapy in general can be successful for aphasic patients in general. This, however, does not answer the question of which forms of functional damage are amenable to improvement. If we reach a precise diagnosis, we also want to know whether the identified damages can be reduced, not simply whether some patients can improve. Single case studies have provided more qualified answers. There are now on record descriptions of successful interventions for many different forms of damage. Many have been described in Chapter 7; the following are selected examples of successfully treated forms of functional damage. This review does not aspire to be complete, nor does it tackle the question of the underlying causes of improvement. Its only aim is to show that for many functional disorders there is evidence that improvement is possible.

Semantic System

Behrmann and Lieberthal (1989) reported results of treatment of a central semantic deficit aimed at the restoration of semantic representations in patient CH (see Chapter 9). The aim of therapy was restoration of the semantic representations of words. After 15 hours of treatment, a significant improvement in the sorting task was noted for the treated items, with generalization to the untreated items in two out of three semantic categories.

Orthographic Input Lexicon

EE, as reported in Chapter 7, was a surface dyslexic patient with damage to the orthographic input lexicon (Coltheart & Byng, 1989). Three therapy programs based on whole-word training were successively implemented, and EE demonstrated good recovery. Coltheart and Byng argued that "these three studies of rehabilitation in acquired dyslexia provide evidence that it is possible to use a whole-word technique to restore at least partially the ability to use the lexical procedure for reading aloud after the use of this procedure has been impaired by neurological damage" (p. 170).

Phonological Output Lexicon

As reported in Chapter 7, two anomic subjects, RBO and GMA, with damage to the phonological output lexicon showed improved naming after specific treatment of words that were consistently produced incorrectly (Miceli et al., 1996). As predicted by the background model of lexical-semantic processing, improvement was restricted to the treated items and no generalization was found to untreated items.

Orthographic Output Lexicon

Behrmann and Herdan (1987) described the case of a bilingual patient with surface dysgraphia. The patient, CCM, had better-preserved reading than writing, and her writing disorder displayed all the symptoms of surface dysgraphia: better writing of nonwords and regular words than of irregular words and impaired homophone writing. Treatment was started with the aim of enhancing the use of the lexical procedure in writing. A posttherapy evaluation revealed a significant improvement in CCM's spelling ability of a group of treated words and a group of untreated words (from 0% to 93% and 83% correct, respectively).

Phoneme-to-Grapheme Conversion

Luzzatti and co-workers (2000) described rehabilitation directly aimed to the phoneme-to-grapheme conversion mechanisms and presented evidence from two Italian patients. RO was a clinically agrammatic patient, 4 years postonset, when rehabilitation of the writing disorder was started. DR was 10 years postonset, and he too presented with Broca aphasia and agrammatism. Both patients benefited greatly from the treatment.

Sentence Level

Sentence-level treatment studies have been less frequent and have proposed less varied interventions than therapy studies for naming disorders. Recently, improvement of sentence comprehension has been demonstrated in many studies (e.g., Jones, 1986; Byng, 1988; Schwartz et al., 1994). Improvement of sentence production has also been demonstrated, although less frequently (e.g., Marshall et al., 1993).

Although by no means exhaustive, this review is probably sufficient to demonstrate that most aphasic disorders have been shown (at least partially) to recover, and it allows us to draw the (provisional) conclusion that all aphasic disorder should be treated.

NEURAL MECHANISMS

How are recovery from brain injury and recovery from language disorders related? Does aphasia therapy effect brain changes? Several studies have been devoted to these questions (for a review, see Robertson & Murre, 1999; Cappa, 2000; Pizzamiglio et al., 2001), but the results have only been descriptive and often contradictory.

The neural mechanisms underlying recovery from aphasia as well as from other cognitive disorders are still an open question. The human central nervous system has only limited potential for regeneration, and in recovery from aphasia the relative contributions of behavioral adaptation and of true neurological recovery is unclear. An important question is whether changes in the organization of the brain are sustained by the left hemisphere zones spared by the lesion or by recruitment of homologous right-hemisphere regions (for reviews, see Cappa & Vallar, 1992; Gainotti, 1993). The possibility of a role for the right hemisphere in recovery from aphasia has been supported since the end of the nineteenth century by clinical observations. Gowers, in describing an aphasic patient, made the following comment: "Loss of speech due to permanent destruction of the speech region in the left hemisphere has been recovered from, and that this recovery was due to supplemental action of the corresponding right hemisphere is proved by the fact that in some cases, speech has been again lost when a fresh lesion occurred in this part of the right hemisphere" (Gowers, 1887, pp. 131–132).

Some indirect evidence that supports transfer of language dominance comes from studies using tachistoscopic or dichotic presentation of linguistic stimuli. A significant left visual field preference for verbal visual stimuli was found in a group of 30 aphasic patients by Moore and Weidner (1974). These same patients also showed a left ear preference on verbal dichotic tests when seen more than 6 months postonset (Moore & Weidner, 1975). A contribution of the right hemisphere to recovery of language in aphasic patients has also been suggested by the results of studies using an evoked potential paradigm (Papanicolaou et al., 1984, 1987).

However, one has to admit that takeover of language functions by the right hemisphere can hardly be considered the rule and that it differs remarkably from one patient to another. With rare exceptions, in fact, global aphasics, who presumably have large lesions destroying all the classic language areas, do not improve substantially. That compensation by the right hemisphere is rare is also suggested by Rasmussen and Milner (1977). Using carotid barbiturate injection, they found that only 12% of adult patients with early left hemisphere damage had right hemisphere speech representation. It is conceivable that this percentage is even smaller in patients who develop left hemisphere lesions at a later age.

A further source of evidence of the role of the right hemisphere in recovery from aphasia is recovered aphasic patients whose language worsen after a second, right-sided insult. These cases are rare and not always sufficiently documented. A few cases, however, are thoroughly documented (Cambier et al., 1983; Lee et al., 1984; Basso et al., 1989; Cappa et al., 1994) and suggest that the right hemisphere was at the root of recovery of language in those subjects. However, although the right hemisphere seems to play a role in recovery from aphasia, the exact nature of that role is still controversial and its contribution varies widely from one patient to another (Gainotti, 1993).

The recent introduction of functional neuroimaging techniques has allowed investigators to study brain activity in vivo and has provided new insights into the cerebral mechanisms of functional recovery. Belin and colleagues (1996), for instance, reported a positron emission tomography (PET) activation study in seven chronic nonfluent aphasics who had undergone successful training with melodic intonation therapy (MIT; Albert et al., 1973). Repetition with natural intonation, which remained poor, extensively activated the right hemisphere. However, in repetition of words with MIT intonation, which had substantially recovered, the right hemisphere was deactivated and activation increased in left frontal areas. The authors argued that the right hemisphere activation reflected "maladaptive" functional reorganization, which is responsible for the persistence of residual deficits; activation of the left frontal areas, on the other hand, was associated with real recovery. The importance of the right hemisphere in recovery, however, was supported by another recent study. Thulborn et al. (1999) conducted a longitudinal study of two patients—one with "expressive" and one with "receptive" aphasia—and reported a progressive shift of activation in the right hemisphere in language tasks concomitant with a behavioral improvement.

In conclusion, notwithstanding the growing literature on imaging studies, there is no unequivocal evidence in favor of either the right or left hemisphere hypothesis in recovery from aphasia. In fact, there is no reason to believe that recovery always occurs either in the left or the right hemisphere. It is more plausible that both hemispheres play a role in recovery, depending on factors such as the site and size of the left-hemisphere lesion. In addition, whether aphasia rehabilitation, besides enhancing recovery, has a qualitative effect on the underlying neural mechanisms,—that is, whether these can vary according to the type of intervention carried out— is an open question. It is my belief that treatment influences the extent of reorganizational processes but not in a qualitatively different manner. Yet not everybody agrees with this assumption.

Thompson and colleagues (2000) demonstrated changes in the pattern of activation in two agrammatic aphasic patients after improvement of their ability to understand and produce sentences and no changes in activation patterns in three untrained (and unrecovered) agrammatic patients. The investigators claimed that changes in activation were therapy-induced. Cardebat and coworkers (2000) reported results of a functional MRI study in an aphasic patient before and after therapy for naming disorders. After therapy, specific left perilesional activation was observed, and the authors claimed that it was associated with the therapy-induced improvement. However, in neither case is this conclusion warranted if by *therapy-induced* the investigators mean that changes would not be the same in spontaneous recovery.

A longitudinal study is required to address this issue. Patients should be examined for the first time after stabilization of the language disorder but before spontaneous recovery, a second time after spontaneous recovery, a third time after a first (effective) therapeutic intervention, and a fourth time after a second (successful) and different therapeutic intervention. Different patterns of activation should be seen if the pattern of activation depends on how recovery has been brought about and not simply if recovery has occurred. I assume that therapy can enhance recovery over and above what would occur spontaneously, but this further recovery is not qualitatively different from that which would occur spontaneously. In other words, aphasia therapy does not induce brain, cognitive, or behavioral changes that could not occur spontaneously in particular situations.

Hopefully, there will come a time when these two levels of investigation—the neural bases of recovery and the implementation of therapy—will find a common ground. However, at this time, it is not unreasonable to ignore the neural mechanisms underlying treatment and focus our efforts on the behavioral changes brought about by rehabilitation.

FACTORS INFLUENCING RECOVERY

Factors influencing recovery can be subdivided into three categories: factors related to the patient (age, sex, education, and so forth), factors related to the injury (etiology, time postonset, severity of the disorders), and factors related to more general cognitive functions, such as attention and memory.

Personal Factors

To my knowledge, no study has tackled the problem of the possible influence of personal factors (age, sex, handedness, educational level) on the effect of rehabilitation. However, they have been studied in relation to spontaneous recovery and, as noted in Chapter 4, we can safely conclude that the most recent investigations have not demonstrated that they have an important role in recovery (for a review, see Cappa, 1998). It seems a sensible hypothesis that their direct influence on the effect of rehabilitation is not very different from their influence on spontaneous recovery, although an indirect influence cannot be excluded. Older aphasic patients, for instance, may be less motivated in aphasia therapy than younger ones. However, until experimental evidence to the contrary is provided, we can keep to the provisional assumption that the influence of personal factors on therapy, if any, is small, and we can temporarily ignore them in our attempt to construe a theory of aphasia therapy.

A further reason for ignoring these factors for the time being is purely practical. If age, for example, had an influence not only on the outcome—younger patients have a somewhat higher probability of recovery—but also had qualitatively different effects on aphasia rehabilitation, we would have to redemonstrate for patients of different ages any conclusion we reached for a group of patients of a given age, which is in itself a Sisyphean task.

Injury-Related Factors

Etiology has not been studied with reference to its effect on rehabilitation, although traumatized patients have demonstrated better spontaneous recovery than vascular patients. Yet, aphasia in traumatized patients is frequently associated with other cognitive disorders, the most frequent being memory and attention disorders. It seems likely that an aphasic patient with memory and/or attention disorders is less amenable to recovery through therapy than an aphasic patient without these accompanying disorders.

As for time postonset, a group of psychologists, linguists, and therapists in Aachen has fine-tuned a treatment regimen "oriented toward the natural course of aphasia" (Huber et al., 1993). They describe three phases of treatment: activation, symptom-specific language training, and consolidation. In the first period after a stroke, when complete restitution of impaired function is possible, "the goal of aphasia therapy is to enhance the evolution of temporarily impaired language function" (p. 56). To reach this goal, all available means are used to activate the patient to respond as communicatively as possible. Although different intervention strategies are used according to the patient's disorders, which must be carefully identified, the techniques employed in this phase are rather generic. More precise interventions are suggested for the second phase. Here the interventions are linguistically based and tailored to the patient's deficit. This phase is continued as long as the patient demonstrates improvement. Finally, the last phase is the consolidation phase, and its aim is to maintain the acquired level of competence rather than to foster further improvement.

Without discussing the intervention strategies themselves, the Aachen proposal deserves comment. Differentiation of the intervention strategies according to time postonset can be an interesting suggestion for patients who enter therapy in the acute phase, soon after onset. However, many patients are first seen long after the acute phase, sometimes years later. Deferred treatment was not found to be less efficacious than nondeferred treatment in a large cooperative VA study (Wertz et al., 1986)—but the delay was of only 12 weeks—and no difference in the effect of rehabilitation was found by Basso and colleagues (1979) between groups of patients who started therapy within 2 months postonset, between 2 and 6 months, and more than 6 months postonset. All patients were rehabilitated at the same aphasia unit, and the therapeutic approach did not differ in the three time periods. By contrast, results of a meta-analysis (Robey, 1998) demonstrated that the difference in the amount of recovery between treated and untreated patients is greater in acute patients than in chronic patients.

To summarize, there is conflicting evidence about whether therapy is less effective if started in the chronic phase, but there are no indications that its effect is qualitatively different. However, it cannot be excluded that an approach that took into account time postonset would have obtained better results (but neither can the opposite hypothesis of a worse result be excluded).

Regarding severity of the disorder, Basso et al.'s (1979) study showed no significant interaction between improvement, severity of the disorder, and rehabilitation. Unexpectedly, Robey's (1998) meta-analysis showed that acute severe aphasic patients, when treated, recover more than acute moderate treated aphasic patients. This result, however, must be considered with caution due to the fact that only three studies entered the meta-analysis on this topic. Again, the only evidence is quantitative, not qualitative.

Cognitive Factors

I am not aware of any study about the relationship between the presence of damage of other cognitive functions, such as memory, attention, or awareness, and the efficacy of aphasia therapy, although it seems highly plausible that without an appreciation of their deficit, patients are unlikely to cooperate with therapy. Furthermore, a limited capacity to deploy attention places restrictions on the duration of therapy sessions, and memory problems can affect learning. Emotional and psychosocial factors can also impact recovery and rehabilitation (e.g., Hemsley & Code, 1996).

To conclude, there is no evidence that any of the personal and injury-related factors can change the effect of therapy, except in reducing the amount of recovery. In all probability cognitive factors do affect therapy, but they are not easily amenable to experimental investigation.

LEARNING

Learning refers to any process that results in the modification of behavior by experience. Studies about learning in normal subjects flourished in the 1940s and 1950s, growing mainly out of the behaviorist tradition in psychology. In the following years, studies on learning were more or less abandoned and investigators became more interested in the other side of the coin: memory. Studies of memory did not develop from the behaviorist approach and have been more in line with cognitive psychology.

At the level of the brain, the most widely adopted model to explain how learning takes place is Hebb's (1949) model. According to Hebb, networks of cells (what he called *cell assemblies*) constitute functional units that under-lie cognitive functions. Hebb argued that coactivated neurons strengthen their synaptic connections. When neurons have been disconnected by a lesion, they may reconnect if they are simultaneously activated, which may happen if both neurons are connected to a functional circuit that is itself frequently activated (Robertson & Murre, 1999). Learning by repeated simultaneous neuronal activation is the result of synaptic strengthening.

Until we know more about how recovery in brain-damaged patients occurs, a rational suggestion seems to be to use data about learning in normal subjects: both adults increasing their knowledge and children acquiring a new capacity. Knowing, for example, how children learn to read can provide suggestions for the rehabilitation of the orthographic input lexicon and the grapheme-to-phoneme conversion mechanisms in aphasic patients. Knowing how adults acquire new words for input and output can help in planning interventions for rehabilitation of the input and output phonological lexicons.

To illustrate, it is now generally agreed that a prerequisite to the acqui-sition of normal reading is phonological awareness, that is, awareness of spoken words as segmentable phonological strings. Children with develop-mental reading disorders have been shown to have poor phonological awareness (e.g., Masterson et al., 1995), but it is unknown whether phono-logical awareness is needed to learn grapheme-to-phoneme conversion rules, lexical reading, or both. However, it seems rational to test phonolog-ical awareness in patients with acquired reading disorders and, if they fail, to treat it before treating the reading disorders.

Basso et al. (1999) recently investigated how normal adults acquire irregular orthographic representations for output, with the aim of checking whether a normal acquisition strategy could be used in the rehabilitation of patients with an acquired disorder of the orthographic output lexicon. Twenty normal controls with no previous knowledge of French were asked to learn the auditory phonological representations of 12 French words, which were irregular according to Italian phoneme-to-grapheme rules. They were then asked to write the words (baseline) and were next presented with the written words, one by one, and shown the corresponding picture until they correctly pointed to the 12 pictures, demonstrating acquisition of the orthographic form of the words for reading. After a filled delay of 10 minutes, the 20 subjects were asked to write the words when shown the pictures, and after a 1-week interval, they were again shown the 12 pictures and asked to write the corresponding words. The number of correct responses at testing varied from 6 to 12 and was significantly different from baseline (p < .00005; mean: 9.7, SD: 1.9). At follow-up 1 week later, the number of correct responses had decreased but was still significantly different from baseline (p <.00005; mean: 7.8, SD: 3.0). Figure 8–1 reports the frequency distribution of the errors made by the 20 subjects at testing and follow-up. These results were interpreted as indicating that knowledge of orthographic representations for reading can support correct spelling, and it was suggested that a patient with damage to the orthographic output lexicon can make use of the same strategy; if the patient learns to pay attention to the orthographic form of the word in reading this can support his or her writing of the same words.

This suggestion appears to have been used in the rehabilitation of a few patients with acquired writing disorders, although not explicitly stated. CCM (Behrmann & Herdan, 1987) was a surface dysgraphic patient with better-preserved reading. Initially, therapy focused on writing; CCM was asked to copy single words and then to spell them aloud. The writing phase was followed by a series of multiple-choice tasks and CCM was asked to select the correct written word from among several alternatives, a task that can be accomplished if the correct representations are held in the orthographic input lexicon and attention is directed to the input representation.

An important issue that has not been expressly studied in aphasic patients is explicitness in the learning process, namely, whether there is a difference between explicit and implicit learning and, if this is the case, which form is more effective. There is no single answer to this question, as shown by some data on recovery from aphasia. In sentence processing rehabilitation, for example, explicit learning has frequently been used

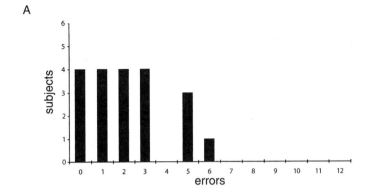

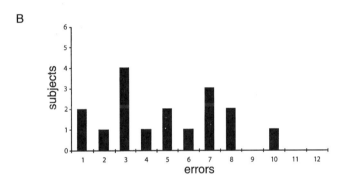

Figure 8–1. Frequency distribution of the errors made by 20 experimental subjects in the acquisition of 12 "irregular" output orthographic representations at testing (A) and follow-up (B) (from Basso et al., 1999).

with positive results. In the studies of Thompson et al. (1993, 1996), for example, patients were explicitly taught to identify the verbs and the roles of the noun phrases, to identify the constituent corresponding to a given question, and to replace it with "What" or "Who" cards, according to the case. However, positive results were also obtained when teaching of the rules was not explicit and the patient was not supposed to gain conscious knowledge of the underlying rules (e.g., Haendiges et al., 1996).

Neither techniques of learning have been frequently explored in aphasia rehabilitation studies. Recently, Wilson and colleagues (1994) applied the technique of errorless learning to a group of severely amnesic patients in a variety of tasks, including such different tasks as learning a list of words, object names, general knowledge, and orientation items. In all cases, errorless learning was superior to trial-and-error learning. It is supposed that errorless learning gives better results because it avoids strengthening the tie between a stimulus and an incorrect response, which is what is supposed to happen in trial-and-error learning.

To sum up, mechanisms of learning have not been extensively studied in brain-damaged patients, but patients have been shown to be able to learn and to utilize the same strategies as normals, even if less efficiently (Tikofsky & Reynolds, 1962, 1963: Edwards, 1965; Brookshire, 1971). Therefore, the same strategies effectively used by normal adults and children are recommended in the rehabilitation of patients with aphasia. Other questions, such as explicit versus implicit learning and the possible advantages of errorless learning, await investigation.

IMPLEMENTATION

The next two chapters illustrate some tasks for the rehabilitation of selective aphasic impairments. Here only some general statements will be reported about what, who, and how long to rehabilitate.

What?

One of the criticisms leveled against traditional therapy is that patients with different disorders have frequently been treated with the same intervention strategies and different intervention strategies have been used to treat the same disorder, making it difficult to relate a specific intervention to a given deficit.

Decades of investigation on aphasia have proven that, without doubt, *aphasia* is a collective name that subsumes many different forms of damage. If we are ready to admit that aphasic patients can present different functional disorders, it logically follows that no single treatment will work for all patients. We saw in Chapter 3 that many approaches to aphasia therapy in the past took into consideration the severity of the disorder but not the qualitative differences among patients. The stimulation approach advocated by Schuell and Wepman, for instance, insisted on auditory stimulation for all patients. The behavior modification approach placed at the core of the intervention the methodology adopted, generally ignoring the content of the therapy.

Global approaches, are still advocated by some. Two such global approaches are the "Holistic Rehabilitation" proposed by Pachalska (1993) and the sociolinguistic perspective described by Armstrong (1993). Nobody would argue that these types of intervention cannot be effective. In fact, each of them may be the most effective for a number of patients. The sociolinguistic approach, for example, has much to recommend it and offers many interesting ideas and suggestions. However, it is presented as a general approach to be used with any aphasic patient but for the majority of patients, other intervention strategies would probably be more adequate, depending on their disorders.

Intervention should be targeted to the underlying damaged processes rather than simply treating the presenting symptoms or looking for a strategy that bypasses the deficit. This seems a logical starting point, and we are now in a position to reach a detailed functional diagnosis for many patients. The advantages of such a diagnosis would be lost should the diagnosis itself not be taken as the starting point of a motivated therapy.

If we choose not to target the identified functional damage directly, the choice of intervention is difficult because no constraints are placed upon it and any type of intervention can be chosen. The reasons for choosing a treatment can be very disparate: because it has been efficacious with another similar patient (but *similar* does not mean that the functional damage was the same) or because it apparently motivates the patient. If we do not constrain at least the choice of our starting point, we will never be able to establish a sound basis upon which to proceed. Many different therapies can be effective for a specific deficit, but until we can establish a clear relationship between the deficit and the intervention, we will not be in a position to suggest the same treatment for a patient presenting with the same deficit. Rarely, however, has it been explicitly stated that therapy must be directed toward the functional damage (e.g., Howard & Patterson, 1989).

It goes without saying that this proposal holds only as long as there is no proof that a direct intervention for a given functional deficit is ineffective, as suggested by Behrmann and McLeod (1995) for letter-by-letter reading (see Chapter 7). If this were the case, indirect interventions would have to be implemented and assessed.

In Chapter 10, however, it will be argued that there are patients, generally severely damaged, for whom spotting the functional damage is either impossible or useless. The therapeutic intervention for such patients is quite different and does not target the functional damage but rather their handicap in daily living.

Who?

The answer is easy: all patients. The fact that it has been so difficult to demonstrate that aphasia therapy is effective is a clear demonstration that it has not been effective for all patients, but we are not in a position to know why it has not been effective. One can offer various reasons, not mutually exclusive, that can all have contributed to the failure of therapy for some patients. The damage was not reversible, the implemented therapy was inadequate or insufficient, the patient presented with associated disorders that rendered recovery impossible, and so forth. The conclusion at this point can only be that we do not know whether therapy will be effective with a given patient since no indisputably negative prognostic factors have been demonstrated. The only reason for denying a patient rehabilitation is that the patient has already been rehabilitated without success or has reached a plateau. Even then, however, it is possible to propose a different intervention that can be efficacious. Many chronic patients who have received what is generally indicated as traditional therapy have been rehabilitated with new and more experimental intervention strategies and have shown significant improvement (e.g., De Partz, 1986; Jones, 1986; Behrmann & Herdan, 1987; Byng, 1988).

How Long?

When reporting results of investigations about the effectiveness of aphasia therapy in Chapter 4, I noted that the effect of therapy was demonstrated when therapy was long-lasting and/or intensive (Hagen, 1973; Basso et al., 1975, 1979; Gloning et al., 1976; Poeck et al., 1989; Mazzoni et al., 1995; Denes et al., 1996b) and that no significant effect was found when rehabilitation was carried out for short periods of time (Vignolo, 1964; Sarno et al., 1970; Levita, 1978; Pickersgill & Lincoln, 1983; Lincoln et al., 1984; Prins et al., 1989). Meta-analyses (Robey, 1998) confirmed that amount of treatment was an important factor in determining the success of the therapy. It seems safe to assume that to be effective, aphasia therapy must be provided for a long time. However, there are descriptions of patients who have benefited from very brief periods of therapy (e.g., Byng, 1988; Marshall et al., 1990; Penn, 1993). The patients described in these investigations were for the most part chronic aphasic patients who had already received traditional therapy and reached a plateau. They can therefore be considered as their own controls when a new type of intervention, generally considered by the authors to be more rationally derived from their impairments, is started. BRB (Byng, 1988), for instance, underwent 6 years of traditional rehabilitation, after which he received a specific program for mapping thematic roles into grammatical relations. Therapy consisted of only two sessions 1 week apart and intervening homework. After this short

period, BRB showed marked improvement in comprehension of the rehabilitated locative sentences and of simple reversible sentences, as well as in
sentence production, which had not been rehabilitated.

The main difference between the type of therapy implemented in the
group studies and that implemented in the single-case studies is that in the
single-case studies therapy was specifically tailored to the patient's functional damage. Hence a possible conclusion appears to be that a nonspecific treatment can be successful if it is provided for a long time, whereas
more specific therapy can be successful even if carried out for a very short
time. This, however, is not the rule. Successful treatment is mostly very long
even when specifically devised for the patient's damage (e.g., De Partz,
1986; Jones, 1986).

In a recent study, Basso and Caporali (2001) compared two therapy
regimens in three pairs of patients matched for age, sex, educational level,
etiology, lesion site, and type and severity of aphasia. The three control
patients underwent rehabilitation 5 days a week for many months (14, 23,
and 20 months, respectively) and the experimental patients practiced 2–3
hours daily with the help of a friend, a family member, or a volunteer,
besides being treated by a speech therapist. Five of the six patients were
treated by the same speech therapist, and the treatment approach did not
differ for the two members of a pair. The study showed that the more
intensive treatment achieved better test results in the three experimental
patients and, more importantly, much better use of the recovered language
in daily life.

Other aspects of implementation, such as whether distributed or
massive exercise is more effective, have not been investigated.

CONCLUSIONS

The statements made in this chapter can be briefly summarized as follows.
It has been argued that, based on cognitive neuropsychological models, we
are now in a position to reach a diagnosis of patients' functional disorders
that in many cases is sufficiently detailed to constrain therapeutic choices
if—as should be the case—therapy directly tackles the underlying functional damage. A further assumption is that all functional disorders and all
patients are amenable to (partial) recovery if treatment is sufficiently long
and intensive. Moreover, until precise data on learning strategies in brain-
damaged patients are available, the learning strategies that have been
demonstrated to work in normal subjects should be used in aphasia

therapy. Finally, since for the time being there is some evidence for the importance of other factors—etiology, age, sex—on recovery but not on therapy, these factors can be ignored, as well as the neurological bases of recovery, and await better knowledge.

This is not a theory of aphasia therapy but only a suggestion for a systematic collection of data in an attempt to extract the crucial variables that affect performance. A theory must be able to explain the known data at the behavioral and neurological levels and to predict new data. A theory of aphasia therapy will not be able to explain why a treatment is efficacious as long as the neural mechanisms of recovery are not better understood. Any treatment, however, efficacious or not, creates new associations in the brain. So the problem is not really to understand how new associations are created but how to create the desired ones. Even if we are not now in a position to understand recovery at the neural level, we can try to understand why different treatments have different results at the behavioral level. In other words, we can try to link logically a treatment with a functional damage. What can and must be done is to collect data based on a motivated hypothesis in order to design a general framework within which all the available data can be analyzed.

At present, a fully articulated theory is not possible. Unless we find a common starting point and some common guidelines, knowledge about aphasia therapy will remain scattered, disconnected, and dispersed. A great concerted effort is essential for the advancement of aphasia therapy.

In this chapter, an important aspect of a theory of aphasia therapy has been overlooked: *what* to do. What to do, however, must be specified for each functional damage, and the next two chapters try to give some answers to this question. Only suggestions, not detailed and specified recipes, are given. They are certainly not the only hopefully effective methods, but they do try to explicit the relationship between the damage and the suggested intervention.

REHABILITATION OF LEXICAL AND SENTENCE DISORDERS

THE QUESTION OF *what* to do has not been dealt with in Chapter 8; it will be taken up in this and the next chapter. An effort will be made to clarify how the suggested treatments are logically compatible with the underlying theory and constrained by it. However, no claim is made that these are the only rational suggestions to be derived from cognitive neuropsychological models, but merely that they take into consideration the model and are constrained by its structure and processes.

Chapter 9 deals with rehabilitation of damage to specific components of the lexicon and briefly reports on a technique—mapping therapy—for sentence-level disorders. The following are not highly structured methods for the reacquisition of a predetermined and limited set of stimuli; they are suggestions offered as guidelines for the implementation of clinical rehabilitation that is supposed to last for many months, and they are targeted to achieve a clinically evident improvement of the patients' language communicative capacities. In outlining them, only the component under discussion will be assumed to be damaged, although this is a very rare occurrence. Many components and/or processes are generally impaired in the same patient within and beyond the lexical system. Some suggestions on how to establish a hierarchy of intervention in case of multiple disorders are also briefly sketched. A further assumption that will be made, as in Chapter 8, is that it is always possible to treat the damaged component/process directly. As an introduction to the suggested rehabilitation of functional disorders not discussed in Chapter 7, such as disorders of the semantic component, a short review of the literature will be presented.

In discussing rehabilitation, the flow of information from the input to the output components will be followed. Some comments on rehabilitation of the sentence-level disorders will close the chapter.

AUDITORY ANALYSIS SYSTEM

In general, the same task used to evaluate the integrity of a component can be used for its treatment. If the patient has a specific deficit in the identification of input phonemes, two phonemes (or, better, two consonant-vowel syllables with the vowel held constant) should be presented orally to the patient, who is required to say whether they are the same or not. In the different pairs, the difference between the two initial phonemes can be initially obvious (/p/ and /r/, for instance) and slowly reduced to a single feature, as in /p/ and /b/, which differ only in sonority.

No direct relationship, however, has been found between phoneme identification impairment and auditory comprehension in general (Basso et al., 1977; Blumstein et al., 1977a, 1977b). A mild impairment at this level of processing can probably be overlooked unless there are special reasons for retraining it, as in the case of word-form deafness and when rehabilitating phoneme-to-grapheme and input-to-output phoneme conversion mechanisms (see below).

ABSTRACT LETTER IDENTIFICATION SYSTEM

The use of computers seems appropriate in cases of damage to the abstract letter identification system. The patient is shown pairs of letters in different fonts and has to say whether they represent the same letter or not. Single letters can then be presented for identification. When the patient is able to identify single letters, he or she is shown two-letter words or nonwords and asked to read them. The duration of exposure can be manipulated as well as the size, character, and font of stimuli. The program progresses from short stimuli exposed for a longer duration to longer stimuli exposed for a shorter duration.

Use of a computer allows the patient to work independently at home. A sufficiently broad and flexible program can be prepared and adapted to each patient's need.

INPUT LEXICONS

There is an amazing paucity of research papers on rehabilitation of word comprehension disorders despite the accuracy with which these have been identified within a psycholinguistic model (e.g., Franklin, 1989). Comprehension disorders have been shown to be the first to recover spontaneously in the largest number of patients (e.g., Basso et al., 1982b) and probably do not need to be rehabilitated in as many patients as production disorders, but the dearth of therapeutic suggestions for damage to the input lexicons is nonetheless surprising.

The classic exercise for word comprehension disorders has always been word–picture matching, which, however, did not distinguish between input lexicon and semantic system disorders. To be correctly performed, word–picture matching requires the substantial integrity of the semantic system and the auditory analysis system (or the abstract letter identification system in case of written words) in addition to integrity of the input lexicon. Moreover, even when the input lexicon is damaged, the patient might be able to select the correct picture, knowing that he or she is being asked to point to a picture on hearing (or seeing) a word, and in many cases the correct picture can be chosen by a process of elimination. When foils are phonologically related in an auditory word–picture matching task, what is trained is the patient's ability to identify single phonemes (as in deciding between *cat* and *mat*) rather than the input lexicon. When foils are semantically related, the exercise taps the semantic system.

In conclusion, word–picture matching is not the most suitable exercise for targeting the input lexicons, and being a very easy task, it would be recommendable only for severely aphasic patients. In the next chapter, however, I will argue that a different approach is more suitable for these patients.

The task of choice for the evaluation of the input lexicons is the lexical decision task, with written stimuli for the orthographic lexicon and spoken stimuli for the phonological lexicon. If the input to the lexicons is not altered by damage to the abstract letter recognition system or the auditory input analysis, known words should be correctly recognized as such, although they acquire meaning only by being processed in the semantic system. The same task can also be used therapeutically, and a patient with damage to the orthographic input lexicon may be asked to recognize which of a series of written stimuli are correctly written and which are not. The same holds for the phonological input lexicon: the patient has to decide whether a heard word is part of his or her lexicon or is new to it.

However, in normal language processing, recognition of a known word also entails comprehension of its meaning, and it seems rational to stimulate the input lexicon not only from the auditory (or visual) analysis system. Concepts can be activated in the semantic system and be made to recirculate in the lexical system and activate the corresponding form in the input lexicons.

An exercise that the patient can do alone is to look up words in a small dictionary containing only frequently used words. The patient has to skip words that are immediately recognized, and those that were not known before the aphasia, and concentrate on those he or she is unsure of. The patient is asked to look at the orthographic form of the unfamiliar word carefully and to read the definition, linking the orthographic form to its meaning in the semantic system. If the patient is asked to read the word aloud, the exercise can also serve to ameliorate the phonological input lexicon since in reading aloud he or she produces the phonological form of the word that serves as an auditory input stimulus. This exercise seems particularly well suited to patients who can recognize a word as such but cannot understand its meaning because of impaired access to the semantic system.

SEMANTIC SYSTEM

Because of its centrality, damage to the semantic component will prevent the correct performance of any task requiring comprehension or production of words. Unfortunately, theories about the structure of the semantic system are far less elaborated than theories about other components of the lexicon. They can only serve as general guidelines in constraining speech therapy. A single semantic system will be assumed here, mainly because it is difficult to see how therapy should be affected by the existence of modality-specific semantic systems. Naturally, all kinds of knowledge (e.g., visual and verbal) must be assessed, and treatment should focus on the impaired knowledge.

In our review of studies on cognitive rehabilitation in Chapter 7, cases of damage to and therapy of the semantic system were not reported because none was included in the papers considered. This attests to the paucity of published cases. Before presenting some personal thoughts, the most frequently cited cases of rehabilitation of semantic disorders and a recently described structured intervention—BOX—will be briefly reported on. It will be seen that semantic therapy can be effective, although not in all cases.

Therapies for the Semantic System

Behrmann and Lieberthal (1989) reported the results of treatment of a central semantic deficit aimed at the restoration of semantic representations. CH was a 57-year-old English-speaking man who suffered a left hemisphere stroke. The therapy study began 2 years postonset. CH had global aphasia with very reduced speech. His comprehension was severely impaired even at the single word level and he performed poorly on tests requiring semantic knowledge, although he could still make gross distinctions of meaning. In a word category sorting task including items from six categories, no difference in performance was found according to the modality of presentation—spoken or written—but a category effect was found, animals being the group most easily categorized. The aim of therapy was restoration of the semantic representations of words. Three categories were selected for treatment (transport, body part, and furniture), and half of the items in these categories were actually treated. The other half were kept for control of a generalization effect. CH was given 15 hours of therapy, 5 hours per category. He was first taught the general features of the category; each item was then introduced individually, and its specific characteristics were illustrated. After treatment, a significant improvement in the sorting task was noted for the treated words, as well as generalization to untreated words in two treated categories and to items of the untreated category food.

Marshall and coworkers (1990) studied the effects of matching a picture with one of four or five semantically related written words in a patient with damage in accessing the phonological lexicon from semantics (patient RS) and two patients with damage to the semantic system (patients IS and FW). The treatment was effective for RS and IS, with no generalization to untreated items, but it failed to help FW.

The investigators underline the fact that a similar therapy program benefited two patients with different disorders and suggest that the task used—semantic discrimination—may be efficacious for different impairments.

Nettleton and Lesser (1991) studied six aphasic patients with severe naming disorders arising at different levels of processing, their aim being to find out whether semantic therapy is appropriate for anomic disorders in general. Two patients had semantic damage, two had a disorder related to the phonological output lexicon, and two had a deficit of the phonological buffer. The phonological output lexicon patients were given phonological therapy, and the remaining four patients were given semantic therapy, which consisted in semantic judgments, category sorting, and word–picture matching with semantic associates. As predicted by the model of lexical processing, phonological therapy was effective for the two phonologically impaired patients and semantic therapy was effective for one of the two semantically impaired patients. Moreover, no significant improvement was found in the two patients with buffer impairment treated with semantic therapy. However, contrary to expectation, in one patient with a semantic disorder the semantic therapy was not effective.

Visch-Brink et al. (1997) described a therapy program (BOX) that, they argue, is directed at the remediation of semantic deficits for aphasic patients with varying degrees of semantic impairment. BOX comprises exercises directed at syntagmatic and paradigmatic relationships, part–whole relationships, semantically anomalous sentence judgment, and semantic definition. BOX differs from the previously described semantic therapies because it focuses on the interpretation of written words, sentences, and texts, without reference to pictures, and attends to the sentence and text levels (for a discussion of BOX, see Visch-Brink et al., 1997, and commentaries therein).

Further Suggestions

As noted earlier, one view of the organization of the semantic system argues that concepts are represented by a bundle of semantic features that univocally describe a given concept and contain all we know about that concept. In other words, if we know that a leopard is a wild carnivorous animal that lives in Africa, looks like a cheetah, and so forth, all this is represented in an amodal code in the semantic system and is part of our concept of *leopard*. Our knowledge of a hammer includes that it is a man-made artifact, used to hit nails, with a handle and heavy head, and that to use it one makes a particular gesture. Our concept of tagliatelle alla bolognese comprises their particular smell and taste. In other words, our knowledge of the visual aspects, function, sensory attributes, associated gestures, category, and so forth of any given concept forms part of our semantic system. This has a direct consequence for the rehabilitation of the semantic system. In fact, neither the stimulus nor the response needs to be verbal: we can use gestures, pictures, or any other form and the patient can respond with gestures, drawings, or anything else; as long as we work on concepts, we work at the level of the semantic system.

This is interesting because pictures are easier than words; in pictures some of the concept's semantic features are visually represented, but the relation between a word and the concept it refers to is arbitrary. The picture of a tiger represents a four-legged animal and it can easily be associated with the picture of a lion, another four-legged animal. The words *tiger* and *lion*, however, are conventionally associated with a tiger and a lion and could just as well mean *fork* and *book*. It is only because we know that they do not, and that they refer to animals, that we can say that they belong to the same semantic category. Severe semantic damage can therefore be tackled more easily by using pictures, but the choice is limited to concrete objects and actions that can be depicted.

That said, we are left with our ingenuity. If the patient's damage is specific to a given class of concepts, it goes without saying that we work on that semantic category. If the damage is general, we can choose any semantic category to start with, and the choice should be based on common sense: start with a category whose items are frequently used and named. We can work on many items simultaneously or on one item at a time. In either case, we should choose a small, well-identified semantic category (e.g., tools, fruits, clothing). The patient can be trained on a subset of its concepts (choosing the ones most frequently encountered), or we can select a single item and try to define and train that specific concept before turning to another one from the same category. Having a clearer idea of any concept helps to clarify meanings of the other items in the same category. If, for instance, one has a clear idea of what a nail is, one will not mistake a screw for a nail, and the concept *screw* will be easily construed from the concept *nail* by simply adding the thread and all that it involves.

Some suggested exercises at the level of a semantic category are category sorting within increasingly specific categories, the odd-one-out exercise, semantic associations, and relatedness judgments. In the odd-one-out exercise, for instance, we can show the patient pictures of an orange, a peach, a banana, potatoes, bread, a fork, and a car. Asked to remove the most incongruous item, the patient should choose the car because all the others have something to do with eating. On being asked which one to remove next, the patient should choose the fork because it is not edible; he or she should then choose the bread (it is neither fruit nor vegetable) and finally the potatoes, leaving just the fruit. In the relatedness judgment task, the patient is shown a picture and then asked to state which of a series of pictures (some related and some unrelated) are related to it. Shown the picture of a spoon, for example, the patient must say whether a fork, bread, table, glass, salad, book, and cat are related to the spoon or not. When these exercises are correctly executed with pictures, it is possible to introduce words and repeat the same exercises with words. It is important to note that up to now, the patient has not been asked to produce words. If damage is limited to the semantic system, he or she will have no difficulty in producing the correct word once the corresponding concept is clear.

An alternative approach is to teach the patient one concept at a time. In my experience, this approach is more effective. One reason for its higher rate of success may be that working on a single concept makes it easier to clarify what the patient knows about the concept and to work specifically on what he or she does not know. The easiest way to ascertain understanding of the concept is to ask the patient to draw the object (artistic competence is unnecessary; all we need is a recognizable object). If the drawing can be recognized and has all the visual defining characteristics, we can safely conclude that the concept is rich enough to sustain the corresponding word. If it is not, we can see what is lacking (or what is wrong) and work on that (a cup without a handle, a screw without thread, a robin with four legs).

To illustrate this type of treatment (and our failure when working on whole categories), the treatment of patient BA with a severe semantic disorder will be briefly reported.

BA (Basso, 1993) was 42 years old when he became a victim of a shooting accident. The bullet entered through his right cheek and exited in the left frontal-temporal region; it was extracted on the same day. A CT scan performed 7 months later showed three lesions in the left hemisphere: frontal-temporal, lenticular, and occipital-parasagittal. BA's speech was abundant, with rare content words and frequent perseverations. Oral and written confrontation naming were equally severely impaired (8 and 7 of 20 answers correct), most of his errors being semantic paraphasias and perseverations. Asked, for instance, to name the picture of a letter, he said "chiusura" (fastening), which was also produced for the six subsequent stimuli (Papagno & Basso, 1996). Perseverations were also present in drawing from memory, as illustrated in Figure 9–1. Oral and written word–picture matching were performed worse (4 and 5 of 20 correct) than naming, but the difference was not significant. Repetition, reading aloud, and writing to dictation were preserved except for some misspellings in

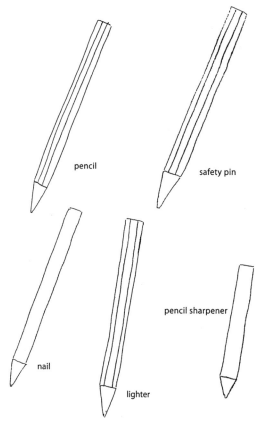

Figure 9–1. Examples of BA's perseveration in a drawing-from-memory task (May 1991) (from Papagno & Basso, 1996).

writing. No perseverations were present in these tasks. The patient scored 10 of 36 on the token test (De Renzi & Faglioni, 1978). He was not apraxic and scored 24 of 36 on Raven's Colored Progressive Matrices (Raven, 1965).

Semantic processing ability was examined further. He was given 10 items in six different categories to name and to point to; naming was preserved for body parts and equally impaired for the other categories. Pointing was worse than naming. In an object and animal decision task he correctly sorted 36 of 40 animals and 26 of 40 objects, rejecting 11 real objects. When asked to draw from memory he generally refused, saying he did not know what the object was. When he agreed to draw, the object was unrecognizable (note that BA was a former draftsman with good drawing ability, which was still evident in copying) or he perseverated on a previously drawn object. To sum up, his most invalidating impairment was at the level of semantic processing, and semantic therapy was started.

The therapy was performed in his home town and consisted in categorization tasks, the odd-one-out tasks, and picture verification tasks. In categorization tasks, two semantic categories—clothing and food—were chosen and the picture of an item from each category was put in front of BA, one on his left and one on his right side. He was then presented with a picture of an item from one of the two categories and asked whether it should go with the item on his right or left side. BA was totally inconsistent in his categorization, and nothing that the therapist could do or say helped him. In the odd-one-out task he was given five pictures, four pertaining to the same category and one pertaining to a distant category (four animals and a piece of furniture, for instance), and he was asked to point to the odd one out. BA remained unable to perform any of these exercises correctly, on which he showed no improvement. Five months later, a control language examination disclosed no change in BA's performance and therapy was discontinued. He was, however, young and motivated, and a few months later therapy was reattempted. The only changes in his performance were a slight reduction in perseveration and a slight recovery of comprehension: he could now point to 42 of 72 pictures. Naming was unchanged.

Semantic processing remained the target of therapy, but this time it was decided that work would be done on one concept at a time rather than on a semantic category. The category of tools was chosen because it is rather limited and tools can easily be handled and drawn. The first tool chosen was a hammer. It was shown to BA, and he was asked to copy it; each part was then discussed and its use explained to the patient, who was then asked to use it and then to pretend to use it with the hammer in full view. Finally, he was asked to pretend to use it without seeing it and then to draw a hammer from memory. BA was generally unable to draw anything resembling a hammer. The hammer was shown again and its use was explained again, and his errors in drawing were discussed. Figure 9–4 illustrates three of BA's attempts to draw a hammer in three different therapy sessions. It took approximately a month of daily rehabilitation before BA could draw a recognizable hammer from memory and pretend to use it. A new tool was then introduced, and the same procedure was followed. During daily therapy sessions from May 1990 to April 1991, three categories were worked on: tools, kitchen utensils, and clothing. After that, recovery proceeded more quickly. A follow-up examination in March 1992 disclosed a mild Wernicke aphasia with rare semantic paraphasias and some word-finding difficulties. BA was now able to describe a picture and sustain

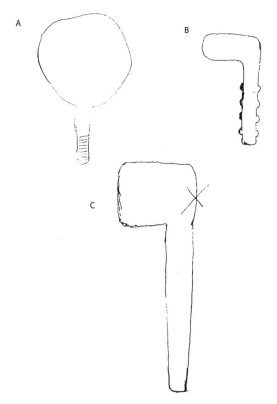

Figure 9–2. Three successive examples of BA's attempts at drawing a hammer from memory at weekly intervals in March 1990.

a conversation; oral and written naming were 85% correct, and he scored 24/36 on the token test.

OUTPUT LEXICONS

Access and Storage Disorders

The question of access and storage disorders was first explored relative to the meaning of words; no mention was made about the usefulness of the same criteria for differentiating access and storage disorders of the form of words. However, although the distinction is not uncontroversial, in aphasia therapy the five criteria described in Chapter 5 have generally been accepted and used to distinguish between disorders of retrieval from the phonological output lexicon and storage disorders of the phonological representations in the output lexicon. It is therefore important to explore the therapeutic implications of such a distinction, namely, how therapy for naming disorders should differ in the case of a deficit of access to preserved phonological representations and a deficit to the stored representations themselves.

One practical problem is immediately evident. How can we translate into practice the five criteria for distinguishing storage and access impairments? Let us consider the consistency criterion since it appears to be the one most frequently accepted and since, in a way, both the rate of presentation and the effect of priming fall under the consistency umbrella. In fact, if a correct response can be given at slower but not at more rapid rates of presentation and if it can be given after a prime but not without it, responses are inconsistent. But when is a response consistent? Does it suffice to have a significant degree of consistency or must consistency be absolute? Moreover, patients who cannot reliably name some pictures and give inconsistent responses to other pictures are frequently seen in clinical practice. Such behavior can be explained by supposing that these patients have both an access and a storage disorder; but which one should be considered first in therapy or should they be treated together?

There is a definite trend in the literature to attribute word-finding difficulties to retrieval disorders rather than to loss of stored representations. Nickels reports that the widely different word-finding difficulties present in the patients she described have been interpreted as problems in accessing phonology from semantics. "In this chapter we have described a number of patterns of speech output, all of which have been attributed to a deficit "between semantics and phonology." There have been reports of patients with deficits attributed to this level who produce semantic errors (Caramazza & Hillis, 1990), phonologically related real-word errors (Best, 1996; Blanken, 1990; Martin et al., 1994), phonologically related nonword errors (Kay & Ellis, 1987), and neologisms (Butterworth, 1979, 1985; Miller & Ellis, 1987). They can show effects of word length in either direction—forward (Friedman & Kohn, 1990), reverse (Best, 1995), or not at all (Kay & Ellis, 1987). They may or may not show effects of frequency (Caramazza & Hillis, 1990; Kay & Ellis, 1987) and imageability (Franklyn, Howard & Patterson, 1995), or may show category-specific effects (e.g., Farah & Wallace, 1992; McKenna & Warrington, 1980; Miceli et al., 1988b)" (Nickels, 1997, p. 161). Nickels is not the only one to consider that anomia is due to damage in retrieving the phonological form of the word. This assumption is implicit in all stimulation therapies based on the principle that language is not lost but inaccessible, as shown by the automatic–voluntary dissociation. Recently, this has been explicitly stated by Le Dorze and Nespoulous. They state, "In conclusion then, anomia in moderate aphasics seems to originate in an intermittent linking address failure needed in the access to formal lexical representations" (Le Dorze & Nespoulous, 1989, p. 398), and Butterworth concludes his review of phonological disorders by saying that "there is little evidence that the storage of phonological information in the lexicon is disturbed in any of the patients in the literature to date" (Butterworth, 1992, p. 283).

One could argue that the question of differentiating between storage and retrieval disorders is not important for therapy because it is far from clear how they would differently constrain the therapeutic choices. If a patient shows a high degree of variability in responses, the therapist will not stubbornly keep asking him or her to name the same few items. On the other hand, if the patient appears to be fairly consistent, he or she will be asked to name the picture that were incorrectly identified and not those correctly named most of the time. How the patient will be asked to name them is another question that does not depend on whether they are lost or inaccessible.

It has been argued that an answer to the question of whether the patient has a retrieval or a storage deficit may come a posteriori from the results of the therapy. If one accepts consistency as a criterion for differentiating access and storage disorders, a logical deduction would be that recovery of treated words only points to a storage disorder, whereas generalization to untreated words is predictable from recovery from an access disorder (e.g., Miceli et al., 1996). This is, however, circular reasoning that runs as follows: access and storage deficits can be differentiated based on consistency of responses; if damage to, say, access to intact phonological representations is diagnosed in a patient and rehabilitation aimed at the access disorder is effective, generalization to untreated items is expected. If, however, the patient recovers treated items only, it is concluded that he or she had a storage and not an access disorder.

To conclude, it is theoretically difficult to distinguish between retrieval and storage disorders, as well as to devise motivated therapeutic interventions aimed at one or the other disorder. Furthermore, generalization results are difficult to interpret. Hence, a practical suggestion is to forget about access versus storage disorders.

Further Suggestions

In most cases, patients rehabilitated for anomia have been required to produce the target words but the strategies used have differed. The techniques most frequently used by therapists are phonemic or semantic cueing (more rarely an orthographic cue), repetition, reading, and word–picture matching (for a review, see Kremin, 1993; Nickels & Best, 1996). Among the facilitation techniques used, the phonemic cue (saying the first phoneme or syllable of the to-be-named word) has been generally found to be the most efficacious, but its facilitating effect is short-lived (Patterson et al., 1983).

In traditional therapy these strategies were used with all anomic patients, with no previous identification of the functional damage. In cognitive rehabilitation the same techniques were used, but intervention was generally preceded by a more accurate functional diagnosis. Investigators, however, did not keep to a specific treatment for a given damage. They used the same technique for patients with different disorders (e.g., Raymer et al., 1993) or different treatments for the same damage (e.g., Le Dorze & Pitts, 1995). Accumulation of knowledge about the structure and the processes of the lexicon should, however, change this state of affairs, and it is hoped that aphasia therapy will become more rationally related to the disorder and more detailed.

Following the assumption that unless recovery has been demonstrated impossible, therapy must be directed at the diagnosed underlying impairment, the aim of therapy in the case of damage to the output lexicons is to restore the phonological and/or orthographic representations (or access to them). In our aphasia unit, we do this by providing the patient with an orthographic cue and by requiring a first written response.

The patient is shown a picture and is asked to name it; if successful, he or she is simply asked to repeat the name once and write it down. If naming is unsuccessful, the patient is asked to write down the name since some patients succeed in writing the first letter(s) of a word they have been unable to name. Generally, however, patients cannot write any of the letters. The therapist then writes the first letter and asks the patient to complete the word without speaking. If successful, the patient is asked to read the word and then the whole procedure is repeated, that is, the patient is asked again to name the picture and then write it down (without being allowed to see the previously written word). When, as is often the case, the patient does not complete the word after the therapist has written the first letter, the therapist writes the second letter and once more asks the patient to complete it without saying the word. The same procedure is followed until the patient completes the written word or, in the case of total failure, copies the entire word written by the therapist. Immediately after writing the word, the patient is asked to say it and then write it without being allowed to copy it.

When the patient produces a correct written response, he or she can then read it through the (undamaged) grapheme-to-phoneme conversion mechanisms. If the word has a regular orthography, the output of the conversion mechanisms corresponds exactly to the phonological representation of the word in the phonological output lexicon, and its production can help strengthen its representation in the phonological lexicon. The great majority of words in languages such as Italian, which have a transparent orthography, can be read through the conversion mechanisms, but the phonology of many English words cannot be correctly produced based on their orthography. This technique will not work in English or French as well as it does in Italian and Spanish.

The orthographic cue has proven to be effective in facilitating naming by patients (Bachy-Langedoch & De Partz, 1989; Henaff Gonon et al., 1989; Best et al., 2000), but it is not the only effective one. Basso et al. (2001) decided to evaluate in normal controls the efficacy of frequently used methods in order to identify the most effective ones. They asked 30 normal controls to learn 30 new words. The "words" were disyllabic neologisms conforming to Italian phonological rules, randomly associated with concepts belonging to different semantic categories (animals, tools, body parts, clothing, fruits, and musical instruments). Sixty pictures were selected and associated with 60 new "words"; 30 were kept as controls and 30 made up the experimental stimuli. Three learning methods frequently used with aphasic patients were chosen: repetition, reading aloud, and orthographic cueing.

Subjects were randomly divided into three groups and assigned to a learning method. Their responses were recorded at baseline, after the learning phase, and at follow-up 1 week later. All subjects learned the 30 words in the learning phase, but the number of trials were significantly lower ($p = .0000$) for the group that learned through the orthographic cue (mean number of trials: 5.1) than for the other two groups, which did not differ from each other (mean number of trials: 7.7 for the repetition group and 7.3 for the reading group). Moreover, at follow-up, the orthographic group remembered a significantly larger number of "words" (16.4) than the other two groups (8.5 in the repetition group and 9.3 in the reading group; $p = .0000$), which did not differ from each other. Figure 9–3 illustrates the mean number of correctly named stimuli by the three groups at baseline and follow-up. No learning of the control pictures had taken place.

The same experimental design was employed with two anomic aphasic patients, RF and MR. Stimuli were 92 and 88 pictures, respectively, that

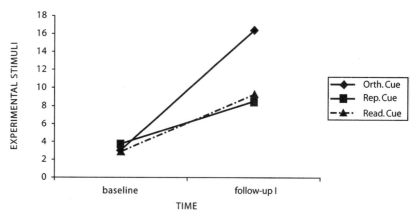

Figure 9–3. Mean number of correctly named stimuli by three control groups following three different learning strategies – repetition, reading aloud, and orthographic cue – at base-line and follow-up (from Basso et al., 2001).

the patients had reliably matched to the spoken word but had not named and for which they always produced an omission. The three therapeutic methods were implemented successively, in random order, for 5 consecutive days each. Neither of the two aphasic patients learned all the words during the therapy period, but all three methods significantly improved their naming. Moreover, both patients correctly named a significantly larger number of words learned through the orthographic cue, and at the last follow-up (12 and 5 weeks after the end of the treatment, respectively) naming accuracy was still significantly different from baseline only for words acquired through the orthographic cueing method. Figure 9–4 illustrates the number of correctly named items at baseline, at the end of treatment, and at follow-ups with each of the three learning methods for patients RF (A) and MR (B).

These results confirmed the effectiveness of the three techniques in normal subjects and in two aphasic patients. The most interesting result was the higher efficacy of the more effortful technique—orthographic cue—compared to the less effortful methods, reading and repetition. The authors argued that their results confirmed the generation effect (Slamecka & Graf, 1978), namely, the advantage in memory of self-produced as opposed to externally presented stimuli, in the group of normal controls and in the two aphasic patients.

Naming to confrontation, although efficacious, is suggested only for severely anomic patients at the beginning of their therapy. There is now sufficient evidence that word-retrieval impairments can be task specific

A

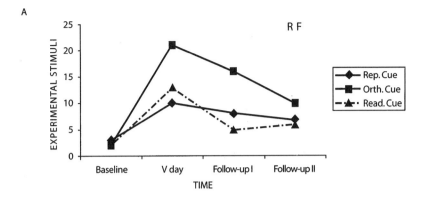

B

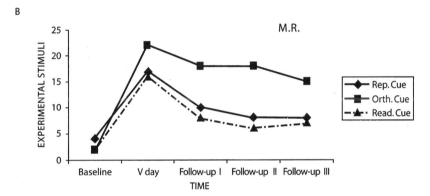

Figure 9–4. Number of correctly named stimuli by patient RF (A) and patient MR (B) following three different learning strategies – repetition, reading aloud, and orthographic cue – at baseline, end of treatment, and follow-ups (from Basso et al., 2001).

(Zingeser & Berndt, 1988; Breen & Warrington, 1994; Denes et al., 1996a; Manning & Warrington, 1996), suggesting that aphasics' naming ability can vary according to the task. Preserved confrontation naming does not guarantee that the patient will use the words he or she can name to confrontation in spontaneous speech (Marangolo et al., 1999) thus stripping the capacity to name of any real communicative value. People do not generally go around naming whatever they see; on the contrary, an item has a greater probability of being named if it is not in view of the speaker.

Further reasons for abandoning confrontation naming tasks as soon as possible are the limited number of picturable words, the advantage of a self-administered exercise, and the necessity of intensive and protracted therapy. What we suggest is that the patient work at home with a small dictionary, as for the input lexicons. The first few sessions, however, must be carried out with the help of the therapist in order to teach the patient how to perform the task. The patient chooses a letter and says all the words he or she can think of that begin with that letter; the patient then says the words again and writes them down (at this stage, misspellings are corrected by the therapist). When the patient cannot think of any more words, he or she rewrites them in alphabetical order and then looks up in the dictionary the first words starting with the letter chosen. As for rehabilitation of the input lexicons, the patient disregards the words that do not seem familiar and searches only for the familiar ones. The patient reads the dictionary definition of the chosen word and, if that word seems important, he or she writes it down with the other ones. In this way, the patient adds a limited number of words per day. On the following day, the first step is to try to remember all the words practiced the day before and write them down. The patient then checks whether any words have been forgotten. Any such words are added to the newly written list, and the patient goes over it again. When this is done, with the help of the dictionary the patient adds a few words. The same is done each day.

In our experience, therapy for anomia is a long-lasting enterprise that requires an enduring and convinced effort on the part of the patient. As an example of how we proceed with therapy for anomia, implementation of aphasia therapy for patient DE will be described. DE is a bilingual right-handed barman with 10 years of formal education, 5 in France and 5 in Italy. In February 1990, when he was 23 years old, he was admitted to a hospital for headache and vomiting. A CT scan showed a left temporal hematoma, and angiography disclosed an arteriovenous malformation (AVM). DE was hemiplegic and aphasic. A month later, after resorption of the hematoma, he was operated on for ablation of the AVM, which was, however, incompletely ablated and bled again in May, when he was reoperated on.

In January 1991, when he was first seen in our aphasia unit, his speech was fluent and abundant but totally devoid of content words, with some stereotypical expressions ("I know it," "slowly slowly," "I would like it") and some nonwords. He was unable to name a picture orally or by writing; reading and writing were totally impossible for both words and nonwords, and comprehension was possible only for a few frequent words and some very simple sentences. He scored 7/36 on the token test. His daily activities were described as follows: "We start, what's its name, that one also, he told me yes. He told yes, I would remember so or nothing. A simple thing but I can't. I don't remember." He had no apraxia and scored 31/36 on Raven's Coloured Progressive Matrices.

Therapy was initially aimed at recovery of auditory comprehension with word–picture matching tasks and at recovery of the transcoding routes. This part of the program was assigned to the patient's mother. She had the patient repeat, write, and read short, easy words and nonwords for 2 hours per day. After 6 months DE could read and write, though rather slowly and mainly through the nonlexical route. Lexical comprehension had also rapidly improved, and in July 1991 the patient's naming disorders were tackled. Initially, this was done by asking DE to name all the objects he could in a given category: fruits, vegetables, kitchen utensils, tools, and so forth. Categories were worked on one at a time, and only when DE demonstrated good recall of a fair number of the objects in the category did the therapist move to a new one. He was asked to work by himself, writing down all the items in a category he could remember and rehearsing them many times during the day. DE was highly motivated and worked very hard without ever slacking. After 4 months, it was decided that this exercise was no longer appropriate for DE. His word-finding difficulties were still very severe, although he could now retrieve some nouns. To work by himself, however, he needed a way of retrieving more words than was possible only by sitting and thinking about them. It was then decided that he would look for words in a dictionary. He was first asked to retrieve all possible words starting with the letter [P] and write them down. As soon as he could remember a new word, he had to put it in his notebook. He worked on this 2–3 hours per day. A month later he had managed to write approximately 150 words, which he could also more or less retrieve if given sufficient time and some cueing, such as the definition of the word or the corresponding picture. He continued with the help of the dictionary, and 4 months later he had written (and could remember when cued) 400 words. DE continued to work at home, 2–3 hours per day, for the following $2\frac{1}{2}$ years, and analyzed words beginning with all the letters in the alphabet. At the end of this period, DE's word-finding difficulties were very mild and his score on a fluency test with semantic (animals) and phonological (letters [P], [L], and [F]) cueing was in the normal range.

Comprehension had improved more rapidly, and in July 1992 his score on the token test was in the normal range, although he still had some difficulties understanding rare words. In a sense, DE's therapy was exceptional because it is rare to find such a highly motivated and cooperative patient. This was probably due to his young age and also to the fact that he was able to see some positive results quickly. Recovery from anomia was regular and, at least initially, evident only for the words beginning with the letter he was working on. DE took a long time to learn new words, but he then rarely forgot the words he had practiced.

DE had always been equally anomic for nouns and verbs, but anomia can be more marked for a specific grammatical class (nouns or verbs) or for a specific type of word (frequent or infrequent, concrete or abstract). The consequence for rehabilitation is that if a specific class of words is impaired, only that class of words will be taken into account in therapy.

Errors

In a confrontation naming task and in spontaneous speech production, the most frequent errors ensuing from damage to the output lexicon (or to a deficit in retrieving representations) are omissions (and/or circumlocutions) and phonological (or orthographic) errors. When there is total failure to retrieve the phonological (or orthographic) form of a word, we have an omission (or a circumlocution if the patient makes an effort to produce the meaning of the sought-for word). When there is partial failure, we have a phonemic (or orthographic) paraphasia. Phonemic (or orthographic) paraphasias do not unequivocally point to damage to the output lexicon. Damage to the buffers, for instance, can also cause phonological (or orthographic) distortions of words. An accurate evaluation of the patient's performance on other tasks (such as repetition of nonwords) can help discriminate between the two levels of damage. Note, however, that this is true for any type of error, and a functional diagnosis requires an in-depth examination.

A few patients have been described with semantic errors in naming tasks, intact semantic representations, and damage between the semantic lexicon and the output lexicon (e.g., Caramazza & Hillis, 1990). Such patients can be compared to normal subjects in a tip-of-the-tongue (TOT) state (Brown & McNeill, 1966; Brown, 1991). In a TOT state, a normal subject is temporarily unable to find the phonological (or orthographic) form of a word in spite of having a normal semantic system. Normal subjects in a TOT state may retain some knowledge of the looked-for word (first phoneme, number of syllables); they can produce an incorrect but phonologically or semantically related word or simply state that they do not remember the word. The incorrect response can be intentional or not. In the first case, the speaker intentionally provides his or her best approximation to the looked-for word; otherwise, the subject is not aware of giving an incorrect response but does recognize that the word is not the target word immediately after having produced it. The same should be true for patients with damage to an output lexicon when they produce a semantic para-phasia, with a very important difference. In normal subjects the TOT state is a temporary phenomenon; in aphasic patients it is, unfortunately, long-lasting. However, aphasic patients should acknowledge that it was not the looked-for word if asked how confident they are that the response is correct since, by definition, the semantic system is undamaged.

Patients who produce semantic errors without damage to the semantic system are rare; omissions are by far the most frequent responses. Why a few patients give an incorrect and semantically related response that they either immediately and spontaneously refuse or rate as wrong if asked is difficult to say. It could be related to the patient's urge to respond: some patients are inclined to respond in any case, while others are more cautious and tend to monitor their responses.

All the patients described in the literature with semantically related errors and damage to the output lexicon have a modality-specific disorder, and the semantic errors are present either in oral (e.g., RGB; Caramazza & Hillis, 1990) or written (e.g., RCM; Hillis et al., 1999) naming. Rehabilitation of such patients does not seem to pose particular problems. Patients must be made aware of their errors and become accus-tomed to block their responses. They must then be taught to look for the response in the undamaged modality and to reproduce it in the damaged modality.

OUTPUT BUFFERS

In describing the structure of the lexical-semantic system, I argued that the buffers are working memory components assigned to the temporary stor-age of lexical or nonlexical representations for successive elaboration. Damage to a buffer will disclose a length effect: shorter stimuli will have a greater chance of being correctly processed than longer ones. The nature of the stimulus—lexical or nonlexical—should have no consequences, both words and nonwords being equally impaired. These observations dictate the first rule of thumb for the rehabilitation of the buffers: words and nonwords can both be utilized, and the stimulus length should be increased in parallel with the patient's recovery.

Things, however, are never quite so simple. Buffers are structured and do not process words as simple left-to-right sequences of phonemes (or graphemes); they specify the serial identities of letters, the consonant–vowel and the syllabic structure (see Chapter 6).

It should therefore be possible to come across a patient with a selective disorder at any of these levels, in which case the intervention program should obviously take this fact into account. In clinical practice, however, it is not possible to study a patient in a sufficiently detailed way to localize such fine-grained functional damage. At the same time, one cannot be sure whether knowing that any of these layers are damaged would allow one to constrain rehabilitation further, except for the obvious consequence of paying more attention to the damaged level. Rehabilitation of all layers occurs in tasks that tap all levels simultaneously, as occurs when the patient is asked to write (or say) a word (or nonword).

As for the choice between words and nonwords, words can be easier, as argued, for instance, by Caramazza et al. (1986) for patient IGR. The length of the stimuli should be such that the patient makes many errors but can sometimes get the answer right; shorter stimuli would be too easy, but longer ones would probably discourage the patient.

To sum up, the exercise of choice for selective damage to an output buffer is dictation (for the orthographic buffer) or repetition (for the phonological buffer) of words and nonwords of such length as to have the patient make a consistent number of errors and some correct responses. This is a very repetitive exercise that does not require the presence of a therapist and can be done by anybody following proper instructions.

CONVERSION RULES

Three conversion rules have been frequently discussed in aphasia literature: (*1*) the input-to-output phoneme conversion; damage to this route prevents the patient from correctly repeating nonwords; (*2*) the grapheme-to-phoneme conversion routine, which allows the patient to read nonwords; and (*3*) the phoneme-to-grapheme conversion routine which allows the patient to write nonwords to dictation. The three conversion rules are functionally independent and can be impaired separately. I shall, however, present a program for the rehabilitation of all three routines at the same time because in clinical practice few patients experience selective disruption of just one of these mechanisms. Furthermore, it costs almost nothing in terms of time or effort to include exercises aimed at the recovery of an unimpaired process. The added advantage is that the exercise is more varied and stimulating.

We always work with nonwords to make sure that only the conversion mechanisms can be used, and the stimuli become longer and more difficult (from an orthographic and phonological point of view) as the impairment gets less severe. The exercise is very simple. If damage to any of the conversion procedures is so severe that the patient cannot repeat, write, or read a single phoneme or letter, the stimulus to be used is a CV syllable but only the initial consonant varies, whereas the vowel is kept constant. The vowel [a] can be used because it is a frequent letter/phoneme whose articulation and recognition are easy in any language. If the patient fails in reading, repeating, or writing the vowel, the therapist immediately provides the correct answer. When single letters and phonemes are mastered, we use CV syllables in which both the vowel and the consonant vary.

The patient is first asked to repeat the syllable; this ensures that he or she has correctly identified the heard phonemes and can translate them into output phonemes. If the patient fails, the stimulus is repeated until the right response is given. The patient is then asked to write the syllable and to check whether the written form corresponds to the spoken one. This step trains phoneme-to-grapheme conversion.

If the patient has made a mistake and does not recognize it, he or she is told so, invited to spot it and read the written syllable aloud (*ta* instead of *da*, for example), drilling grapheme-to-phoneme conversion. When the patient succeeds in reading what has erroneously been written, he or she is asked to repeat what should have been written. If the patient fails, the therapist says it once more and invites the patient to repeat, write it, and look for the difference with what was previously written incorrectly. When the syllable is written correctly and the patient has checked that it corresponds to what he or she had heard and repeated, a new stimulus is given and the whole procedure starts again. When four or five syllables are written, the patient is asked to read them in random order. Note that this is the first time the patient is really asked to read because reading immediately after writing the stimulus is in most cases a repetition.

When the patient is able to translate most of the syllables, two-syllable nonwords (CVCV) are used and tasks to enhance the patient's phonological awareness are presented. After correct repetition of the stimulus, the patient is asked to repeat the stimulus slowly and to concentrate on the order of the syllables. He or she is then asked to repeat the nonword, one syllable at a time, and then to repeat either the first or the second syllable in isolation. When the therapist is certain that the phonology of the to-be-written stimulus is clear to the patient, the therapist asks the patient to write it down. Oral reading is requested when four to five nonwords are written to make sure that the patient is really reading and not repeating.

With this exercise, we simultaneously train the auditory analysis system, all conversion procedures, and phonological awareness held to be important for reading acquisition (e.g., Masterson et al., 1995) and generally impaired in phonological dyslexic patients (see the special issue of *Cognitive Neuropsychology*, v. 13, n. 6, 1996). The program can be easily carried out at home by the patient with the help of anybody instructed by the therapist who has enough time and motivation to work regularly with the patient.

An advantage of a language like Italian is that its orthography is fairly transparent. Very few phonemes must be rendered by two letters, and very few letters correspond to more than one phoneme. Languages such as English or French have less transparent orthographies, and the rehabilitation of conversion rules (except input-to-output phoneme conversion) is more complex.

MULTIPLE DISORDERS

Up to now, we have only considered damage to a single component. In clinical practice, this is a very rare occurrence. Some examples of multiple disorders and some suggestions for their treatment follow.

Let us consider a patient with damage to the semantic system and any one (or more) of the lexicons. The semantic system is a central component necessary for the comprehension and production of words, whether in the orthographic or the phonological code, whereas the input and output lexicons are peripheral with respect to the semantic system and are specific for phonology and orthography. Logically, it follows that damage to the semantic system will prevent the normal functioning of the output lexicons (which receive abnormal inputs) and nullify the effect of the normal functioning of the input lexicons because their output cannot be processed normally. On the other hand, damage to any of the four lexical components will be restricted to a single modality (input or output) and a single code (phonology or orthography). This being the case, damage to these levels cannot be considered equivalent and rehabilitated in any order. It seems more sensible to treat the semantic system first since improvement of the semantic system has positive consequences for comprehension and production of auditory and written language. On the other hand, prior improvement of an input lexicon will not allow the patient to understand words because of damage to the semantic system. Similarly, prior improvement of an output lexicon will not allow the patient to produce correct words, even if the phonological (or orthographic) representations are restored. A damaged semantic system will send an altered signal to the output lexicon, and the patient will probably produce a semantic paraphasia instead of an anomia he or she could have produced because of co-occurring damage to the output lexicon.

For example, a patient with damage to the semantic system *and* the output phonological lexicon requested to name the picture of a glass could try to activate the incorrect phonological form for *bottle*. He or she would not be able to find it because of damage to the output lexicon and could give no response or produce a phonological paraphasia for the word *bottle*. Prior recovery of the phonological lexicon impairment would result in the patient's producing the correct phonological form for the incorrectly activated form: *bottle* for *glass*, for example. Prior recovery of the semantic system would also not allow the patient to produce the correct word orally but he or she could produce it in writing. Successive recovery of the phonological output lexicon would allow the patient to produce the correct word both orally and in writing. The same line of reasoning is valid for damage to the semantic system and an input lexicon.

In this example we have apparently applied a simple rule: first retrain the more central component. However, the following example will show that this rule cannot be generalized and that more peripheral components must sometimes be trained first. Imagine a patient with damage to an output lexicon and the corresponding buffer, such as the phonological output lexicon and buffer. Damage to the buffer will prevent the patient from correctly saying, reading, and repeating words and nonwords, depending on their length. Damage to the lexicon will disrupt or make inaccessible (some) phonological representations. Previous recovery of the lexicon would allow the patient to select the correct word but not to produce it because of the coexistent damage to the buffer. Previous recovery of the buffer, on the other hand, would allow the patient to correctly produce those words for which the phonological representation in the lexicon is available, and to repeat and read all regular words.

A further practical reason suggests previous recovery of the buffer. Rehabilitation of the lexicon is in fact made difficult by the coexisting deficit to the buffer, which prevents the patient from producing correct responses, depending on the severity of the buffer deficit. Rehabilitation of the buffer can be carried out independently of the integrity of the lexicon by using nonword stimuli.

When no suggestion can be derived from the structure of the lexicon, therapy should be planned to be of the greatest benefit to the patient.

SENTENCE LEVEL

Sentence-level problems are very frequent in aphasia and are the most salient diagnostic sign of agrammatism. Compared to the number of treatment options for naming disorders, sentence-level disorders have rarely been tackled, and before the cognitive neuropsychological approach flourished, treatment was confined to sentence production and consisted mainly in reestablishing a single sentence type through repeated practice at its actual production (Holland & Levy, 1971; Helm-Estabrooks et al., 1982; Kearns & Salmon, 1984). The HELPSS method (Helm-Estabrooks et al., 1982), illustrated in Chapter 3, is a perfect example of a form of treatment that presents the patient with repeated opportunities to produce grammatically correct sentences, focusing on the sentence structures that the patient cannot produce. Kearns and Salmon's (1984) intervention has a more limited scope but is in the same vein: repeated production of the correct sentence structure. The authors treated two agrammatic chronic patients, who were taught to produce the third-person singular auxiliary *is* in sentence contexts using action pictures (e.g., *boy is drinking*). At the end of treatment the patients were better at producing the auxiliary *is* in trained and untrained sentences, but there was no generalization to the use of *is* as copula (e.g., *man is tall*).

Recently, sentence-level treatments have benefited from contributions from psycholinguistic studies. In Chapter 7 treatments based on Garrett's model of sentence production (Mitchum et al., 1993; Mitchum & Berndt, 1994; Haendiges et al., 1996) and on Chomsky's government-and-binding theory (Thompson et al., 1993, 1996) were described. The mapping hypothesis and mapping therapy are illustrated here.

The Mapping Hypothesis

During the 1970s, it was discovered that many agrammatic patients also suffer from impaired comprehension and that their problems emerge mainly with sentences that cannot be understood merely by processing the meaning of the content words. The sentence "The boy is eating an apple" can be understood by simply combining the meanings of the words "boy," "apple," and "eating" because boys can eat apples but apples cannot eat boys. To understand a reversible sentence, such as "Mary is kicking John," one must also make use of syntax in order to know who is the doer (Mary) and who undergoes the action (John) since the meaning of the whole sentence cannot be construed from the lexical content alone. Agrammatic patients were shown to have difficulties interpreting sentences in which word order and grammatical morphemes must be processed, such as reversible and passive sentences. It was initially argued that they had a parsing deficit and were unable to identify the phrase boundaries and generate a syntactic representation of sentences (Caramazza & Zurif, 1976; Schwartz et al., 1980b; Berndt & Caramazza, 1981).

The *asyntactic* comprehension hypothesis was soon challenged by a series of influential papers. Linebarger et al. (1983) showed that four agrammatic patients were remarkably accurate in detecting grammatical violations in spoken sentences. In a grammaticality judgment task they were able to detect, among others, violations of strict subcategorization (*The policeman was talking a woman) and of phrase structure rules (*The gift my mother is very nice). This high level of performance in complex syntactic analysis of sentences contrasted with the patients' very poor performance on picture-pointing tasks of sentence comprehension. The investigators argued that the patients were still able to construct a syntactic representation of the sentence, as shown by their accuracy in detecting grammatical violations, but were unable to exploit it for comprehension, as shown by their inability to select the corresponding picture. This interpretation was termed the *mapping hypothesis.*

The mapping hypothesis distinguishes two variants that address different aspects of patients' performance, a lexical and a procedural version. Patients with a lexical impairment have lost specific verbs' thematic information; they may still retain the core meaning of the verbs but not their thematic structure.

It is argued that the verb's semantic information specifies more than the core meaning of the verb; it also dictates the number of arguments involved and their role in the event. Thus the core meaning of *kill* is to cause death; it is a two-argument verb, and the thematic roles involved are an agent (causing the killing) and a patient (undergoing the killing). If a patient still understands the core meaning of *kill* but has lost information about its thematic grid, he or she will have nothing to map onto syntax and will have problems understanding sentences such as "The thief killed the old lady" unless he or she makes use of knowledge of the world, where it is more probable for a thief to kill an old lady than vice versa. The lexical version of the mapping hypothesis argues that patients with a lexical impairment in verb processing and impoverished verb entries cannot assign the verb's thematic roles to syntax and have problems understanding simple, reversible subject-verb-object (SVO) structures, as did patients in Schwartz et al.'s (1980b) study.

Patients with a procedural mapping impairment, on the other hand, can still retain the verb's thematic structures and can understand canonical structures; they are unable to use the procedures to map them onto their grammatical roles in moved-argument structures. Schwartz et al. (1987) provided an account that focuses on the procedures necessary to achieve a correct interpretation of the correctly parsed input. They used a plausibility judgment. Two basic anomalies were examined in the study: structure-based and lexical. In the structure-based sentences the anomaly consisted in a thematic role reversal (e.g., "The puppy dropped the little boy" versus "The little boy dropped the puppy"); in the lexical condition the anomalies could not be rectified by a simple reversal of the two noun phrases (e.g., "The spoon ate the table"). In both conditions there were basic ("The puppy dropped the little boy"), padded ("The puppy ran around excitedly and accidentally dropped the little boy onto the wet grass, which upset Louise"), and moved-argument sentences ("It was the little boy that the puppy dropped"). The subjects were 6 agrammatic patients, 4 anomic and 2 conduction aphasic, and 10 right-hemisphere brain-damaged patients. They had to judge whether the spoken sentence did or did not convey a plausible meaning. Padded sentences were judged as well as basic ones by the six agrammatic patients and the two conduction aphasic patients, but their performance dropped when arguments were moved from their canonical positions.

Schwartz et al. (1987) argued that to judge the plausibility of padded sentences, one has to parse the sentences at least for their major grammatical functions. The agrammatic patients' selective vulnerability to moved-argument manipulations is attributed by the authors to the nontransparency in these sentences from syntactic functions to thematic roles, which complicates the mapping operation. When the translation is syntactically transparent, as in simple SVO sentences, patients may be able to succeed. However, when the thematic structure of the verb no longer projects directly from the verb, and transmission of thematic roles is indirect and is dictated by general procedures that indicate how the movement must be bridged, as in passive sentences, patients fail. Put briefly, Schwartz et al.'s claim is that aphasic patients' difficulty in interpreting sentences with moved arguments relates to mapping and not to parsing.

An important aspect of the mapping hypothesis for treatment is that the mapping deficit is assumed to be central to production and comprehension. Impaired knowledge of verbs' thematic structure, for example, would result in impaired comprehension and production of sentences. The central nature of the underlying deficit leaves the therapist free to choose to train either one or the other, with the expectation that in case of success, both comprehension and production will improve.

The mapping hypothesis has given rise to many therapy programs for comprehension and production. In the lexical variant, studies focused on stressing the centrality of the verb and its relationships with the nouns in the sentence; in the procedural variant, therapy attempted to link sentence structure to sentence meaning (for a review, see Marshall, 1995; Mitchum et al., 2000).

A very interesting therapeutic proposal comes from Schwartz et al. (1995). They agree that agrammatism is not a unitary disorder and that it does not make sense to treat all agrammatic patients alike. Yet, they argue that it is not necessary for therapy to take into consideration minor differences in the patients' performance. According to the authors, "practical and economic constraints in the treatment environment preclude such an endeavor, at least in the U.S." (p. 94), but this is not the only reason. They argue, in fact, that not all the differences that emerge from a theory-driven evaluation can influence therapy outcome and they advocate a "middle-course" treatment, which is equally distant from an undifferentiated treatment for all agrammatic patients and a completely individualized treatment.

A review of agrammatic production leads them to isolate several levels of possible deficit and to promote a three-module therapy program. The first module should target morphosyntactic production, the second verb retrieval and mapping rules, and the third assignment of thematic roles.

An attempt to specify better treatment of the second module—verb retrieval and mapping rules—is proposed here. Mapping disorders are frequent enough to justify elaboration of a therapeutic program and, at the same time, they are sufficiently restricted to justify the use of a single adaptable and flexible approach.

If the program encompasses all the main necessary steps going from the interpretation and comprehension of a verb's thematic structure to its mapping onto grammatical roles in sentences with moved arguments, the program could be used with patients believed to have a mapping problem, whether it be at the lexical or the procedural level. The program should be run from the beginning to the end with all patients supposed to benefit from it, even if a specific and more restricted damage was diagnosed. The cost for having patients do things at which they are not impaired would be very low since this part of the treatment can be abandoned quickly. The advantage is that if a mild impairment at any of these levels had gone unnoticed, running the appropriate level of the program would disclose it and reinforce the patient's capacity.

The most difficult thing is to envisage the rational steps of such a program and their succession. Only a very sketchy hypothesis is offered here.

If, as has been proposed, the mapping procedures are used in both production and comprehension, improvement in either comprehension or production would also be reflected in the other modality. Generalization from sentence comprehension to sentence production has in fact been reported (Jones, 1986; Marshall et al., 1993; Byng et al., 1994; Schwartz et al., 1994).

Except for verb retrieval, the whole program tackles comprehension and uses metalinguistic tasks such as identification of the verb in a sentence or explicit teaching of verbs' thematic structure. It remains unclear whether patients successfully rehabilitated with a mapping therapy have reacquired normal, automatic mapping processes or a conscious strategy.

The program consists of the following steps:

1. Comprehension of the core meaning of verbs: the patient is asked to point to the correct verb among loosely semantically related alternatives and then among closely semantically related alternatives.
2. Explanation of the difference between nouns and verbs and the fact that verbs always have a thematic grid (except for meteorological verbs), whereas concrete nouns do not.
3. Verb retrieval. Most agrammatic patients have a more or less evident reduction in verb retrieval. Verb retrieval can be drilled by the patient alone, with the help of a dictionary and with only occasional help from the therapist. It should be performed throughout the therapy program since it takes effort and time to overcome the anomia, even partially.
4. Parsing simple SVO sentences and comprehension of simple reversible sentences.
5. Answering questions about who is doing what to whom in SVO sentences.
6. For languages with a rich verb morphology, morphological training should also be introduced in the program.
7. Grammaticality judgments on sentences that violate the verb's argument structure ("John is eating at an apple"), as well as identification of the error and its correction.
8. Given a simple SVO sentence, the patient is required to ask *wh-*questions relative to a specified argument.
9. Identification of the verb's thematic roles in passive sentences to facilitate their comprehension.

CONCLUSIONS

In suggesting therapy for lexical disorders, an effort has been made to relate the task to the underlying deficit. This is not always easy or possible since reference models are not always sufficiently detailed. The level of detail of the therapeutic interventions is constrained by the level of detail of the reference model of the normal cognitive structure. The interventions targeted to lexical disorders and to sentence disorders have a different degree of specificity because models of lexical processing are more detailed than models of sentence production and comprehension. Both types of models, however, are cognitively inspired.

The next chapter reports on a therapeutic approach for severely impaired aphasic patients that moves away from the principles of cognitive neuropsychology and from the kinds of treatment described here.

10

SEVERE APHASIA AND PRAGMATICS

THUS FAR THE LEVEL OF PRAGMATICS has been neglected. The modern use of the term *pragmatics* can be traced back to Charles Morris (1938) and his syntax-semantics-pragmatics trichotomy. *Syntax* refers to the study of the relations among signs, *semantics* to the study of the relations between signs and the objects they refer to, and *pragmatics* to the study of the relations between signs and their users.

The interest in pragmatics is not new among clinicians, and a pragmatic approach to aphasia rehabilitation has been described in Chapter 3. Lately, an ever-increasing number of clinicians have shown an interest in the pragmatic aspects of communication in aphasic patients. Lesser and Milroy (1993), for example, dedicated much of their book *Linguistics and aphasia. Psycholinguistic and pragmatic aspects of intervention* to pragmatics, illustrating its theoretical aspects and its applications to aphasia. They underlined the necessity of an analytic framework to interpret aphasic spoken language and maintained that conversation analysis is the most systematic approach to this end. They illustrated five important advantages of a conversation analysis approach. The first is that in conversation analysis there is only a minimum prior imposition of analytic categories, and everything that takes place between conversationalists is relevant. Secondly, conversation analysis is a suitable tool for describing the conversational ability of aphasic patients, which is generally impaired. Thirdly, conversation analysis takes into consideration the role of the patient's interlocutor as well as the patient's verbal behavior. Fourthly, it analyzes the conversational contributions in their sequential context rather than each one separately. Finally, the success or failure of the interaction is taken into consideration, not the appropriateness of the patient's behavior.

Interest in pragmatics has produced many observational schedules (Penn, 1985; Prutting & Kirchner, 1987; Gerber & Gurland, 1989). Lesser and Milroy (1993) proposed a checklist for the analysis of a conversational sample that helps identify the problems the patient and his or her partner experience in a conversation. The five conversational procedures considered in the checklist are turn-taking, repair, embedding of sequences, routines, and discourse markers.

Examples of pragmatic interventions can be found in Green (1984), Holland (1991), Penn (1993), and Aten (1996), among others. Pragmatic approaches are in general more comprehensive and less prescriptive than cognitive and psycholinguistic approaches. Cognitive rehabilitation endeavors to restore the functioning of an impaired aspect of language; pragmatic therapy endeavors to augment impaired language use, mostly by teaching compensatory and productive strategies and by discouraging possible maladaptive strategies. In Conversational Coaching (Holland, 1991), for example, a short script is chosen and practiced by the therapist and the patient, and the therapist suggests which strategies the patient should use to better convey the intended message. A family member is then called in, and the patient has to communicate to him or her the content of the script while they are both videotaped. The videotape is then projected and discussed by the patient and the family member with the therapist, who indicates which strategies were successful and why and encourages the patient and the family member to use them in everyday conversation. Unsuccessful strategies are identified and discouraged.

The efficacy of this approach is even more difficult to evaluate than that of other, more structured approaches. Some clinicians (e.g., Penn, 1993) argue that it enhances the communicative efficiency of all patients. However, no two aphasic patients are alike, and it is inconceivable that the same intervention can be the best one for all patients even if it is beneficial for all of them. As Strauss Hough and Pierce (1994) aptly state, "Emphasis on pragmatic issues to the exclusion of remediating other aspects of disordered language is a disservice to our aphasic patients" (p. 246), and Holland (1991) suggests combining the pragmatic approach with other approaches.

This chapter is made up of three parts. Firstly, an attempt will be made to identify the patients for whom the pragmatic approach can be efficacious. Secondly, some of the main pragmatic topics will be discussed. Finally, some guidelines for treatment will be illustrated.

PATIENT SELECTION

Two groups of patients are good candidates for the pragmatic approach. First of all, as with any type of intervention, patients with an identifiable disorder of the specific behavior targeted by the approach—in this case, a disorder of language use—should be selected for this type of therapy.

However, patients with a primary deficit of language use, though good candidates for the pragmatic approach, are rare and difficult to identify. There are data in the literature pointing to the fact that the level of pragmatics is generally preserved in left-hemisphere-damaged aphasic patients (Wilcox et al., 1978; Kadzielewa et al., 1981; Foldi et al., 1983; Foldi, 1987; Van Lanckner & Kempler, 1987; Huber, 1990; Holland, 1991), whereas it is frequently disrupted in nonaphasic right-hemisphere-damaged patients (Brownell et al., 1986; Foldi, 1987; Stemmer et al., 1994; Sabbagh, 1999).

Moreover, to disentangle a primary deficit of language use from a deficit secondary to other impairments such as anomia or comprehension impairments is not easy. Not unexpectedly, in fact, any language disorder affects language use. A normal person speaking an imperfectly known second language will encounter some difficulty using the second language because of, say, limited comprehension or reduced vocabulary. The foreign speaker may, however, make the best use of his or her knowledge of the language, demonstrating that he or she has no difficulty in language use. Treating this level when it is not primarily impaired can be broadly compared to teaching someone who is unable to play any instrument to follow the conductor's instructions or, more generally, to follow the rules of a game the person is unable to play.

There is a second group of good candidates for such an approach, which is much larger and easily identifiable. The cognitive approach requires a detailed and thorough investigation of the functional damage and a careful choice of the possible intervention strategies. Not always, however, is it possible to locate the patient's functional damage and theoretically justify a cognitive intervention. With extensive disruption of language, the task of attributing each symptom to a given underlying impairment is very difficult and sometimes impossible. Not all the symptoms of aphasia have in fact been explained on the basis of a model of normal processing. Perseveration, stereotypical utterances, and jargon—probably multilevel impairments—are but some examples of symptoms for which no straightforward interpretation has been advanced. But even if it were possible to locate all of the patient's symptoms on a functional model, the analysis of the language deficit of a globally aphasic patient, impaired in all language behaviors, will show that all cognitive functions are impaired. Such a conclusion would be of no help in guiding the choice of therapeutic intervention.

In a global aphasic we can decide, for example, to start with semantic therapy, as did Behrmann and Lieberthal (1989). Even if we succeed in improving the patient's functioning, he or she will not be able to use the newly recovered semantic knowledge because of damage to the input and output lexicons and multiple disorders at the sentence level. Or consider training of the sublexical procedures; this seems unwarranted in a patient with multiple and severe damages to the lexical-semantic system and the sentence level. A theoretically motivated starting point is difficult to locate in these severely aphasic patients, and one should look for a different theoretical justification on which to base a rationale choice for therapy.

The World Health Organization's (WHO) International Classification of Impairment, Disability and Handicap (World Health Organization, 1980) can be of some help in deciding what to do with severe patients. WHO's definitions encompass the disease and how it affects the whole person, changing his or her ability to participate in society. *Impairment* refers to the damage at the level of the organ. *Disability* is defined as the difficulty in carrying out everyday activities and *handicap* as the limitations brought about by the disability in relation to a person's role in society, such as the ability to earn a living and have normal social interactions. Applied to aphasia, we may consider that damage to the orthographic output lexicon, for example, is the impairment; writing difficulties are the consequent disability; and the impossibility of doing any job requiring the ability to write is the handicap. When location of the impairment is impossible or does not constrain the choice of the intervention, it seems sensible to look for the handicap.

Cognitive rehabilitation is a bottom-up process that begins with the identification of the impairment and works up by trying to remediate it. If successful, recovery from the impairment should also lead to total or partial recovery from the disability and the handicap. The pragmatic approach is a top-down process that begins with the identification of the handicap or disability and works down to the impairment. It must not be forgotten that for all aphasic patients the final goal of rehabilitation is the recovery of language, particularly of the communicative function of language, even when the immediate goal is the recovery of a specific damaged function, such as the recognition of letters.

PRAGMATICS

Pragmatics lacks an agreed-upon definition and its boundaries are not clearly determined, but everyone would agree that its main characteristic is an active conception of language as being used. A viable definition for practical use in aphasiology is that *pragmatics* refers to the study of the use of situated language. The main topics in pragmatics are concepts such as deixis, presupposition, conversational implicature, and speech acts.

Deixis

Deictic expressions are those expressions that take an important part of their meaning from the situation in which they are uttered and are interpretable only in the context of the utterance in which they occur. Personal pronouns, verb tense, and words such as *here* and *now*, for example, are directly related to the circumstances in which they occur. Deixis has an egocentric organization, and the anchorage point is the speaker. One must refer to the time, the place, and the person speaking to understand deictic expressions such as "yesterday," "you," "in half an hour," "near," and so forth.

Presupposition

Presupposition is the information carried by a proposition that goes beyond the linguistic message but that the listener can easily presuppose. The proposition "It was Peter who arrived last night" presupposes that someone arrived last night, whereas the proposition "Peter arrived last night" does not. Presuppositions, as well as deixis, are mainly based on conversation because conversationalists have to present information according to the interlocutor's knowledge. The proposition "It was Peter who arrived last night" can only be said to someone who already knows that someone arrived; otherwise, the more neutral form "Peter arrived last night" should have been used.

Conversational Implicature

An important aspect of conversation is the notion of conversational implicature developed by Grice (1975) that allows one to account for the discrepancy between what is actually said and what the speaker meant. Implicatures do not follow logically from what is said but they are based on shared knowledge, and the participants are entitled to draw the implicatures because they collaborate in a cooperative endeavor. In the following exchange taken from Levinson (1983)—"Where is Charles?" "There is a yellow VW in front of Ann's house"—apparently the response has little to do with the question unless one draws some conversational implicatures: that Charles has a yellow VW, that he knows Ann, and that the speaker is suggesting that Charles is at Ann's house. Conversational implicatures are obviously typical of conversation.

Speech Acts

Finally, the speech act theory emphasizes the act accomplished by a proposition. By uttering a sentence, people do things, and each sentence performs a speech act. Sentences can have, for example, the force of an assertion ("John has a gun"), a request ("Does John have a gun?"), or a warning ("John has a gun!"). To understand the meaning of the sentence, the listener has to go beyond its linguistic content and identify the speech act it performs.

Certain conditions must be fulfilled if the speech act is to be carried out felicitously. Every speech act has specific felicity conditions. The act of questioning, for example, can be said to be felicitous only if the speaker does not know the response to the question and believes that the listener does. In aphasia therapy, therapists sometimes pose questions to which they already know the response, contravening the felicity conditions for questioning. This is sometimes difficult to avoid, but the therapist can and should pretend not to know the response and behave accordingly.

Speech acts must not be confused with the content of the sentence uttered. The speech act identifies the specific function of the sentence, the reason the sentence has been uttered; and the propositional content refers to what the speaker asks, asserts, or promises. The speech act in the sentence "Did Mark read the book?" is a question, and the propositional content is about Mark reading a book. The speaker expects the listener to know that Mark is reading (or has the intention of reading) a book, and he or she is asking whether or not Mark has done so.

THE STRUCTURE OF CONVERSATION

Conversation is the fundamental and primary type of language use. It is the most widely diffuse type of familiar discourse in which two or more participants take turns speaking and listening. It is the prototype of language use and the form in which we all learn our native tongue. In addition, conversation is a type of interactive discourse in which many pragmatic concepts, such as deixis, presupposition, speech acts, and conversational implicatures, are centered.

Communication is not a matter of logic or truth but of cooperation. It is not confined to what a speaker says, but to what he or she says *given the circumstances in which he or she is speaking and the listener's expectations.*

A conversation is a collaborative endeavor in which participants alternate between the roles of speaker and listener and each participant recognizes a common goal. What the conversationalists say is at any moment determined by the common final goal. Each proposition is designed to serve a specific function: informing the listeners, questioning them about a fact, or promising them something are some of the speech acts that can be performed by uttering a proposition. The function each proposition serves is critical to communication.

Listeners cooperate with speakers. They interpret the sentences they hear in the belief that the speaker is telling the truth and does not leave out anything necessary for the understanding of the intended message. Listeners are expected to recognize the function served by the proposition and act accordingly: receive information, respond to a question, and acknowledge a promise.

A conversation can be described as an action toward a common goal and, like any other collaborative action, can be analyzed in a series of successive actions. When talking with a salesperson, for instance, we do not start the conversation by simply asking for what we want to buy. The conversation starts with some sort of greetings or remarks; after that, we can move on to the central part of the conversation and ask for what we want. The conversation ends with salutations. If one of the interlocutors does not open (or close) the conversation correctly, the other interlocutor will get the impression of incompleteness (or bad manners).

According to Grice (1975), a conversation is guided by some general principles or conversational maxims. All together, the conversational maxims express the cooperation principle, which is at the root of any collaborative act performed by two or more people, regardless of whether the act is linguistic or not, such as changing a tire, cooking, or building an airplane. In order to communicate accurately and efficiently, speakers observe some conventions in what they say and how they express it, and listeners interpret what they hear on the assumption that speakers adhere to these conventions. Acceptance of these conventions or maxims is not conscious; rather, the maxims are similar to a reference point that helps the listener interpret the speaker's meaning and choose what to say. Conversationalists do not have explicit knowledge of the maxims; they behave accordingly without intention.

The conversational maxims proposed by Grice are the maxim of quality (make your contribution one that is true), the maxim of quantity (make your contribution as informative as necessary), the maxim of relation (be relevant), and the maxim of manner (be perspicuous). Grice expressed the maxims as imperatives, but they are not intended as orders; they describe the conventions that the speaker and listener (automatically) observe in speaking and understanding.

Adhering to the cooperation principle allows the speaker to be parsimonious in giving out information because the listener will "reconstruct" the whole body of information simply by applying the cooperative principle and its four subprinciples to what the speaker has actually said. The listener knows that the speaker believes that what he or she says is true and does not say things for which he or she has inadequate evidence (maxim of quality). The listener also knows that the speaker has said all that he or she needs to know (maxim of quantity) and that all that has been said is relevant to the current topic (maxim of relation). Finally, the speaker makes it easy to understand what he or she is saying by avoiding obscurity and by being brief and orderly (maxim of manner).

People can intentionally violate the cooperative principle and tell lies or be obscure and long-winded. However, if the listener does not make the assumption of cooperation, much of what the speaker says will become difficult to understand even if the speaker adheres to the cooperative principle. Sometimes the rules are intentionally broken in order to obtain a given effect. If both speaker and hearer are looking at an abstract picture and the speaker says "What a wonderful picture! So marvelously drawn and so meaningful," the listener would probably understand that what the speaker means is that he or she does not like the picture.

SHARED KNOWLEDGE AND CONTEXT

For a conversation to run smoothly, interlocutors utilize common knowledge and the situational and linguistic contexts. Use of all these devices renders the speaker's task much easier because the speaker can omit a large part of what he or she wants to say. Conversely, the listener has to do more than simply take in what the speaker says. The listener has to reintegrate what the speaker says with what he or she has skipped. Contrary to common belief, in a conversation the work is evenly distributed between the listener and the speaker.

Shared Knowledge

When they start a conversation, participants presuppose that they share some common knowledge based on their belonging to certain groups (ethnic or cultural, for instance) or based on previous common experiences. Not all the information necessary to understand what we say is expressed verbally because an important part is considered to be already known by the interlocutor. To really understand what we are told, it is necessary to go beyond the literal meaning of the sentences addressed to us and complete them with what we know. If one knows nothing about the new European currency, for instance, it would be difficult to understand the sentence "The introduction of the Euro should boost the EU economy." The listener would understand that something should boost the economy in Europe but would not know what should boost it—a new currency—and would be totally unable to understand why that should be.

Besides this sort of common knowledge, which corresponds to what we know about the world, when we speak we also utilize a different sort of knowledge: what we know about our interlocutor and what he or she knows about us. To understand the role of this knowledge in our choice of words and sentences, we can think about how much more fast-flowing a conversation is with a close friend than with a stranger. With a friend, a few words may suffice to make ourselves understood because we have many common experiences; with a stranger we only share knowledge about the world, and we have to give more information (using more words) in order to convey the same meaning.

Brenneise-Sarshad et al. (1991) examined the effect of the listener's knowledge on aphasics' production. The aphasic patients produced more words and more information units when talking with naive listeners than when talking with more knowledgeable listeners, suggesting that aphasic patients are sensitive to the amount of shared information. However, it is common to encounter patients who are unable to automatically evaluate what the interlocutor knows and who fail to break away from their own point of view. They are unable to decentralize and give information that is important for the listener. They frequently use, for instance, proper names

("Mary") instead of the role of the intended person ("my wife") even when they speak with someone who does not know their wife's name (or whether they are married at all).

Some breakdowns in normal conversations are due to the fact that the speaker has not correctly evaluated what the listener knows and gives insufficient information. If someone says "I got three yesterday," thinking that the interlocutor knows that the speaker went fishing when in fact he or she does not, communication breaks down and necessitates a repair ("Three what?" "Fish! I went fishing") before proceeding.

Situational Context

Another resource used by the speaker is the situational context. Words that clearly refer to the situational context include *here, there, this* and so forth, which can be understood only by someone in the same situational context. If one says "Give me those peaches," *those* can be understood only by someone who can see the peaches. The same sentence can have different meanings, depending on the situation in which it is said. "Are you thirsty?", for instance, when said while eating, may be an offer of something to drink, and a plausible response would be "My glass is still full, thank you"; if spoken on a hot sunny day while rock climbing, it may be a request for information to evaluate possible dehydration.

Linguistic Context

Finally, linguistic context, the verbal information given before (or after) a target linguistic unit, is very important. The most common example of linguistic context is the use of pronouns. To understand what a pronoun stands for, one has to know what has been said before. In the sentence "I met Anthony yesterday; he was going to the cinema with John," *he* stands for Anthony and can only be understood by considering what has been said before.

In conclusion, listeners must go beyond virtually every word they hear and look for what is really meant. Much of what is understood about an utterance does not come from what is directly said but from what is inferred by the listener.

PROPOSITIONAL CONTENT

Propositional content refers to what is said explicitly by the speaker. The propositional content of the sentence "What time is it?" refers to current time, and the speech act is a question; the propositional content of the sentence "I went to the movies yesterday" refers to the speaker's going to the movies, and the speech act is an assertion. "Mary gave me a book" refers to someone called Mary giving a book to the speaker, and again it is an assertion.

When the speaker has decided on the propositional content to be communicated, he or she has to decide how to express it. In general, part of what the speaker says is already known by the listener, and part of it is new and corresponds to what the speaker predicates about it. The part already known by both conversationalists is frequently called *given* information and corresponds to what the listener is expected to be able to identify uniquely; the *new* information specifies what the speaker predicates about it.

Sentences frequently contain elements that allow the listener to distinguish between given and new information, and the listener has to identify which elements carry the given information and which carry the new information. One of the most frequently used conventions is the type of article: an indefinite article is used to introduce new information and a definite article to refer to given information.

Given information is frequently placed at the beginning of the sentence as the subject. In the sentence "Mary made the cake," *Mary* is generally understood as the given information that can be uniquely identified by both speakers, and the new information predicated about Mary is that she made the cake. In the sentence "The cake was made by Mary," it is the cake that can be uniquely identified and corresponds to the given information, and the new information predicated of the cake is that it was made by Mary. In the sentence "John arrived very late last night," *John* is the given information—that is, what people are talking about—and that he arrived very late is what the speaker predicates about John and is new information for the listener.

REHABILITATION

The following pages will illustrate how a theory of conversation can help guide the therapist's[1] behavior during conversation/rehabilitation with a severely aphasic patient. It is difficult to describe this type of treatment because it is based mainly on the interaction between the therapist and the patient and not on tasks, as with rehabilitation of lexical and sentence-level

---

[1] In this section, the therapist is assumed to be female and the patient male.

disorders. Here any response given by the patient is accepted, and the therapist must adjust his or her behavior to the patient's response. The underlying rationale for this type of treatment is the same as for the other treatments described: it is supposed that if the therapist succeeds in having frequent verbal exchanges with the patient, the patient's capacity to participate will improve and gradually he will be able to produce more information and to understand interlocutor better.

The first strong recommendation to therapists is not to be directive. Ulatowska et al. (1992) studied speech acts in a group of aphasic patients and observed that many speech acts were preserved. However, Wilcox and Davis (cited in Strauss Hough & Pierce, 1994), comparing the communicative effectiveness of aphasic patients in individual therapy and unstructured group therapy, observed that the therapists retained their directive role in both situations and did not give patients the opportunity to demonstrate their intent to communicate.

The second recommendation is to build a conversational exchange as close as possible to the kind of natural conversation the patient may want to sustain in his or her daily life. In the course of treatment, the conversation/rehabilitation must be conducted so as to make the patient progress from passive to active participation. Right from the start of treatment and regardless of how poor the active participation of the patient may be, the patient's and the therapist's conversational behavior must be *ecological*, that is, as similar as possible to normal conversational behavior.

As stated before, a conversation between normal conversationalists is a collaborative endeavor that generally runs more or less smoothly with a few repairs. The aphasic patient, however, has a limited capacity for language use, and the burden of maintaining a normal conversation will rest mainly on the therapist. To do this, the therapist should know what goes on in a normal conversation.

We can look at the conversation between therapist and patient as if it were a conversation between two interlocutors, one of whom is eager to chat while the other is not, or as a conversation made difficult for other reasons, such as inadequate knowledge of the language by one of the interlocutors. Let's imagine that the interlocutor who is eager to chat (or the one who is speaking her mother tongue) is the therapist and that the second interlocutor, who is reluctant to speak (or who does not know the language used), is the patient. The first interlocutor may start by greeting the second, who does not respond, either because he does not want to or is unable to do so. It is conceivable that the first interlocutor will repeat her greetings until the addressee gives some signs of acknowledgment (nodding his head, muttering). She will then proceed to ask the addressee, for instance, how he is feeling or to say something about the weather. Should the addressee fail to respond again (because he does not want to or because he has not understood), in a normal conversation the speaker would repeat her question and also use gestures if she supposes that the listener has not understood her. She is likely to continue in this way until she elicits an answer, and she will not dispute the addressee's response, whatever it is, but would proceed with the conversation. A similar conversation can easily be sustained even with a severely aphasic patient. However, to transform this conversation into a therapy session, the therapist must use the conversation as a tool to increase the patient's language capacity.

The therapist's behavior as a listener and as a speaker will be considered separately, but before trying to engage in a conversation with an aphasic patient, the therapist must make sure that the patient can sustain the correct attitude, namely, that he or she can take turns in speaking and listening.

Turn-Taking

If one analyzes a conversation, it soon becomes clear that interlocutors exchange their roles continually, from listener to speaker and vice versa. When this does not happen, we would speak more of a monologue than of a conversation. Many aphasic patients are no longer able to exchange their role normally: some have reduced spontaneous speech and do not actively intervene in a conversation; they may respond whenever interrogated but do not take any initiative. Others, with abundant speech, may have a tendency to speak without listening to the interlocutor. In both cases, turn-taking does not occur normally.

The therapist has to use different strategies, depending on whether the patient does not speak or does not listen. In the first case, she has to ask some relevant questions (about the patient's illness, his work, or his family, for example) so as to make it evident that she is waiting for an answer, and she has to encourage the patient to give a response, either verbally or through any other communicative channel. At this point, it is not necessary that the response be correct. Once a response is given, the therapist must underline that a response was exactly what she wanted, but if the response was not correct, the therapist must find a gentle way of offering the patient the correct response before going on with another relevant question. If, for instance, she has asked whether the patient is married (which she knows he is) and he answers "no," the patient has correctly taken his turn, which was the therapist's goal, but the response was wrong and the therapist should signal it to the patient without making it evident that her previous question had not fulfilled the felicity conditions because she already knew the response. In this example she may say, "Oh, I thought the lady waiting outside might be your wife" and then go on. The conversation must proceed for a certain number of pairs of turn-taking and must not stop after each question/response pair, as was usually the case in the traditional confrontation naming or pointing task, where each pair was independent of the preceding one.

In the case of a patient who speaks a lot without letting his interlocutor speak and without listening to her when she succeeds in saying something, the therapist must adopt a different approach but the immediate goal is the same: to accustom the patient to turn-taking. She must first have the patient stop speaking and listen to her; he can then resume the role of speaker for a short time, after which he will again be interrupted and the therapist will speak, and so on. The therapist's aim at this point is to get the patient involved in something that, like a normal conversation, is constructed little by little, with alternating contributions of the patient and the therapist.

Many severely aphasic patients do not have a problem with turn-taking and the therapist can, from the start, pay attention to the communicative intention and the content of their messages.

The Therapist in the Role of Speaker

When the therapist acts as a speaker, the patient acts as a listener and the therapist's job is to facilitate his role. We have seen that understanding is not an easy process and that the listener has quite a job to do. He has to recognize the speaker's communicative intention, identify the given information, and understand what is predicated about it. Finally, he has to behave accordingly to the speaker's communicative intention. Acting as a speaker, the therapist must facilitate all these operations as much as she can and be careful not to violate the conversation rules. Let us start with the communicative intention.

The linguistic acts that may be important in the rehabilitation of severely aphasic patients are few: questions, communications, and requests for action (orders). Other linguistic acts, such as promising or warning, for example, are rarely used in aphasia therapy at this point. Speakers of the language have no difficulty in identifying the linguistic act and behaving adequately, but things may go differently with severely aphasic patients, although Boller and Green (1972) demonstrated that aphasic patients understand the communicative intention of the speaker better than they understand the propositional content of the message. There are, however, patients who are impaired at this level. In these cases, the therapist must express her communicative intention in such a way as to make it easy for the patient to identify it. This can be done by simply stating "Now I want to ask you something" or "I want you to do something" and then pose the question or the request.

In helping the patient distinguish between given and new information, a good rule of thumb while speaking with very severe aphasics is first to single out what is already known (what we are talking about) and put the new information at the end of the sentence: "The cake, did *Mary* make it?". The therapist should proceed with the new information only when she is reasonably certain that the patient has identified what she is talking about (the given information) and will pay attention to what follows, which is the new information.

Finally, to facilitate comprehension of the propositional context, the most important maxim for the therapist when she acts as the speaker is the maxim of manner and its four submaxims: avoid obscurity of expression, avoid ambiguity, be brief, and be orderly.

Here are some further strategies that can be useful in talking with a severe aphasic. The therapist should always catch the patient's attention whenever she changes the topic. This can be done by simply stating that she is going to talk about something else. She should also avoid open questions ("What did you do yesterday?), which are too difficult for aphasic patients at this stage, and ask only closed question ("Did you go out yesterday?"). Finally, she should make use of all communicative channels—facial mimicry, gestures, prosody, and so forth—and not rely solely on language.

The role of prosody in the auditory comprehension of aphasic patients has received much attention. Recent research has confirmed its role and has found it to be more important in severe than in moderate aphasics (Kimelman, 1999).

Therapists sometimes unknowingly break the felicity conditions of speech acts, particularly in questioning. Many of the questions therapists ask are infelicitous because they already know the response. This is sometimes unavoidable, but the therapist must do her best not to let the patient understand that she already knows the response. If the patient understands that the therapist already knows the response, he may become confused, and instead of answering the question, he will try to work out why he was asked something the therapist already knew.

In brief, in order to make herself understood by the patient, the therapist must explicitly state her communicative intention, separate the known part from the new part of her message, express herself in a simple way, and stress prosody.

The Therapist in the Role of Listener

Let's now consider what the therapist's attitude should be when she acts as a listener. It is important that the therapist behave as if the patient were a normal conversationalist and make all the possible conversational implicatures to find out how the patient's contribution may be related to what was previously said, as she would do in a conversation with a normal interlocutor.

Whenever the patient answers a question, the therapist must behave as if the question were understood and, more importantly, as if what the patient has said is a possible answer to her question. In reality, the patient's answer may or may not be adequate to the question; if adequate, it may or may not be correct ("Do you have any children?" "yes/no"; both answers are adequate, but only one is correct). An adequate response, regardless of whether it is correct, requires the therapist to proceed with the conversation: "Do you have children?" "Yes." "Oh, how many?"

Often, however, the patient's reply is not immediately associated with the question, but it is important that the therapist continue the conversational game. One of the maxims of the cooperation principle at the root of a conversation is the maxim of relation: what the speaker says is pertinent to the topic of the conversation. In other words, a response must always be considered pertinent to the question. Taking this assumption for granted, if the patient answers "Mary" in response to the question "Do you have children?", the therapist must search for a possible relation between the question and the answer. In this case, a plausible relationship is easy to see: the patient has a daughter, and her name is Mary. The therapist must proceed from this assumption. If the conversation took place in a normal setting, there would be no doubt that this was what the speaker intended. With an aphasic patient, it is always possible that this is not the case and the therapist must ask for confirmation ("Ah, you have a daughter, Mary; is this correct?"). It is not always easy for the therapist to find a link between her question and the patient's answer, but she has to behave as if the link existed.

In daily life, when we do not understand what we are told, we ask for clarification. The therapist should do the same and offer some possible interpretations ("Do you have any children?" "London." "What do you mean by London? Do you have children in London?" or "Do you have any children?" "Yesterday." "I'm afraid I didn't understand what you mean. Do you mean that one of your children came to see you yesterday?"). The therapist often has to stretch her imagination to find a possible link between what she says and what the patient replies. She must, however, be the one to shoulder the burden of not having understood without telling the patient that he was wrong ("Sorry, I didn't understand what you meant there," not "I asked you whether you have any children, not where you live"). The therapist goes on asking questions as long as the patient's response is clearly inadequate and she finds no relation between her question and the patient's answer ("Do you have any children?" "Bread"). A clearly inadequate response generally indicates that the patient has not understood or that he has been unable to respond. When the conversation breaks down, the therapist must make sure that her question has been understood, as she would do in any normal conversation, and help the patient give a response.

Therapists frequently fail to try to understand why the patient gives a certain answer; they simply ignore it, as if it were incorrect and not pertinent to the question. Needless to say, in a normal setting they would not behave this way. In a normal conversation, when we do not understand why our interlocutor says something, we ask for clarification, but we do not ignore it lest we be considered rude.

A second important recommendation for the therapist is to always check whether she has understood correctly. Rephrasing what she has understood and asking the patient for confirmation can achieve this. Otherwise, it is possible to go on for many turn-takings based on a misunderstanding.

To sum up, in a conversation with a severe aphasic, when the patient is in the role of the speaker, the therapist must accept everything he says and try to relate it to the topic of conversation, asking for confirmation of her interpretation. Only when she receives clearly contradictory answers is she allowed to make the patient notice the incongruity, reminding him of what he had previously said and underlining the fact that it is impossible for both answers to be correct. "You told me before you had two sons; do you remember? Now it seems you are telling me that you do not have any. Let me get this clear; do you have any children or not?" This is a subtle way of letting the patient know that he made a mistake and allowing him correct it.

The therapist can use almost anything to start the conversation: how the patient is dressed, the traffic, whether he likes cooking, the weather, an apple, what he takes at breakfast, mountains, and so forth. It must not be forgotten that the conversation will not proceed quickly and that in a session even very few exchanges (8–10) can be considered a good result.

CONCLUSIONS

In this chapter, a conversational treatment for severe aphasia has been outlined. This is nothing new since conversation forms the basis of many pragmatic approaches. In general, however, pragmatic approaches have aimed at developing strategies of functional communication in the patient and his or her significant others, as described, for example, in the Conversational Coaching approach (Holland, 1991). Amelioration of the patient's linguistic impairments can be a side effect of therapy, but it is not the aim of the intervention. As stated by Holland, "pragmatic approaches are not designed to change the aphasia symptom-complex necessarily, but merely to provide a framework within which the patient is expected to accommodate and compensate" (Holland, 1991, p. 205). By contrast, the aim of the conversation therapy described here is to achieve linguistic improvements, possibly to the point where a more precise diagnosis of the patient's disorders is possible—an essential prerequisite for therapy appropriate to the functional disorder.

11

FINAL REMARKS

WHAT THIS BOOK HAS ATTEMPTED TO DO IS to establish the connection between research and therapy of aphasia. Taking as a starting point the beginning of scientific aphasiology in the second half of the nineteenth century, the currents of thought about the nature of aphasia and how these have influenced clinicians and their ways of thinking about rehabilitation have been illustrated.

In the nineteenth century, the prevailing opinion was that language consists of different abilities (speaking, understanding, reading, and writing) that were related to different brain areas and could be differently impaired. This school of thought did not yield any therapeutic intervention of interest, and therapy was inspired by standard school teaching. The early twentieth century saw the fall of the associationist models and the rise of the holistic school. Aphasia therapy took root after World War I in German-speaking countries but became more widespread after World War II, mainly in the United States. Therapy was mainly inspired by the holistic school, which envisioned just one form of aphasia. The approach varied according to the severity of the deficit and tended to focus on the treatment of comprehension disorders. Two of the most outstanding representatives of this school—Hildred Schuell and Joseph Wepman—are still frequently referred to, and their methods, though partially modified, are still in use, especially in the United States.

In the years following World War II, linguistics played an important role in aphasia therapy, and principles from pragmatics stressing the role of communication formed the foundations of a new approach to aphasia therapy, the pragmatic approach.

It was around this time that Luria published his works in Russian. Traumatized patients were studied, evaluated, and treated according to the principles of the functional approach, which became widely known in the Western countries after the publication of Luria's works in English (Luria, 1963, 1964, 1970).

In the 1970s, Norman Geschwind and the Boston school relaunched a classification of the aphasias, based on refined knowledge of the anatomy of the brain, and Goodglass and Kaplan (1972) elaborated an objective method of evaluating aphasic disorders—the Boston Diagnostic Aphasia Examination, which is probably the most widely used standardized test for aphasia. Treatment followed in these lines and was based on the clinical diagnosis—Broca aphasia, Wernicke aphasia, and so forth—and on an analysis of the language disorder that took into consideration the linguistic level of breakdown: phonological, lexical, and syntactic.

In those same years, psychologists with an interest in cognition started to use data from brain-damaged patients to study the functional organization of normal cognition. This brought about an important change both in the way patients were studied and in the reference model, which was no longer the brain but the functional structure of normal cognitive functioning. Data from single patients became the basis for cognitive neuropsychological research, and group studies lost the privileged status they had enjoyed in the previous decades with the introduction of the methods of experimental psychology in neuropsychology.

Cognitive neuropsychology has fostered a new approach to the study of aphasia and provided us with proper tools—such as models of the functional structure and processing of the lexicon—for reaching a precise functional diagnosis. Its influence was initially magnified mainly because, in the euphoria of the first years, it was thought that identification of the patient's functional damage would by itself make therapy more closely tailored to the patient's disorders. Therapy, however, starts after the damage has been identified. A precise identification of the functional damage restricts the number of rational therapeutic choices, and this is of great advantage to aphasia therapy. However, not many new ideas about implementation of therapy came from early cognitive neuropsychology.

Since the 1960s, a huge amount of research has been carried out with the aim of verifying the efficacy of aphasia therapy, and most clinicians consider that this has now been satisfactorily demonstrated. More precise questions about aphasia therapy, such as which treatment to use and for whom, are now being asked.

At the moment, the main research topic in aphasia therapy seems to be the development of a theory of therapy, which would pull together all the loose threads and, above all, render explicit what is generally implicit in therapy.

This last chapter is concerned with some important fields of research and some aspects of therapy that have thus far been overlooked. Any attempt to cover exhaustively even a single area of neuropsychology is doomed to failure due to the vastness of the literature. Any book is a selection performed by the authors and reflects their choices, and this book is no exception.

NEGLECTED TOPICS

Imaging Studies

A major breakthrough in the study of the neural bases of language (and of cognitive functions in general) was the development of neuroimaging methods—positron emission tomography and functional magnetic resonance imaging—that provide an opportunity to investigate functional activation in normal and brain-damaged subjects engaged in cognitive tasks.

One of the first issues to be addressed was whether the regions of the brain related to damage of specific language functions in aphasic patients are activated in normal subjects performing a task based on these same functions. In other words, the issue is whether, for example, perisylvian areas, which are generally damaged in patients with impaired repetition, are activated in normal subjects performing phonological tasks. Studies of this kind have generally proved to be in good agreement with lesion studies.

In brain-damaged patients, regional brain metabolism has been studied in the resting state, namely, when patients are not engaged in any particular task. An important use of this procedure is in follow-up studies that provide a means of tracking the modifications in brain functions and correlating them with recovery.

Recent technical advances have now made it possible to study single patients, thereby avoiding the problems related to group studies, where one important source of variance is related to the different lesions (for a review, see Cappa, 2000; Pizzamiglio et al., 2001).

The wealth of new data following the introduction of imaging studies in neuropsychology initially led to the belief that it was possible to uncover the brain mechanisms of language, that is, the algorithm controlling the neural activity that produces, for example, the understanding of a sentence. This is still a very distant goal, but functional imaging techniques have dramatically improved recently and imaging studies are furthering our understanding of the brain correlates of language. Furthermore, activation studies in aphasic patients are very promising tools for fostering our understanding of recovery mechanisms.

Connectionist Modeling

A recent approach to the investigation of mental architecture is connectionist modeling, which provides a useful framework for the study of normal and impaired cognitive processes. Connectionist networks consist of a large number of neuron-like units interconnected by weighted connections that determine the amount and direction of activation from one unit to another. Connectivity can be unidirectional, in which case the network is called *feedforward*, or bidirectional, in which case it is called *interactive*. Three main units can be distinguished: input units, output units, and hidden units with efferent and afferent projections within the system. Repeated presentation of a stimulus causes strengthening of the associations between the units and results in learning. Connectionist models do not learn explicit rules but rather acquire connection strengths that allow the network to behave as though it knew the rules. Rules and representations emerge from interactions between units. A concept, for example, is not stored as such but emerges when a particular pattern of activation fires; it is the ability to regenerate that pattern of activation that is stored.

Neural networks were initially used to simulate the activity of the normal cognitive system, but the effects of a local lesion on a cognitive task have also been simulated. In Seidenberg and McClelland's (1989) seminal work on parallel distributed processing, the reading process was simulated. The authors trained a network to associate phonological and orthographic representations, providing an account of how readers recognize and pronounce letter strings. Reading disorders, such as surface and deep dyslexia, were among the first to be simulated by damaged connectionist networks (see Plaut & Shallice, 1994, for a review).

The most important contribution of connectionist models to aphasia therapy is the importance given to the concepts of learning and relearning. Wilson and Patterson (1990) suggested that connectionist or parallel distributed processing (PDP) models can be used to explore intervention strategies. "Clearly, we would not try to argue that all of the many issues in design of rehabilitation programme are about to be solved by PDP models. We merely suggest that much might be learned by simulating, within working computational models (and without any ethical considerations), various forms of damage followed by various regimen of re-learning" (p. 256).

THE PROCESS OF THERAPY

Thus far, the first steps the therapist must go through when first confronted with a patient have been described: he or she must locate the damage and decide on the tasks and goals of therapy. As argued before, locating the impairment is a necessary starting point, and the subsequent selection of tasks reflects the therapist's choice about how to treat the damage, but the actual therapy process has yet to begin. You may know exactly what is wrong with the engine of your car and be able to select the right tools, but unless you are a good mechanic, you will not be able to repair it. Similarly, a therapist has not finished working when he or she has tested the patient, identified the damage, and decided on what to do. Therapy must then be implemented, and the therapist's personality as well as that of the patient will play an important role in their subsequent interactions.

Throughout the book, aphasia therapy has been described as though it and the tasks assigned to the patient were more or less one and the same. Only in describing the pragmatic approach based on a conversation with the patient has some attention been paid to the interaction between patient and therapist. In reality, what happens between the therapist and the patient, which—following Byng (1993)—will be called the *process of therapy*, is of far greater importance than one can infer from what has been written thus far. The process of therapy is much more difficult to define and to describe than the tasks implemented, and this could explain why it is only rarely mentioned (but see Byng, 1995). A frequent criticism leveled against aphasia therapy is that it is implicit (e.g., Howard & Hatfield, 1987; Byng, 1995). One reason for this state of affairs may be that therapy is an interactive process and not the mechanical application of a predefined behavior.

Some therapeutic programs specify the range of permitted responses from the patient and how the therapist should act given the patient's response. But no one can guarantee that the patient will not give an unforeseen response, in which case the therapist has to decide on the spot how to behave. Actually, the therapist's behavior is predetermined only in controlled experimental settings. In clinical practice, it is highly unusual for a therapeutic program to follow a rigid schema. The therapist's behavior is shaped by the aphasic person's behavior, and it continually changes according to the aphasic's responses.

Everyone would agree that even if they start from the same diagnosis and the same choice of tasks, treatment of the same patient would not be carried out in exactly the same way by any two therapists. The therapist immediately reacts to the patient with his or her facial expression, tone of voice, smile, and so on and must take in what the patient has said and frame the next request accordingly. How the therapist reacts to the patient's responses has a great influence on the patient's performance. Therapists are well aware of this, but how they react is not easily expressed in words or even known at a conscious level.

The relationship between therapist and patient is basic to therapy. Byng (1995) describes the process of therapy as "an essentially interactive process in which the therapist and the person with aphasia should be equal partners" (p. 10). One could argue that it is the therapist's role to adapt to the patient because it is the therapist who is the undamaged person and the one who has the leading role in their relationship. It is not up to the patient to adapt his or her behavior to the therapist's mood or to the therapist's willingness to maintain the relationship. On the other hand, the therapist should be able to sustain the interest, attention, and collaboration of the patient throughout each session. In this sense, they are not equal partners; the therapist should keep in step with the patient, whereas the patient may or may not do the same with the therapist.

One of the most important tools the therapist uses to maintain contact with the patient and gain insight into what the patient is striving to say is attentive listening. Today listening is not a very cultivated art. People are keen to speak, but nobody seems to have either the time or the inclination to listen to others, especially if they have difficulty expressing themselves. In Chapter 10, the importance of listening in a conversation, and the fact that it is not a passive process but one that requires participation and interest for the conversation to proceed smoothly, was mentioned. However, it is not sufficient to apply Grice's cooperative principle and to make all the necessary inferences and conversational implicatures to relate what the patient says to the topic of the conversation; attentive listening is something different—vaguer and less easily defined.

Therapists should listen to patients in more than a superficial way. They should listen to them in order to understand what they want to say but are unable to express. Aphasic patients cannot express correctly the intended message; they can only give some hints, more or less detailed depending on the severity of the disorder. Therapists should reconstruct the intended message by a clever, creative, and constant use of inferences, repeatedly asking the patient for confirmation. They should be able to empty their minds of any preconceived idea about what the patient will say and should not impose their mental schemes or interpret what the patient says based on what they believe. It is sometimes dangerous to offer a suggestion because it may be wrong and may divert the patient from what he or she was trying to say.

Therapists must be ready to grasp any signal coming from the patient, be sensitive to any change, and be receptive. They must be very attentive and open to what the patient is actually saying without being biased by their previous knowledge about the patient. They must be able to perceive the patient's mood and convey their affectivity. They must not press the patient, but a long silence can be wearing, and therapists must fill it with the constant but silent assertion that they are interested in what the patient is trying to say.

THE THERAPEUTIC CONTRACT

Whenever rehabilitation has been dealt with in this book, I tried to make it clear that aphasia therapy cannot be delivered to a patient[1] who passively receives it. Being given therapy is not quite the same as being given a pill or an injection; the patient must be an active participant. At the Brussels Neuropsychological Rehabilitation Unit the active participation of the patient is explicitly required, and patients are asked to sign a therapeutic

[1] The word *patient* stresses the passivity of the role since the etymology of the word indicates someone who endures something. Lately, the *British Medical Journal* has questioned whether the word *patient* should be kept, and alternatives such as *client* and *user* have been offered (Neuberger, 1999). An interesting interpretation of the word *patient* came from one of the responses to the *British Medical Journal*. According to O. Basso, the word *patient* means "one who endures a doctor or other health professionals." This is because one is merely ill until a representative of the health profession appears. Only then does he or she become a patient. Thus, contrary to common belief, a patient is not someone enduring an illness but someone enduring a doctor!

contract with the unit (Seron & De Partz, 1993). The contract serves multiple purposes, the first and most important of which is to emphasize the fact that patients are responsible adults who can make commitments on their own and that they are actively engaged in their therapy. A second aim of the contract is to make explicit the goals of therapy and its time schedule. Finally, the coherence and the efficacy of therapy can be monitored.

This is an interesting suggestion but not one that is always practical. Severely aphasic patients will probably be unable to fully understand what they are being asked to sign and may be unwilling to do so. However, the patient must participate actively in therapy and cannot be left out of the decision to undertake it or not. This should be clearly explained to the patient and his or her family, as well as the therapist's opinion about the utility of therapy and what its realistic goals are. The therapist must gain the patient's confidence and collaboration, but the final decision should be left to the patient and those close to him or her. In this way, their active and conscious collaboration should be assured.

THE REALITY

This is all very well, but has it anything to do with what actually happens? Unfortunately, not much. Katz and colleagues (2000) investigated access, diagnostic procedures, and treatment of aphasic patients in Australia, Canada, the United Kingdom, and the United States. The impetus for the study was the worldwide restructuring of health care systems. Clinicians are becoming less involved in controlling access to health care and are substituted for by administrators whose task is to reduce costs by a more "rational" administration of resources.

The authors developed a 37-item questionnaire and distributed it to 394 speech-language clinicians on professional organizations' membership lists in the four countries selected. The return rate was 44%. There were eight areas of inquiry: access to care, diagnostic procedures, group treatment, number and duration of sessions, limitations of the number of sessions, termination of treatment, follow-up, and resumption of therapy. Respondents generally felt that aphasic patients have access to therapy. They reported that the most widely used test for evaluating the aphasic disorder is the Boston Diagnostic Aphasia Examination, which is the most or the second most frequently used test in all countries except the United Kingdom, where informal language tests are used most frequently. Other widely used tests are the Western Aphasia Battery and the Boston

Naming Test (Kaplan et al., 1983). Time dedicated to testing was evaluated to be two or three sessions, but the length of sessions varied between acute (within a year) and chronic (more than a year) patients. It averaged 30 minutes in acute patients and 1 hour in chronic patients. The reported number of therapy sessions was more varied: from 1 to 5 sessions in Australia and the United Kingdom to 16 to 20 sessions in Canada and the United States in acute patients. Interestingly, regardless of the small number of therapy sessions, only 14% of the respondents reported limitation of the number of sessions as a cause for interrupting therapy. Other reasons were achievement of the goal (the most frequent reason) or reaching a plateau. Group treatment was available in approximately 40% of the clinics, generally one session per week. Finally, half of the respondents declared that they treated patients after discharge only "Some of the time" or "Never." However, according to 64% of the respondents, resumption of treatment for former patients was possible.

No published data exist about the situation of aphasia therapy in Italy. In my experience, Italian aphasic patients rarely have the chance to be admitted to a rehabilitation center or to be hospitalized in places where speech therapists work. When they do get therapy, it can last longer than Katz's et al. (2000) report for Canadian and United States patients. Hospitalization in a rehabilitation center, for example, lasts for 2 months, with daily rehabilitation, which can be continued on an outpatient basis.

As the study by Katz et al. (2000) and the Italian situation point out, there is a yawning gap between what is suggested by aphasia research and what actually happens. These results should, however, be interpreted with caution due to the small number of respondents in the Katz et al. study and the absence of published data in Italy. Research on aphasia therapy efficacy has clearly stated that the duration and intensity of therapy are important factors for recovery (see Chapter 4). In most of the studies where no effect of therapy was found, therapy was offered for only short periods of time. The current situation seems purposely created to confirm the futility of aphasia therapy, and unless this practice is altered, aphasia therapy will soon be denied to everybody.

However, what is most striking about the responses to Katz et al.'s questionnaire is the fact that only 14% of respondents complained about the limitation imposed on therapy, whereas the most frequent response was that the goal of therapy was reached. This makes one wonder about what the goal of therapy could possibly have been; it is unlikely to have been a general improvement in the patient's disorder and that, after such a small number of therapy sessions, the patient's ability to communicate improved.

If this were the case, it would not have been so difficult to demonstrate the efficacy of aphasia therapy! It almost seems as though speech therapists may be the first group of practitioners not to believe in the theoretical or practical possibility that the patient's language disorder can be improved in a meaningful way and that they are the first to declare themselves beaten.

CONCLUSIONS

This book has been written with two goals in mind: firstly, to show the clear relationship between research on aphasia and aphasia therapy, and, secondly, to demonstrate how knowledge of the past can enrich our present knowledge. New ideas do not come out of the blue but are built up from previous ideas and new knowledge.

Much criticism has been leveled against aphasia therapy as it was conducted in the past (e.g., Howard & Hatfield, 1987). I hope to have shown that the criticism is unjustified if it refers to the past, when the bases for a detailed and theoretically driven intervention were not present. We are now in a position to offer more rational interventions tailored to the patient's specific deficits, and therapy should not be conducted today as it was in the past.

Knowledge, however, is never definitive; what is true today will change tomorrow. All the disciplines that contribute to our knowledge about aphasia and its therapy are constantly evolving, and the way we consider aphasia and implement therapy should change at the same pace. Nothing of what is being done today or has been done in the past enjoys any special status. It has been and will be substituted for by something else, hopefully something more "correct."

Yet, when treating patients, we cannot wait for further knowledge without doing anything. We can perform well in any situation and at any moment as long as we apply current knowledge with intelligence, competence, and ingenuity.

Appendix 2 briefly recounts Dr. Ignaz Semmelweis' (1818–1865) commitment to the battle against puerperal fever at a time when its causes were unknown. Semmelweis found an effective treatment that was not accepted by his contemporaries. It was based on insight; "scientific" knowledge came later. What has aphasia therapy to do with Semmelweis and puerperal fever? Nothing, but the lesson we can draw from Semmelweis is important. He had not discovered the cause of childbed fever. In his time, histology was in its infancy and bacteria were unknown. However, he did treat puerperal fever successfully. Aphasia therapy cannot do more. The underlying causes will probably always be a mystery, as will the structure of the normal function.

It is presumptuous to say that what we do now is better than what was done in the past. What is done should always be the best that can be done with reference to current knowledge. The more knowledge we have, the better we should do, but we cannot wait for the ultimate truth (and do we really know the ultimate truth about childbed fever?) to act. I hope that this book has clarified these topics and demonstrated how research on aphasia and aphasia therapy have taken advantage of other disciplines—mainly linguistics and psychology—and how they have gone hand in hand.

1

SYSTEMATIC SAMPLING AND CASUAL OBSERVATION: TWO APOLOGUES

THE FOLLOWING APOLOGUES illustrate an important aspect of group and single-case studies by comparing systematic sampling and casual observation. The first apologue is set in the Soviet Union and takes place in the years of Chernobyl's nuclear power plant disaster. In April 1986, the chain reaction went out of control, one of the Chernobyl reactors exploded, and a large amount of radioactive material was released in the atmosphere. The second apologue is set in China in the years of Mao Zedong's long march. In October 1934, Mao Zedong and approximately 100,000 men moved westward. Throughout their journey, which lasted many months and during which they covered 6,000 miles, they fought against the Nationalist forces under Chiang Kai-shek.

THE SINGLE-CASE-APPROACH APOLOGUE

For some decades, disagreement had been growing among geneticists about the growth of upper and lower limbs: the debate was centered on whether their growth is controlled by a single gene or two different genes. Sustainers of the single-gene hypothesis argued that giants and dwarfs generally have upper and lower limbs of congruent length. Sustainers of the double-gene hypothesis argued that there are two genes, but that these may be metabolically similar and chromosomically so close that a single noxious agent would probably damage both.

The clarification came from Kiev, the holy city. In its monastery lived a pious monk dedicated to the solitary study of biology and theology. The idea that the human appearance has the wonderful harmony that we all appreciate every day not because of a divine decision taken once and for all and materialized in a single gene, but because of a choice that divine providence puts into practice each time a new creature is born, appeared to him more consonant to the idea of the might and freedom of God. Two genes that can be manipulated, he surmised, are more respectful of divinity.

He had in fact the proof that there are at least two genes for the growth of the limbs. And, by extrapolation, he deduced that there are genes specialized for any part of the body—the mouth, the nose, the eyes, maybe one for the right and one for the left eye, and so on. So, at each new conception, God, as is proper for Him, has unlimited freedom to decide the human appearance.

Here is the proof.

A week after the explosion of Chernobyl's nuclear reactor, when townspeople became aware of the danger and of the impotence of the authorities to protect them, a multitude of fugitives invaded the monastery. Among them was a young woman who some months later delivered a beautiful child with blond hair and blue eyes. Unfortunately, with the passing of time the child slowly became deformed, assuming a monkey-like appearance, with short legs and normal arms.

The pious monk took this as proof that divine providence had not abandoned the Russian Church and that it had revealed the mystery of the two genes through him, its humble servant. What else could he think of the monkey-like child if not that the radiation had compromised the legs' gene, leaving unharmed the arms' gene? The event, highly unlikely when the level of radioactivity is normal, had become possible by the explosion of the nuclear reactor.

The prior, however, did not want to worsen the tension with the state authorities and also hoped that two American journalists who were in Ukraine for a report on Chernobyl would hear nothing of the news. He forbade the monk to talk about his discovery. Difficult though it was, the monk had to follow his vow of obedience and keep the discovery to himself.

A few months later, a man in his mid-thirties with disproportionately short legs arrived at the monastery. He came from Novosibirsk, where he had chosen to work, for ideological (and monetary) reasons, first at the construction and then the running of the thermal power station. He had come to see his mother, a refugee from Chernobyl. She was still living in the monastery, where she was much appreciated for her selfless dedication to helping others.

The monk was now sure that there were two genes. Besides the case caused by Chernobyl, he could rely on a confirmation: a man born in normal circumstances. He pressed the prior, who could no longer conceal the truth and discreetly informed the Ukraine Academy of Sciences.

The Academics were quite interested and decided to carry out an ample and systematic investigation as soon as they could find the necessary money. They kept their word. Ten years later, the research came to an end. Three further similar cases had been found in the Soviet Union: two near Moscow and the last one at Alma Ata. Of these new cases, one was a brother of the man from Novosibirsk, but the other two were unrelated, had never lived in the same parts of the country, and had had nothing to do with nuclear enterprises.

The finding was published by the Academy of Science and convinced most of the geneticists that the genes for the growth of the human body are many and that they are specialized for the various parts of the body. No less important, the monastery received financial support for the restoration of the roof and the old wing.

Some, albeit few, geneticists of the old school and a young mathematician specialized in the theory of probability were not convinced. The mathematician was uncertain about the conclusions because he still believed it possible that the five cases were the result of causes that had not been considered by the researchers. However, no specific cause could be suggested, and the reasons for doubting appeared to everybody so vague and generic that they soon disappeared from the reported evidence of the five cases. The discussion came to an end, to the satisfaction of many and the ill-concealed bitterness of the few who could not understand the *thoughtlessness* (they really used this word) with which assertions in the realm of science were accepted without considering their objections and giving up the possibility of measuring the risk of their assertion.

Only the prior knew the truth, but he wisely decided not to reveal it. The prior had kept in touch with the old woman. During his conversations with her, he learned how hard it had been for her to raise her four children, particularly the first two, when the people at Chernobyl used to live together—two families of four people in two small rooms ("young people of today do not realize how hard was life before the nuclear reactor!"). To make life a little easier, and especially to make sure her children would grew up strong and healthy, she discovered how to obtain suitable nourishment from cow's milk and wheat flour, how to lull the children to sleep with local herbs, and how to swaddle them so that they would not feel the cold but still be able to express all their infantile restlessness by moving their heads and arms. Not their legs! It is good for the children not to walk until they are 3 or 4 years old, when the locomotor apparatus has developed and cannot be damaged by falls. Her rearing had produced good results, not only with her own children but also with another child she had nursed in Alma Ata, where she had gone after becoming a widow. When she was finally able to settle down in Moscow with a sister of hers, her neighbors— he a foreman and she an engineer—gave her their newborn child to rear. The prior then remembered how, years before, immediately after the atomic disaster, the old woman had helped the mother of the monkey-like child to rear him. He began to suspect that the five men with short legs were among the seven children reared by the old woman, and he soon found out that this was the case. He understood then that the crippled legs were caused by the swaddling. However, he did not express his thoughts. The financial support for the final repairs might come to an end! He trusted divine providence. God would know how long scientists should believe in two genes!

APOLOGUE ON THE RANDOMIZED CONTROLLED TRIAL

After the vicissitudes of a bloody and exhausting long march, when the end seemed near, the renovation of Chinese society became inevitable and necessary. Among other decisions, Mao Zedong had to decide whether to use the scarce remaining resources to train doctors and build hospitals and dispensaries suited to traditional Chinese medicine or to Western medicine.

One evening he was in his cave in the town of Liu Ling with an old local doctor, Han Ying-lin, and the Oxford graduate David John Sommerville, M.D., who was known to them as Song En-li. Song En-li had been fascinated by the new man whose maxims were to be regrouped in a small red booklet and had followed him since the time of Shangai, organizing the medical care of the Fourth and Eighth Armies after the rebellion at the Kuo Min-tang.

Mao asked the two doctors to describe the advantages of their relative methods. Han Ying-lin had no difficulty finding someone to testify in favor of traditional medicine. He called for Li Yang-ching, a young woman who had not only been saved by him but had also delivered a child without any pain, using only millenary techniques. This experience was also supported by a dozen other people who came from nearby caves.

Song En-li, for his part, filled the cave with some 15 peasant-soldiers whom he had cured of dysentery, peritonitis, abscesses, bone fractures, and so on.

The debate went on all night. At dawn it showed no signs of abating and indeed looked as if it might even endanger the harmony between the locals, who appreciated traditional medicine, and the soldiers, who were convinced that Song En-li had cured them well and feared being obliged to use only needles and herbs. For this reason, the gathering was brought to an end and everybody went back to their usual activities.

Mao Zedong was left by himself. He fell asleep and slept for 2 hours. When Captain Li Huang-fu awoke him, he found himself having to make a quick decision about how to spend the small amount of money he had left. There were many urgent needs—6 bicycles to ensure the liaisons, 4 wagons to carry the harvest to town, 10 chickens eaten by the soldiers on their arrival, seeds, and many other things besides—but one of the most compelling had to do with the purchase of medicines to control an epidemic of dysentery. Their stocks of herbs and disinfectant were clearly insufficient. Mao was perplexed and thought that for the time being he would accept both types of medicine, and he assigned 500 yen for the herbs and 500 for the disinfectant. But he remained thoughtful all day, concerned that he might have wasted part of his money and endangered both the sowing and the harvest and the advancing of the march.

The debate of the previous night had shown that it was very difficult to decide whether it would be better to spend money and time on either traditional or Western medicine, having as the only evidence the two doctors' personal beliefs.

He sought Captain Li Huang-fu's advice. Considering their geographical position, they agreed on a plan, which seemed to offer the only reasonable way of deciding between traditional and Western medicine.

The town of Liu Ling lies in the Shentsi region, a vast, hilly, and scarcely inhabited region. Because of the frequent incursions by bandits, the peasants had been obliged to live in fortified villages that were practically isolated because of the great distances between them.

Mao Zedong and Li Huang-fu decided to test the two medicines by applying each one in a village. They easily found two villages that were similar in number of inhabitants, age, male female ratio, occupations, diet, and outrages endured. They decided to stay in the region for approximately 2 years (the Long March had been exhausting, and a long rest was necessary) and to assign one village to Han Ying-li and his traditional medicine and the other one to Song En-li and his Western medicine. Two thousand yen were given to each of the doctors for their expenses, and they were publicly reminded that both Confucius and Hippocrates had ordered the doctors to do all in their power to cure their patients.

At the end of the 2 years, Li Huang-fu would count the number of dead people and their age, the felicitous births, and the number of days of dysentery. They would then be able to make a decision based on sound data about which medicine was more efficacious.

APPENDIX

2

SEMMELWEIS

IGNAZ SEMMELWEIS WAS BORN IN BUDA in 1818 and received his medical degree in Vienna in 1844. In January 1846 he received his degree in obstetrics, and in February of the same year he was appointed assistant in one of the two obstetric clinics at Marie Thérèse Hospital, directed by Dr. Johann Klein. The chief of the other clinic was Dr. Wolfgang Bartch.

At that time, childbed fever was raging through Europe and up to 25–30% of hospitalized women died from puerperal infection. The causes were unknown. The medical board appointed by Louis XVI during the puerperal epidemic in Paris in 1774 came to the conclusion that the cause was the milk, and all obstetric clinics were closed and the wet nurses removed. Other suggested causes were overcrowding, poor ventilation, and miasma.

Vienna was no better or worse than any other city in Europe, with, however, a peculiarity: the percentage of women dying in Dr. Klein's clinic was twice that of women dying in Dr. Bartch's clinic. This fact was known, and women tried not to enter Dr. Klein's clinic. Semmelweis decided to fight the childbed fever starting from the only known fact: in Dr. Klein's clinic there was a larger number of deaths, and the only obvious difference between the two clinics was that in Klein's clinic medical students were taught, whereas in Bartch's clinic midwives were taught. Semmelweis asked students to go to Bartch's clinic and midwifes to Klein's. A reversal was immediately noted: more women died in Bartch's clinic, and he asked to have the midwifes back. Dr. Klein could no longer ignore the fact but ascribed it to foreign students, who were expelled. As the number of students was reduced, the number of deaths also diminished for a short time, but it soon returned to the previous level.

Semmelweis noted a second fact. The women who were hospitalized in the clinic, even in periods of epidemic but after delivery, generally survived. He reached the conclusion that the cause of death was something carried by the medical students who examined women during labor after coming directly from the dissection room. Without knowing why, he asked the students to wash their hands before entering the maternity ward. This change was not welcomed and was soon abandoned.

The death of a surgeon from a wound infection incurred during a dissection impressed Semmelweis with its similarity to what happened in puerperal fever. He reasoned that the students carried the infection from the corpses to the delivering women, and he ordered the students to wash their hands in a solution of chlorinated lime before entering the maternity ward whenever they came from the dissection room. The mortality rate dropped to 12%. It was a victory but not the final one. Semmelweis, unsatisfied, pursued his research.

A few months later, an unfortunate experience allowed him to better understand the cause of puerperal fever. He had examined a woman with cancer of the uterus; without washing his hands, he then examined five pregnant women. They all died of childbed fever a few days later. Semmelweis understood that it was not something from the corpses but the hands themselves that caused the fever. He ordered every one entering the maternity ward to wash their hands in a solution of chlorinated lime. With this procedure, the mortality rate dropped to less than 2%.

The medical world, however, was not ready for his discovery, and the general reaction was adverse. Semmelweis addressed several open letters to prominent obstetricians all over Europe, but his doctrine was rejected. The puerperal fever raged for many years after Semmelweis' discovery until, in 1882, Pasteur identified *Streptococcus pyogenes*, one of the causes of puerperal fever. Had Semmelweis' contemporaries accepted his ideas, regardless of the lack of theoretical explanations, many lives would have been saved.

REFERENCES

Alajouanine Th. *L'aphasie et le langage patologique*. Paris: Baillière & Fils, 1968.

Albert ML, and Bear D. Time to understand: A case study of word deafness with reference to the role of time in auditory comprehension. *Brain 97*: 373–384, 1974.

Albert ML, Goodglass H, Helm NA, Rubens AB, and Alexander MP. *Clinical aspects of dysphasia*. Wien: Springer-Verlag, 1981.

Albert ML, Sparks RW, and Helm NA. Melodic intonation therapy for aphasia. *Archives of Neurology 29*: 130–131, 1973.

Aliminosa D, McCloskey M, Goodman-Schulman R, and Sokol SM. Remediation of acquired dysgraphia as a technique for testing interpretations of deficits. *Aphasiology 7*: 55–69, 1993.

Allport AD, and Funnel E. Components of the mental lexicon. *Philosophical Transactions of the Royal Society of London B295*: 397–410, 1981.

Anderson SW, Damasio AR, and Damasio H. Troubled letters but not numbers. *Brain 113*: 749–766, 1990.

Ardila A. Errors resembling semantic paralexias in Spanish-speaking aphasics. *Brain and Language 41*: 437–445, 1991.

Arguin M, and Bub D. Single-character processing in a case of pure alexia. *Neuropsychologia 31*: 435–458, 1993.

Arguin M, and Bub D. Pure alexia: Attempted rehabilitation and its implications for interpretation of the deficits. *Brain and Language 47*: 233–268, 1994.

Armstrong EA. Aphasia rehabilitation: A sociolinguistic perspective. In AL Holland and MM Forbes (Eds.) *Aphasia treatment. World perspectives.* San Diego: Singular Publishing Group, 1993, pp. 263–290.

Assal G, Buttet J, and Jolivet R. Dissociations in aphasia: A case report. *Brain and Language 13*: 223–240, 1981.

Aten JL. Functional communication treatment. In R Chapey (Ed.), *Language intervention strategies in adult aphasia*, 3rd ed. Baltimore: Williams & Wilkins, 1996, pp. 292–303.

Aten JL, Caligiuri MP, and Holland AL. The efficacy of functional communication therapy for chronic aphasic patients. *Journal of Speech and Hearing Disorders 47*: 93–96, 1982.

Auerbach SH, and Alexander MP. Pure agraphia and unilateral optic ataxia associated with a left superior parietal lobule lesion. *Journal of Neurology, Neurosurgery and Psychiatry 14*: 430–432, 1981.

Auerbach SH, Allard T, Naeser M, Alexander MP, and Albert ML. Pure word deafness: Analysis of a case with bilateral lesions and a defect at the prephonemic level. *Brain 105*: 271–300, 1982.

Bachy-Langedock N, and De Partz M-P. Coordination of two reorganization therapies in a deep dyslexic patient with oral naming disorder. In X Seron and G Deloche (Eds.), *Cognitive approaches in neuropsychological rehabilitation.* Hillsdale, NJ: Lawrence Erlbaum Associates, 1989, pp. 211–247.

Badecker W, and Caramazza A. Morphological composition in the lexical output system. *Cognitive Neuropsychology 8*: 335–367, 1991.

Baillarger J. *Recherches sur les maladies mentales.* Paris: Masson, 1865.

Basser LS. Hemiplegia of early onset and the faculty of speech with special reference to the effects of hemispherectomy. *Brain 85*: 427–460, 1962.

Basso A. *Il paziente afasico.* Milan: Feltrinelli, 1977.

Basso A. Approaches to neuropsychological rehabilitation: Language disorders. In MJ Meier, AL Benton, and L Diller (Eds.), *Neuropsychological rehabilitation.* London: Churchill Livingstone, 1987, pp. 294–314.

Basso A. Prognostic factors in aphasia. *Aphasiology 6*: 337–348, 1992.

Basso A. Two cases of lexical-semantic rehabilitation. In FJ Stachowiak (Ed.), *Developments in the assessment and rehabilitation of brain-damaged patients.* Tubingen: Gunter Narr Verlag, 1993, pp. 259–262.

Basso A, Burgio F, and Prandoni P. Acquisition of output irregular ortho-graphic representations in normal adults: An experimental study. *Journal of the International Neuropsychological Society 5*: 405–412, 1999.

Basso A, Capitani E, and Moraschini S. Sex differences in recovery from aphasia. *Cortex 18*: 469–475, 1982a.

Basso A, Capitani E, and Vignolo LA. Influence of rehabilitation of language skills in aphasic patients: A controlled study. *Archives of Neurology 36*: 190–196, 1979.

Basso A, Capitani E, and Zanobio ME. Pattern of recovery of oral and written expression and comprehension in aphasic patients. *Behavioural Brain Research 6*: 115–128, 1982b.

Basso A, and Caporali A. Aphasia therapy or the importance of being earnest. *Aphasiology 15*: 307–332, 2001.

Basso A, Casati G, and Vignolo LA. Phonemic identification defect in aphasia. *Cortex 13*: 84–95, 1977.

Basso A, and Chialant D. *I disturbi lessicali nell'afasia*. Milan: Masson, 1992.

Basso A, Corno M, and Marangolo P. Evolution of oral and written confrontation naming errors in aphasia. A retrospective study on vascular patients. *Journal of Clinical and Experimental Neuropsychology 18*: 77–87, 1996.

Basso A, Faglioni P, and Vignolo LA. Etude controlée de la rééducation du langage dans l'aphasie: comparaison entre aphasiques traités et non-traités. *Revue Neurologique 131*: 607–614, 1975.

Basso A, Gardelli M, Grassi MP, and Mariotti M. The role of the right hemisphere in recovery from aphasia. Two case studies. *Cortex 25*, 555–566, 1989.

Basso A, Lecours AR, Moraschini S, and Vanier M. Anatomoclinical correlations of the aphasias as defined through computerized tomog-raphy: Exceptions. *Brain and Language 26*: 201–226, 1985.

Basso A, Marangolo P, Piras F, and Galluzzi C. Acquisition of new "words" in normal subjects: A suggestion for the treatment of anomia. *Brain and Language 77*: 45–59, 2001.

Basso A, Taborelli A, and Vignolo LA. Dissociated disorders of speaking and writing in aphasia. *Journal of Neurology, Neurosurgery and Psychiatry 41*: 556–563, 1978.

Bastian HC. *A treatise on aphasia and other speech defects*. London: Lewis, 1898.

Baxter DM, and Warrington EK. Neglect dysgraphia. *Journal of Neurology, Neurosurgery and Psychiatry 46*: 1073–1078, 1983.

Baxter DM, and Warrington EK. Category specific phonological dysgraphia. *Neuropsychologia 23*: 653–666, 1985.

Baxter DM, and Warrington EK. Ideational agraphia: A single case study. *Journal of Neurology, Neurosurgery and Psychiatry 49*: 369–376, 1986.

Baxter DM, and Warrington EK. Transcoding sound to spelling: Simple or multiple sound unit correspondence? *Cortex 23*: 11–28, 1987.

Bay E. Principles of classification and their influence on our concepts of aphasia. In AVS De Reuck and M O'Connor (Eds.), *Ciba Foundation symposium on disorders of language.* London: Churchill Livingston, 1964, pp. 122–139.

Beaton A, Guest J, and Ved R. Semantic errors of naming, reading, writing, and drawing following left-hemisphere infarction. *Cognitive Neuropsychology 14*: 459–478, 1997.

Beauvois M-F, and Dérouesné J. Phonological alexia: Three dissociations. *Journal of Neurology, Neurosurgery and Psychiatry 42*: 1115–1124, 1979.

Beauvois M-F, and Dérouesné J. Lexical or orthographic agraphia. *Brain 104*: 21–49, 1981.

Beauvois M-F, and Dérouesné J. Recherche en neuropsychologie et rééducation: Quels rapports? In X Seron and C Laterre (Eds.), *Rééduquer le cerveau.* Bruxelles: Pierre Mardaga, 1982, pp. 163–189.

Beauvois M-F, Saillant B, Meininger V, and Lhermitte F. Bilateral tactile aphasia: A tactoverbal dysfunction. *Brain 101*: 381–401, 1978.

Behrmann M, and Byng S. A cognitive approach to the neurorehabilitation of acquired language disorders. In DI Margolin (Ed.), *Cognitive neuropsychology in clinical practice.* New York: Oxford University Press, 1992, pp. 327–350.

Behrmann M, and Herdan S. The case for cognitive neuropsychological rehabilitation. *Die Suid-Afrikaanse Tydscift vir Kommunikasieafwykings 34*: 3–9, 1987.

Behrmann M, and Lieberthal T. Category-specific treatment of a lexical-semantic deficit: A single case study of global aphasia. *British Journal of Disorders of Communication 24*: 281–299, 1989.

Behrmann M, and McLeod J. Rehabilitation of pure alexia: Efficacy of therapy and implications for models of normal word recognition. *Neuropsychological Rehabilitation 5*: 149–180, 1995.

Behrmann M, Plaut DC, and Nelson J. A literature review and new data supporting an interactive account of letter-by-letter reading. *Cognitive Neuropsychology 15*: 7–51, 1998.

Behrmann M, and Shallice T. Pure alexia: A nonspatial visual disorder affecting letter activation. *Cognitive Neuropsychology 12*: 409–454, 1995.

Belin P, Van Eeckhout PP, Zilbovicius M, Remy P, François C, Guillaume S, Chain F, Rancurel G, and Samson Y. Recovery from nonfluent aphasia after melodic intonation therapy: A PET study. *Neurology 47*: 1504–1511, 1996.

Benson DF. *Aphasia, alexia, and agraphia*. New York: Churchill Livingstone, 1979.

Benson F, and Ardila A. *Aphasia. A clinical perspective*. New York: Oxford University Press, 1996.

Benton A. Neuropsychology: Past, present and future. In F Boller and J Grafman (Eds.), *Handbook of neuropsychology*, Vol. 1. Amsterdam: Elsevier Science Publishers, 1988, pp. 3–27.

Berndt RS, and Caramazza A. Syntactic aspects of aphasia. In MT Sarno (Ed.), *Acquired aphasia*. London: Academic Press, 1981, pp. 157–181.

Berndt RS, and Mitchum C. Approaches to the rehabilitation of "phonological assembly": Elaborating the model of non-lexical reading. In MJ Riddoch and GW Humphreys (Eds.), *Cognitive neuropsychology and cognitive rehabilitation*. Hove UK: Lawrence Erlbaum Associates, 1994, pp. 503–526.

Berndt RS, Mitchum C, Haendiges AN, and Sandson J. Verb retrieval in aphasia. Characterizing single word impairments. *Brain and Language 56*: 68–106, 1997.

Best WM. A reverse length effect in dysphasic naming. When elephant is easier than ant. *Cortex 31*: 637–652, 1995.

Best WM. When racquets are baskets but baskets are biscuits, where do the words come from? A single-case study of formal paraphasic errors in aphasia. *Cognitive Neuropsychology 13*: 443–480, 1996.

Best WM, Hickin J, Herbert R, Howard D, and Osborne F. Phonological facilitation of aphasic naming and predicting the outcome of treatment for anomia. *Brain and Language 74*: 435–438, 2000.

Bisiacchi P, Cipolotti L, and Denes G. Impairment in processing meaningless verbal material in several modalities: The relationship between short-term memory and phonological skills. *Quarterly Journal of Experimental Psychology 41A*: 293–319, 1989.

Blanken G. Formal paraphasias: A single case study. *Brain and Language 38*: 534–554, 1990.

Blumstein SE, Baker E, and Goodglass H. Phonological factors in auditory comprehension in aphasia. *Neuropsychologia 15*: 19–30, 1977a.

Blumstein SE, Cooper WE, Zurif EB, and Caramazza A. The perception and production of voice-onset time in aphasia. *Neuropsychologia 15*: 371–383, 1977b.

Boller F, and Green E. Comprehension in severe aphasics. *Cortex 8*: 382–394, 1972.

Borgo F, and Shallice T. When living things and other "sensory quality" categories behave in the same fashion: A novel category specification. *Neurocase 7*: 201–220, 2001.

Brain WR. *Speech disorders*. London: Butterworths, 1961.

Breedin S, Saffran E, and Schwartz M. Semantic factors in verb retrieval: An effect of complexity. *Brain and Language 63*: 1–31, 1998.

Breen K, and Warrington EK. A study of anomia: Evidence for a distinction between nominal and propositional language. *Cortex 30*: 131–145, 1994.

Brenneise-Sarshad R, Nicholas LE, and Brookshire RH. Effects of apparent listener knowledge and picture stimuli on aphasic and non-brain-damaged speakers' narrative discourse. *Journal of Speech and Hearing Research 34*: 168–176, 1991.

Brindley P, Copeland M, Demain C, and Martyn P. A comparison of the speech of ten Broca's aphasics following intensive and non-intensive periods of therapy. *Aphasiology 3*: 695–707, 1989.

Broca PP. Remarques sur le siège de la faculté de la parole articulée, suivies d'une observation d'aphémie (perte de parole). *Bulletin de la Société d'Anatomie (Paris) 36*: 330–357, 1861.

Broca PP. Sur le siége de la faculté du language articulé. *Bulletin d'Anthropologie 6*: 377–393, 1865.

Broida H. Language therapy effects in long term aphasia. *Archives of Physical Medicine and Rehabilitation 58*: 248–253, 1977.

Brookshire RH. Effects of delay of reinforcement on probability learning by aphasic subjects. *Journal of Speech and Hearing Research 14*: 92–105, 1971.

Brown AS. A review of the tip-of-the-tongue experience. *Psychological Bulletin 109*: 204–223, 1991.

Brown AS, and McNeill D. The "tip-of-the-tongue" phenomenon. *Journal of Verbal Learning and Verbal Behavior 5*: 325–337, 1966.

Brown JW. *Aphasia, apraxia, and agnosia*. Springfield, IL: Charles C. Thomas, 1972.

Brownell HH, Potter HH, and Bihrle AM. Inference deficits in right-brain-damaged patients. *Brain and Language 27*: 310–321, 1986.

Bub D, Black S, Howell J, and Kertesz A. Speech output processes and reading. In M Coltheart, G Sartori, and R Job (Eds.), *The cognitive neuropsychology of language*. Hove, UK: Lawrence Erlbaum Associates, 1987, pp. 79–110.

Bub D, Cancelliere A, and Kertesz A. Whole-word and analytic translation of spelling-to-sound in a non-semantic reader. In KE Patterson, J Marshall, and M Coltheart (Eds.), *Surface dyslexia*. Hove, UK: Lawrence Erlbaum Associates, 1985, pp. 15–34.

Bub D, and Kertesz A. Deep agraphia. *Brain and Language 17*: 146–165, 1982a.

Bub D, and Kertesz A. Evidence for lexicographic processing in a patient with preserved written over oral single word naming. *Brain 105*: 697–717, 1982b.

Butfield E, and Zangwill OL. Re-education in aphasia: A review of 70 cases. *Journal of Neurology, Neurosurgery and Psychiatry 9*: 75–79, 1946.

Butterworth B. Hesitation and the production of verbal paraphasias and neologisms in jargon aphasia. *Brain and Language 8*: 133–161, 1979.

Butterworth B. Lexical representation. In B Butterworth (Ed.), *Language production*, Vol. 2. New York: Academic Press, 1983, pp. 257–294.

Butterworth B. Jargon aphasia: Processes and strategies. In SK Newman and R Epstein (Eds.), *Current perspectives in dysphasia*. London: Academic Press, 1985, pp. 61–96.

Butterworth B. Disorders of phonological encoding. *Cognition 42*: 261–286, 1992.

Byng S. Sentence processing deficits: Theory and therapy. *Cognitive Neuropsychology 5*: 629–676, 1988.

Byng S. Hypothesis testing and aphasia therapy. In AL Holland and M Forbes (Eds.), *Aphasia treatment. World perspectives*. San Diego, CA: Singular Publishing Group. 1993, pp. 115–130.

Byng S. What is aphasia therapy? In C Code and D Müller (Eds.), *Treatment of aphasia: From theory to practice*. London: Whurr Publishers Ltd, 1995, pp. 1–17.

Byng S, Nickels L, and Black M. Replicating therapy for mapping deficits in agrammatism: Remapping the deficit? *Aphasiology 8*: 315–342, 1994.

Cambier J, Elghozi D, Signoret JL, and Henin D. Contribution de l'hémisphère droit au language des aphasiques: Disparition de ce language après lésion droite. *Revue Neurologique 139*: 55–63, 1983.

Caplan D. *Neurolinguistics and linguistic aphasiology*. Cambridge: Cambridge University Press, 1987.

Cappa S. Spontaneous recovery from aphasia. In B Stemmer and HA Whitaker (Eds.), *Handbook of neurolinguistics*. San Diego, CA: Academic Press, 1998, pp. 535–545.

Cappa S. Neuroimaging of recovery from aphasia. *Neuropsychological Rehabilitation 10*: 365–376, 2000.

Cappa S, Miozzo A, and Frugoni M. Glossolalic jargon after a right hemisphere stroke in a patient with Wernicke's aphasia. *Aphasiology 8*: 83–87, 1994.

Cappa S, and Vallar G. The role of the left and right hemispheres in the recovery from aphasia. *Aphasiology 6*: 354–372, 1992.

Cappa S, and Vignolo LA. "Transcortical" features of aphasia following left thalamic hemorrhage. *Cortex 15*: 121–130, 1979.

Caramazza A. The logic of neuropsychological research and the problem of patient classification in aphasia. *Brain and Language 21*: 9–20, 1984.

Caramazza A. On drawing inferences about the structure of normal cognitive systems from the analysis of patterns of impaired performance: The case for single-patient studies. *Brain and Cognition 5*: 41–66, 1986.

Caramazza A. The interpretation of semantic category-specific deficits: What do they reveal about the organization of conceptual knowledge in the brain? *Neurocase 4*: 265–272, 1998.

Caramazza A, and Hillis AE. Where do semantic errors come from? *Cortex 26*: 95–122, 1990.

Caramazza A, and Hillis AE. Lexical organization of nouns and verbs in the brain. *Nature 349*: 788–790, 1991.

Caramazza A, and Hillis AE. For a theory of remediation of cognitive deficits. *Neuropsychological Rehabilitation 3*: 217–234, 1993.

Caramazza A, Hillis AE, Rapp BC, and Romani C. The multiple semantic hypothesis: Multiple confusions? *Cognitive Neuropsychology 7*: 161–190, 1990.

Caramazza A, and McCloskey M. The case for single-patient studies. *Cognitive Neuropsychology 5*: 517–528, 1988.

Caramazza A, and Miceli G. The structure of graphemic representations. *Cognition 37*: 243–297, 1990.

Caramazza A, Miceli G, and Villa G. The role of the (output) phonological buffer in reading, writing and repetition. *Cognitive Neuropsychology 3*: 37–76, 1986.

Caramazza A, Miceli G, Villa G, and Romani C. The role of the graphemic buffer in spelling: Evidence from a case of acquired dysgraphia. *Cognition 26*: 59–85, 1987.

Caramazza A, and Shelton JR. Domain-specific knowledge systems in the brain. The animate–inanimate distinction. *Journal of Cognitive Neuroscience 10*: 1–34, 1998.

Caramazza A, and Zurif E. Dissociation of algorithmic and heuristic processes in language comprehension: Evidence from aphasia. *Brain and Language 3*: 572–582, 1976.

Cardebat D, Léger M, Puel M, Aithamon B, Touyeras B, Boulanouar K, and Démonet J-F. A functional MRI study of language therapy in a conduction aphasic patient. *Brain and Language 74*: 392–394, 2000.

Carlomagno S, and Parlato V. Writing rehabilitation in brain-damaged adult aphasics: A cognitive approach. In X Seron and G Deloche (Eds.), *Cognitive approaches in neuropsychological rehabilitation.* Hillsdale, NJ: Lawrence Erlbaum Associates, 1989, pp. 175–209.

Charcot J. *Differenti forme d'afasia. Lezioni fatte nella Salpêtrière nel semestre d'estate dell'anno 1883.* Milan: Vallardi, 1884.

Chomsky N. *Syntactic structures.* The Hague: Mouton, 1957.

Chomsky N. *Some concepts and consequences of the theory of government and binding.* Cambridge, MA: MIT Press, 1982.

Cicerone KD, Dahlberg C, Kalmar K, Langenbahn DM, Malec JF, Bergquist TF, Felicetti T, Giacino JT, Harley JP, Harrington DE, Herzog J, Kneipp S, Laatsch L, and Morse PA. Evidence-based cognitive rehabilitation: Recommendations for clinical practice. *Archives of Physical Medicine and Rehabilitation 81*: 1596–1615, 2000.

Collignon R, Hécaen H, and Angelergues G. A propos de 12 cas d'aphasie acquise chez l'enfant. *Acta Neurologica et Psychiatrica Belgica 68*: 245–277, 1968.

Coltheart M. Aphasia therapy research: A single-case study approach. In C Code and DJ Müller (Eds.), *Aphasia therapy.* London: Edward Arnold, 1983, pp. 194–202.

Coltheart M. Editorial. *Cognitive Neuropsychology 1*: 1–8, 1984.

Coltheart M, and Byng S. A treatment for surface dyslexia. In X Seron, and G Deloche (Eds.), *Cognitive approaches in neuropsychological rehabilitation.* Hillsdale, NJ: Lawrence Erlbaum Associates, 1989, pp. 159–174.

Coppens P, Lebrun Y, and Basso A. (Eds.). *Aphasia in atypical populations.* Mahwah, NJ: Lawrence Erlbaum Associates, 1998a.

Coppens P, Parente MA, and Lecours AR. Aphasia in illiterate individuals. In P Coppens, Y Lebrun, and A Basso (Eds.), *Aphasia in atypical populations.* Mahwah, NJ: Lawrence Erlbaum Associates, 1998b, pp. 175–202.

Costlett HB, Gonzalez-Rothi L, Valenstein E, and Heilman KM. Dissociation of writing and praxis: Two cases in point. *Brain and Language 28*: 357–369, 1986.

Cuetos F, Valle-Arroyo F, and Suarez M-P. A case of phonological dyslexia in Spanish. *Cognitive Neuropsychology 13*: 1–24, 1996.

Damasio H. Neuroanatomical correlates of the aphasias. In MT Sarno (Ed.), *Acquired aphasia* (2nd ed.). San Diego, CA: Academic Press, 1991, pp. 45–71.

Damasio H, and Damasio A. The anatomical basis of conduction aphasia. *Brain 103*: 337–350, 1980.

Damasio H, Grabowski T, Tranel D, Hichwa RD, and Damasio AR. A neural basis for lexical retrieval. *Nature 380*: 499–505, 1996.

Darley FL. Treat or neglect? *Asha 21*: 628–631, 1979.

Darley FL. *Aphasia*. Philadelphia: W.B. Saunders Company, 1982.

David RM, Enderby P, and Bainton D. Treatment of acquired aphasia: Speech therapists and volunteers compared. *Journal of Neurology, Neurosurgery and Psychiatry 45*: 957–961, 1982.

David RM, Enderby P, and Bainton D. Speech therapists and volunteers—Some comments on recent investigations of their effectiveness in the treatment of aphasia. Response to T. R. Pring. *British Journal of Disorders of Communication 18*: 73–77, 1983a.

David RM, Enderby P, and Bainton D. Treatment of acquired aphasia: Speech therapists and volunteers compared. Reply. *Journal of Neurology, Neurosurgery and Psychiatry 46*: 692–693, 1983b.

Davis G, and Wilcox M. *Adult aphasia rehabilitation: Applied pragmatics*. Windsor: NFER-Nelson, 1985.

Davis L, Foldi NS, Gardner H, and Zurif E. Repetition in the transcortical aphasias. *Brain and Language 6*: 226–238, 1978.

Dejerine JJ. Sur un cas de cécité verbale avec agraphie suivi d'autopsie. *Mémoires-Société Biologie 3*: 197–201, 1891.

Dejerine JJ. Contribution à l'étude anatomo-clinique des différentes variétés de cécité verbale. *Mémoires-Société Biologie 4*: 61–90, 1892.

Denes G, Meneghello F, Vallese F, and Vanelli L. Task-dependent noun retrieval deficit: An experimental case study. *Neurocase 2*: 35–42, 1996a.

Denes G, Perazzolo C, Piani A, and Piccione F. Intensive versus regular speech therapy in global aphasia: A controlled study. *Aphasiology 10*: 385–394, 1996b.

De Partz M-P. Reeducation of a deep dyslexic patient: Rationale of the method and results. *Cognitive Neuropsychology 3*: 149–177, 1986.

De Partz M-P. Deficit of the graphemic buffer: Effects of a written lexical segmentation strategy. *Neuropsychological Rehabilitation 5*: 129–147, 1995.

De Renzi E, and Faglioni P. Normative data and screening power of a shortened version of the Token Test. *Cortex 14*: 41–49, 1978.

De Renzi E, and Vignolo LA. The Token Test: A sensitive test to detect receptive disturbances in aphasics. *Brain 85*: 556–578, 1962.

Dérouesné J, and Beauvois M-F. Phonological processing in reading: Data from alexia. *Journal of Neurology, Neurosurgery and Psychiatry 42*: 1125–1132, 1979.

Dérouesné J, and Beauvois M-F. The "phonemic" stage in the nonlexical reading process: Evidence from a case of phonological alexia. In KE Patterson, JC Marshall, and M Coltheart (Eds.), *Surface dyslexia*. Hove, UK: Lawrence Erlbaum Associates, 1985, pp. 399–457.

Devlin JT, Gonnerman LM, Andersen ES, and Seidenberg MS. Category-specific semantic deficit in focal and widespread brain damage: A computational account. *Journal of Cognitive Neuroscience 10*: 77–94, 1998.

Dubois J, Hécaen H, and Marcie P. L'agraphie "pure." *Neuropsychologia, 7*, 271–286, 1969.

Ducarne de Ribaucourt B. *Rééducation sémiologique de l'aphasie*. Paris: Masson, 1986.

Edwards AE. Automated training for a "matching-to-sample" task in aphasia. *Journal of Speech and Hearing Research 8*: 39–42, 1965.

Elbert T, Pantev C, Weinbruch C, Rockstroh B, and Taub E. Increased cortical representation of the fingers of the left hand in string players. *Science 270*: 305–307, 1995.

Ellis AW, Miller D, and Sing G. Wernicke's aphasia and normal language processing: A case study in cognitive neuropsychology. *Cognition 15*: 111–144, 1983.

Ellis AW, and Young AW. *Human cognitive neuropsychology*. Hove, UK: Lawrence Erlbaum Associates, 1988.

Farah MJ, and Wallace MA. Semantically-bounded anomia: Implications for the neural implementation of naming. *Neuropsychologia 30*: 609–621, 1992.

Fitz-Gibbon CT. In defense of randomised controlled trials, with suggestions about the possible use of meta-analysis. *British Journal of Disorders of Communication 21*: 117–124, 1986.

Fodor JA. *The modularity of mind*. Cambridge, MA: MIT Press, 1983.

Foldi NS. Appreciation of pragmatic interpretation of indirect commands: Comparison of right and left hemisphere brain-damaged patients. *Brain and Language 31*: 88–108, 1987.

Foldi NS, Cicone M, and Gardner H. Pragmatic aspects of communication in brain-damaged patients. In S Segalowitz (Ed.), *Language functions and brain organization*. New York: Academic Press, 1983, pp. 51–86.

Franklin SE. Dissociations in auditory word comprehension; evidence from nine fluent aphasic patients. *Aphasiology 3*: 189–207, 1989.

Franklin SE, Howard D, and Patterson K. Abstract word anomia. *Cognitive Neuropsychology 12*: 549–566, 1995.

Friedman RB, and Kohn SE. Imparied activation of the phonological lexicon: Effects upon oral reading. *Brain and Language 38*: 278–298, 1990.

Froeschels E. Ueber die Behandlung der Aphasien. *Archiv fur Psychiatrie und Nervenkrankheiten 53*: 221–261, 1914.

Froeschels E. Zur Behandlung der motorischen Aphasie. *Archiv fur Psychiatrie und Nervenkrankheiten 56*: 1–19, 1916.

Funnell E. Phonological processing in reading: New evidence from acquired dyslexia. *British Journal of Psychology 74*: 159–180, 1983.

Gainotti G. The riddle of the right hemisphere's contribution to the recovery of language. *Journal of Disorders of Communication 28*: 227–246, 1993.

Gainotti G. Development of the concept of aphasia. In G Denes and L Pizzamiglio (Eds.), *Handbook of clinical and experimental neuropsychology*. Hove, UK: Psychology Press, 1999, pp. 135–154.

Gainotti G. What the locus of brain lesion tells us about the nature of the cognitive defect underlying category-specific disorders: A review. *Cortex 36*: 539–559, 2000.

Gainotti G, Silveri MC, Villa G, and Miceli G. Anomia with and without lexical comprehension disorders. *Brain and Language 29*: 18–33, 1986.

Gall F. *Sur les fonctions du cerveau et sur celles de chacune de ses parties*. Paris: Baillière, 1825.

Garrett MF. The analysis of sentence production. In GH Bower (Ed.), *The psychology of learning and motivation*, Vol. 9. New York: Academic Press, 1975, pp. 133–177.

Garrett MF. Levels of processing in sentence production. In B Butterworth (Ed.), *Language production*, Vol. 1. New York: Academic Press, 1980, pp. 177–220.

Garrett MF. Production of speech: Observation from normal and pathological language use. In AW Ellis (Ed.), *Normality and pathology in cognitive functions*. London: Academic Press, 1982, pp. 19–76.

Gerber S, and Gurland GB. Applied pragmatics in the assessment of aphasia. *Seminars in Speech and Language 10*: 263–281, 1989.

Gernsbacher MA. Resolving 20 years of inconsistent interactions between lexical familiarity and orthography, concreteness, and polysemy. *Journal of Experimental Psychology: General 113*: 256–281, 1984.

Geschwind N. The paradoxical position of Kurt Goldstein in the history of aphasia. *Cortex 1*: 214–224, 1964.

Geschwind N. Disconnection syndromes in animals and man. *Brain 88*: 237–294, 585–644, 1965.

Geschwind N. Wernicke's contribution to the study of aphasia. *Cortex 3*: 449–463, 1967.

Geschwind N. *Selected papers on language and the brain* (edited by RS Cohen and MX Wartofsky) Boston: D. Reidel Publishing Company, 1974.

Gleason JB, Goodglass H, Green H, Ackerman N, and Hyde MR. The retrieval of syntax in Broca's aphasia. *Brain and Language 2*: 451–471, 1975.

Gloning I, Gloning K, and Hoff H. Aphasia. A clinical syndrome. In L Halpern (ed.), *Problems of dynamic neurology*. Jerusalem: Hebrew University, 1963, pp. 63–70.

Gloning K, Trappl R, Heiss WD, and Quatember R. Prognosis and speech therapy in aphasia. In Y Lebrun and R Hoops (Eds.), *Recovery in aphasics*. Atlantic Highlands, NJ: Humanities Press, 1976, pp. 57–62.

Goldberg E. *Contemporary neuropsychology and the legacy of Luria*. Hillsdale, NJ: Lawrence Erlbaum Associates, 1990.

Golden CJ, Hammeke TA, and Purisch AD. *The Luria-Nebraska neuropsychological battery*. Los Angeles: Western Psychological Services, 1980.

Goldstein K. *Language and language disturbances*. New York: Grune & Stratton, 1948.

Goodglass H. *Understanding aphasia*. San Diego CA: Academic Press, 1993.

Goodglass H, and Hunter M. A linguistic comparison of speech and writing in two types of aphasia. *Journal of Communication Disorders 3*: 28–35, 1970.

Goodglass H, and Kaplan E. *The assessment of aphasia and related disorders*. Philadelphia: Lea and Febiger, 1972 (2nd ed. 1983).

Goodman RA, and Caramazza A. Aspects of the spelling process: Evidence from a case of acquired dysgraphia. *Language and Cognitive Processes 1*: 263–296, 1986.

Gowers WR. *Lectures on the diagnosis of diseases of the brain.* London: Churchill, 1887.

Green G. Communication in aphasia therapy: Some of the procedures and issues involved. *British Journal of Disorders of Communication 19*: 35–46, 1984.

Greener J, Enderby P, and Whurr R. Speech and language therapy for aphasia following stroke (Cochrane review). In: *The Cochrane Library*, Issue 4. Oxford: Update software, 1999.

Greenwald ML, Raymer AM, Richardson ME, and Rothi LJG. Contrasting treatments for severe impairments of picture naming. *Neuropsychological Rehabilitation 5*: 17–49, 1995.

Grice P. Logic and conversation. In P Cole and J Morgan (Eds.), *Syntax and semantics 3: Speech acts.* London: Academic Press, 1975, pp. 41–58.

Gutzmann H. Heilungsversuche bei centromotorischer und centrosensoricher Aphasie. *Archiv fur Psychiatrie und Nervenkrankheiten 28*: 354–378, 1896.

Haendiges AN, Berndt RS, and Mitchum CC. Assessing the elements contributing to a "mapping" deficit: A targeted treatment study. *Brain and Language 52*: 276–302, 1996.

Hagen C. Communication abilities in hemiplegia: Effect of speech therapy. *Archives of Physical Medicine and Rehabilitation 54*: 454–463, 1973.

Hanson WR, and Cicciarelli AW. The time, amount, and pattern of language improvement in adult aphasics. *British Journal of Disorders of Communication 13*: 59–63, 1978.

Hanson WR, Metter JF, and Riege WH. The course of chronic aphasia. *Aphasiology 3*: 19–29, 1989.

Hartman J, and Landau WM. Comparison of formal language therapy with supportive counseling for aphasia due to acute vascular accident. *Archives of Neurology 24*: 646–649, 1987.

Hatfield FM. Looking for help from linguistics. *British Journal of Disorders of Communication 7*: 64–81, 1972.

Hatfield FM, and Patterson KE. Phonological spelling. *Quarterly Journal of Experimental Psychology 35A*: 451–468, 1983.

Hatfield FM, and Shewell C. Some applications of linguistics to aphasia therapy. In C Code and DJ Müller (Eds.), *Aphasia therapy.* London: Edward Arnold, 1983, pp. 61–75.

Head H. *Aphasia and kindred disorders of speech*. Cambridge: Cambridge University Press, 1926.

Hebb DO. *The organization of behavior. A neuropsychological theory*. New York: John Wiley & Sons, 1949.

Hécaen H, and Albert ML. *Human Neuropsychology*. New York: John Wiley & Sons, 1978.

Hécaen H, and Lanteri-Laura G. *Evolution des connaissances et des doctrines sur les localisations cérébrales*. Paris: Desclée de Brouwer, 1977.

Heilman KM, Tucker DM, and Valenstein E. A case of mixed transcortical aphasia with intact naming. *Brain 99*: 415–426, 1976.

Helm NA, and Barresi B. Voluntary control of involuntary utterances: A treatment approach for severe aphasia. *Clinical Aphasiology 10*: 308–315, 1980.

Helm-Estabrooks N, and Albert M. *Manual of aphasia therapy*. Austin, TX: Pro-Ed, 1991.

Helm-Estabrooks N, Emery P, and Albert M. Treatment of Aphasic Perseveration (TAP) program. *Archives of Neurology 44*: 1253–1255, 1987.

Helm-Estabrooks N, Fitzpatrick PM, and Barresi B. Responses of an agrammatic patient to a syntax stimulation program for aphasia. *Journal of Speech and Hearing Disorders 46*: 422–427, 1982.

Helmick JW, and Wipplinger M. Effects of stimulus repetition on the naming behavior of an aphasic adult: A clinical report. *Journal of Communication Disorders 8*: 23–29, 1975.

Hemsley G, and Code C. Interactions between recovery in aphasia, emotional and psychosocial factors in subjects with aphasia, their significant others and speech pathologists. *Disability and Rehabilitation 18*: 567–584, 1996.

Henaff Gonon MA, Bruckert R, and Michel F. Lexicalization in an anomic patient. *Neuropsychologia 27*: 391–407, 1989.

Henschen SE. *Klinische und pathologische Beitrage zur Pathologie des Gehirns*. Stockholm: Almqvist und Wiksell, 1922.

Hier DB, and Mohr JP. Incongruous oral and written naming. *Brain and Language 4*: 115–126, 1977.

Hillis AE, and Caramazza A. Mechanisms for accessing lexical representations for output: Evidence from a category-specific semantic deficit. *Brain and Language 40*: 106–144, 1991.

Hillis AE, and Caramazza A. Converging evidence for the interaction of semantic and sublexical phonological information in accessing lexical representations for spoken output. *Cognitive Neuropsychology 12*: 187–227, 1995.

Hillis AE, Rapp B, and Caramazza A. When a rose is a rose in speech but a tulip in writing. *Cortex 35*: 337–356, 1999.

Hillis AE, Rapp B, Romani C, and Caramazza A. Selective impairment of semantics in lexical processing. *Cognitive Neuropsychology 7*: 191–243, 1990.

Holland AL. Some clinical applications of behavioral principles to clinical speech problems. *Journal of Speech and Hearing Disorders 32*: 11–16, 1967.

Holland AL. Case studies in aphasia rehabilitation using programmed instruction. *Journal of Speech and Hearing Disorders 35*: 377–390, 1970.

Holland AL. *Communicative abilities in daily living*. Baltimore: University Park Press, 1980.

Holland A. Pragmatic aspects of intervention in aphasia. *Journal of Neurolinguistics 6*: 197–211, 1991.

Holland AL, and Forbes M. *Aphasia treatment. World perspectives*. San Diego, CA: Singular Publishing Group, 1993.

Holland AL, and Levy C. Syntactic generalization in aphasia as a function of relearning an active declarative sentence. *Acta Symbolica 2*: 34–41, 1971.

Howard D. Beyond randomised controlled trials: The case for effective studies of the effects of treatment in aphasia. *British Journal of Disorders of Communication 21*: 89–102, 1986.

Howard D, and Franklin S. *Missing the meaning. A cognitive neuropsychological study of processing words by an aphasic patient*. London: MIT Press, 1988.

Howard D, and Hatfield FM. *Aphasia therapy. Historical and contemporary issues*. Hillsdale, NJ: Lawrence Erlbaum Associates, 1987.

Howard D, and Patterson K. Models for therapy. In X Seron and G Deloche (Eds.), *Cognitive approaches in neuropsychological rehabilitation*. Hillsdale, NJ: Lawrence Erlbaum Associates, 1989, pp. 39–64.

Howard D, Patterson KE, Franklin S, Morton J, and Orchard-Lisle VM. Variability and consistency in picture naming by aphasic patients. In FC Rose (Ed.), *Recent advances in neurology, 42: Progress in aphasiology*. New York: Raven Press, 1984, pp. 263–276.

Howard D, Patterson K, Franklin S, Orchard-Lisle V, and Morton J. Treatment of word retrieval deficits in aphasia: A comparison of two therapy methods. *Brain 108*: 817–829, 1985.

Huber W. Text comprehension and production in aphasia: Analysis in term of micro- and macrostructure. In Y Joanette and H Brownell (Eds.), *Discourse ability and brain damage: Theoretical and empirical perspectives*. New York: Springer Verlag, 1990, pp. 154–179.

Huber W, Poeck K, Springer L, and Willmes C. Treatment of acquired aphasia: Speech therapists and volunteers compared. Letter to the editor. *Journal of Neurology, Neurosurgery and Psychiatry 46*: 691–692, 1983.

Huber W, Poeck K, and Willmes C. The Aachen test. In FC Rose (Ed.), *Progress in aphasiology*. New York: Raven Press, 1984, pp. 291–303.

Huber W, Springer L, and Willmes K. Approaches to aphasia therapy in Aachen. In AL Holland and FF Forbes (Eds.), *Aphasia treatment. World perspectives*. San Diego, CA: Singular Publishing Group, 1993, pp. 55–86.

Jackson JH. On affections of speech from disease of the brain. *Brain 1*: 304–330; *2*: 203–222, 323–356, 1878.

Jackson JH. *Selected writings of John Hughlings Jackson*. New York: Basic Book, 1958.

Jakobson R. Towards a linguistic typology of aphasic impairments. In AVS de Reuck and M O'Connor (Eds.), *Disorders of language*. London: Churchill Livingstone, 1964, pp. 21–42.

Jones EV. Building the foundation for sentence production in a non-fluent aphasic. *British Journal of Disorders of Communication 21*: 63–82, 1986.

Kaas JH. Plasticity of sensory and motor maps in adult mammals. *Annual Review of Neuroscience 14*: 137–167, 1991.

Kadzielewa D, Dabrowska A, Nowakowska M, and Seniow J. Literal and conveyed meaning as interpreted by aphasics and nonaphasics. *Polish Psychological Bulletin 12*: 57–62, 1981.

Kaplan E, Goodglass H, and Weintraub S. *Boston naming test*. Philadelphia: Lea & Febiger, 1983.

Katz RB, and Goodglass H. Deep dysphasia: Analysis of a rare form of repetition disorder. *Brain and Language 39*: 153–185, 1990.

Katz RC, Hallowell B, Code C, Armstrong E, Roberts P, Pound C, and Katz L. A multinational comparison in aphasia management practices. *International Journal of Language and Communication Disorders 35*: 303–314, 2000.

Kay J, and Ellis AW. A cognitive neuropsychological case study of anomia: Implications for psychological models of word retrieval. *Brain 110*: 613–629, 1987.

Kay J, and Hanley R. Simultaneous form perception and serial letter recognition in a case of letter-by-letter reading. *Cognitive Neuropsychology 8*: 249–273, 1991.

Kay J, Lesser R, and Coltheart M. *Psycholinguistic assessment of language processing in aphasia*. Hove, UK: Lawrence Erlbaum Associates, 1992.

Kearns KP, and Salmon SJ. An experimental analysis of auxiliary and copula verb generalisation in aphasia. *Journal of Speech and Hearing Disorders 49*: 152–163, 1984.

Kenin M, and Swisher LP. A study of pattern of recovery in aphasia. *Cortex 8:* 56–68, 1972.

Kertesz A. *The Western aphasia battery*. New York: Grune & Stratton, 1982.

Kertesz A, and McCabe P. Recovery patterns and prognosis in aphasia. *Brain 100*: 1–18, 1977.

Kertesz A, and Phipps JB. Numerical taxonomy of aphasia. *Brain and Language 4*: 1–10, 1977.

Kimelman MDZ. Prosody, linguistic demands, and auditory comprehension in aphasia. *Brain and Language 69*: 212–221, 1999.

Kinsbourne M, and Rosenfield DB. Agraphia selective for written spelling: An experimental case study. *Brain and Language 1*: 215–225, 1974.

Klippel M (Ed.). Discussion sur l'aphasie. *Revue Neurologique 16*: 611–636, 974–1023, 1025–1047, 1908.

Kohn SE, Lorch M, and Pearson D. Verb finding in aphasia. *Cortex 25*: 57–69, 1989.

Kremin H. Is there more than ah-oh-ah? Alternative strategies for writing and repeating lexically. In M Coltheart, G Sartori, and R Job (Eds.), *The cognitive neuropsychology of language*. Hillsdale, NJ: Lawrence Erlbaum Associates, 1987, pp. 295–335.

Kremin H. Therapeutic approaches to naming disorders. In M Paradis (Ed.), *Foundations of aphasia rehabilitation*. Oxford: Pergamon Press, 1993, pp. 261–292.

Kremin H, and Basso A. Apropos the mental lexicon: The naming of nouns and verbs. In FJ Stachowiak (Ed.), *Developments in the assessment and rehabilitation of brain-damaged patients. Perspectives from a European concerted action*. Tubingen: Gunter Narr Verlag, 1993, pp. 233–242.

Kremin H, Hahn-Barma V, Guichart-Gomez E, and Dubois B. Preserved picture naming in spite of impaired semantic comprehension: A case study. *Brain and Language 79*: 41–43, 2001.

Kucera H, and Francis WN. *Computational analysis of present-day American English*. Providence, RI: Brown University Press, 1967.

Kussmaul A. *Die Störungen der Sprache*. Leipzig: Vogel, 1877.

Laiacona M, and Capitani E. A case of prevailing deficit of nonliving categories or a case of prevailing sparing of living categories? *Cognitive Neuropsychology 18*: 39–70, 2001.

Leal MG, Farrajota L, Fonseca J, Guerriero M, and Castro-Caldas A. The influence of speech therapy on the evolution of stroke patients (Abstract). *Journal of Clinical and Experimental Neuropsychology 15*: 399, 1993.

Lecours AR, Chain F, Poncet M, and Nespoulous J-L. Paris 1908: The hot summer of aphasiology or a season in the life of a chair. *Brain and Language 32*: 105–152, 1992.

Le Dorze G, and Nespoulous J-L. Anomia in moderate aphasia: Problems in accessing the lexical representation. *Brain and Language 37*: 381–400, 1989.

Le Dorze G, and Pitts C. A case study evaluation of the effects of different techniques for the treatment of anomia. *Neuropsychological Rehabilitation 5*: 51–65, 1995.

Lee H, Nakada T, Deal JL, Lynn S, and Kwee IL. Transfer of language dominance. *Annals of Neurology 15*: 304–307, 1984.

Legh-Smith JA, Denis R, Enderby PM, Wade DT, and Langton-Hewer R. Selection of aphasic stroke patients for intensive speech therapy. *Journal of Neurology, Neurosurgery, and Psychiatry 50*: 1488–1492, 1987.

Leischner A, and Lynk HA. Neure Erfahrungen mit der Behandlung von Aphasien. *Nervenartz 38*: 199–205, 1967.

Lendrem W, and Lincoln NB. Spontaneous recovery of language in patients with aphasia between 4 and 34 weeks after stroke. *Journal of Neurology, Neurosurgery and Psychiatry 48*: 743–748, 1985.

Lesser R. Aphasia: Theory-based intervention. In MM Leahy (Ed.), *Disorders of communication: The science of intervention*. New York: Taylor and Francis, 1989, pp. 189–205.

Lesser R, and Milroy L. *Linguistics and aphasia. Psycholinguistic and pragmatic aspects of intervention*. London: Longman, 1993.

Levinson SC. *Pragmatics*. Cambridge: Cambridge University Press, 1983.

Levita E. Effects of speech therapy on aphasics' responses to the Functional Communication Profile. *Perceptual and Motor Skills 47*: 151–154, 1978.

Lhermitte F, and Dérouesné J. Paraphasies et jargonaphasie dans le language oral avec conservation du language écrit. *Revue Neurologique 130*: 21–38, 1974.

Lichtheim L. On aphasia. *Brain 7*: 433–484, 1885.

Lincoln NB, McGuirk E, Mulley GP, Lendrem W, Jones AC, and Mitchell JRA. Effectiveness of speech therapy for aphasic stroke patients: A randomized controlled trial. *Lancet 1*: 1197–1200, 1984.

Linebarger M, Schwartz M, and Saffran E. Sensitivity to grammatical structure in so-called agrammatic aphasics. *Cognition 13*: 361–392, 1983.

Lomas J, and Kertesz A. Patterns of spontaneous recovery in aphasic groups: A study of adult stroke patients. *Brain and Language 5*: 388–401, 1978.

Loonen MCB, and van Dongen HR. Outcome one year after onset. In IP Martins, A Castro-Caldas, HR van Dongen, and A van Hout (Eds.), *Acquired aphasia in children*. Dordrecht: Kluwer Academic Publishers, 1991, pp. 185–200.

Luria AR. *Restoration of function after brain injury*. Oxford: Pergamon Press, 1963.

Luria AR. Factors and forms of aphasia. In AVS de Reuck and M O'Connor (Eds.), *Ciba foundation symposium on disorders of language*. London: Churchill Livingstone, 1964, pp. 143–161.

Luria AR. *Traumatic aphasia*. The Hague: Mouton, 1970.

Luria AR, Nyadin VL, Tsvetkova LS, and Vinarskaya EN. Restoration of higher cortical function following local brain damage. In PJ Vinken and GW Bruyn (Eds.), *Handbook of clinical neurology*, Vol. 3. Amsterdam: North-Holland Publishing Company, 1969, pp. 368–433.

Luzzatti C, Colombo C, Frustaci M, and Vitolo F. Rehabilitation of spelling along the sub-word-level routine. *Neuropsychological Rehabilitation 10*: 249–278, 2000.

Mackenzie C. An aphasia group intensive efficacy study. *British Journal of Disorders of Communication 26*: 275–291, 1991.

MacMahon MKC. Modern linguistics and aphasia. *British Journal of Disorders of Communication 7*: 54–65, 1972.

Manning L, and Warrington EK. Two routes to naming: A case study. *Neuropsychologia 34*: 581–600, 1996.

Marangolo P, Basso A, and Rinaldi MC. Preserved confrontation naming and impaired sentence completion: A case study. *Neurocase 5*: 213–221, 1999.

Marie P. Révision de la question de l'aphasie: la troisième circonvolution frontale gauche ne joue aucun rôle spécial dans la fonction du langage. *Semaine Médicale 26*: 241–247, 1906.

Marie P, and Foix Ch. Les aphasies de guerre. *Revue Neurologique 25*: 53–87, 1917.

Marks M, Taylor M, and Rusk HA. Rehabilitation of the aphasic patient: A summary of three years' experience in a rehabilitation setting. *Archives of Physical Medicine and Rehabilitation 38*: 219–226, 1957.

Marshall J. The mapping hypothesis and aphasia therapy. *Aphasiology 9*: 517–539, 1995.

Marshall J, Pound C, White-Thompson M, and Pring T. The use of picture-word matching tasks to assist word retrieval in aphasic patients. *Aphasiology 4*: 167–184, 1990.

Marshall J, Pring T, and Chiat S. Sentence processing therapy: Working at the level of the event. *Aphasiology 7*: 177–199, 1993.

Marshall JC, and Newcombe F. Syntactic and semantic errors in paralexia. *Neuropsychologia 4*: 169–176, 1966.

Marshall JC, and Newcombe F. Patterns of paralexia: A psycholinguistic approach. *Journal of Psycholinguistic Research 2*: 175–199, 1973.

Marshall RC, Tompkins C, and Phillips DS. Improvement in treated aphasia: Examination of selected prognostic factors. *Folia Phoniatrica 34*: 305–315, 1982.

Marshall RC, Wertz RT, Weiss DG, Aten JL, Brookshire RH, Garcia-Bunuel L, Holland AL, Kurtzke JF, LaPointe LL, Milianti FJ, Brannegan R, Greenbaum H, Vogel D, Carter J, Barnes NS, and Goodman R. Home treatment for aphasic patients by trained nonprofessionals. *Journal of Speech and Hearing Disorders 54*: 462–470, 1989.

Martin N, Dell GS, Saffran EM, and Schwartz MF. Origins of paraphasias in deep dysphasia: Testing the consequences of a decay impairment to an interactive spreading activation model of lexical retrieval. *Brain and Language 47*: 609–660, 1994.

Martin N, and Saffran EM. A computational account of deep dysphasia: Evidence from a single case study. *Brain and Language 43*: 240–274, 1992.

Martins IP, and Ferro JM. Recovery from aphasia and lesion size in the temporal lobe. In IP Martins, A Castro-Caldas, HR van Dongen, and A van Hout (Eds.), *Acquired aphasia in children*. Dordrecht: Kluwer Academic Publishers, 1991, pp. 171–184.

Masterson J, Hazan V, and Wiijayatilake L. Phonemic processing problems in developmental phonological dyslexia. *Cognitive Neuropsychology 12*: 233–259, 1995.

Mazzoni M, Vista M, Geri E, Avila L, Bianchi F, and Moretti P. Comparison of language recovery in rehabilitated and matched, non-rehabilitated aphasic patients. *Aphasiology 9*: 553–563, 1995.

McCarthy R, and Warrington E. A two-route model of speech production. *Brain 107*: 469–485, 1984.

McCloskey M. The future of cognitive neuropsychology. In B Rapp (Ed.), *The handbook of cognitive neuropsychology*. Philadelphia: Psychology Press, 2000, pp. 593–610.

McCloskey M, Badecker W, Goodman-Schulman RA, and Aliminosa D. The structure of graphemic representations in spelling: Evidence from a case of acquired dysgraphia. *Cognitive Neuropsychology 11*: 341–392, 1994.

McGlone J. Sex differences in the cerebral organization of verbal function and cognitive impairment in stroke. Age, sex, aphasia type and laterality differences. *Brain 100*: 775–793, 1977.

McGlone J. Sex differences in human brain asymmetry: A critical survey. *Behavioral Brain Sciences 3*: 215–263, 1980.

McKenna P, and Warrington EK. Testing for nominal dysphasia. *Journal of Neurology, Neurosurgery, and Psychiatry 43*: 781–788, 1980.

Meikle M, Wechsler E, Tupper A, Benenson M, Butler J, Mulhall D, and Stern G. Comparative trial of volunteer and professional treatments of dysphasia after stroke. *British Medical Journal 2*: 87–89, 1979.

Miceli G. The processing of speech sounds in a patient with cortical auditory disorder. *Neuropsychologia 20*: 5–20, 1982.

Miceli G, Amitrano A, Capasso R, and Caramazza A. The treatment of anomia from output lexical damage: Analysis of two cases. *Brain and Language 52*: 150–174, 1996.

Miceli G, Benvegnù B, Capasso R, and Caramazza A. The independence of phonological and orthographic lexical forms: Evidence from aphasia. *Cognitive Neuropsychology 14*: 35–70, 1997.

Miceli G, and Capasso R. Semantic errors as evidence for the independence and the interaction of orthographic and phonological word forms. *Language and Cognitive Processes 12*: 733–764, 1997.

Miceli G, Capasso R, and Caramazza A. Sublexical conversion procedures and the interaction of phonological and orthographic lexical forms. *Cognitive Neuropsychology 16*: 557–572, 1999.

Miceli G, and Caramazza A. Dissociation of inflectional and derivational morphology. *Brain and Language 35*: 24–65, 1988.

Miceli G, Gainotti G, Caltagirone C, and Masullo C. Some aspects of phonological impairment in aphasia. *Brain and Language 11*, 159–169, 1988a.

Miceli G, Giustolisi L, and Caramazza A. The interaction of lexical and non-lexical processing mechanisms: Evidence from aphasia. *Cortex 27*: 57–80, 1991a.

Miceli G, Laudanna A, and Burani C. *Batteria per l'Analisi dei Deficit Afasici.* Milan: Associazione per lo Sviluppo delle Ricerche Neuropsicologiche, 1991b.

Miceli G, Silveri C, and Caramazza A. Cognitive analysis of a case of pure dysgraphia. *Brain and Language 25*: 187–212, 1985.

Miceli G, Silveri C, Nocentini U, and Caramazza A. Patterns of dissociation in comprehension and production of nouns and verb. *Aphasiology 2*: 351–358, 1988b.

Miceli G, Silveri C, Villa G, and Caramazza A. On the basis for agrammatics' difficulty in producing main verbs. *Cortex 20*: 207–220, 1984.

Michel F, and Andreewsky E. Deep dysphasia: An analog of deep dyslexia in the auditory modality. *Brain and Language 18*: 212–223, 1983.

Miller D, and Ellis AW. Speech and writing errors in "neologistic jargonaphasia": A lexical activation hypothesis. In M Coltheart, R Job, and G Sartori (Eds.), *The cognitive neuropsychology of language.* Hillsdale, NJ: Lawrence Erlbaum Associates, 1987, pp. 253–271.

Miller N. Acquired speech disorders: Applying linguistics to treatment. In K Grundig (Ed.), *Linguistics in clinical practice.* New York: Taylor and Francis, 1989, pp. 281–300.

Milner B, Branch G, and Rasmussen T. Observations on cerebral dominance. In AVS Reuck and M O'Connor (Eds.), *Ciba foundation symposium on disorders of language.* London: Churchill Livingstone, 1964, pp. 200–214.

Miozzo M, and Caramazza A. Varieties of pure alexia: The case of failure to access graphemic representations. *Cognitive Neuropsychology 15*: 203–238, 1998.

Mitchum CC. Treatment generalization and the application of cognitive neuropsychological models in aphasia therapy. In: *Aphasia treatment: Current approaches and research opportunities.* NIDCD Monograph. Bethesda, MD: National Institute of Deafness and Other Communication Disorders, 1992, pp. 99–116.

Mitchum CC, and Berndt RS. Diagnosis and treatment of "phonological assembly" in acquired dyslexia: An illustration of the cognitive neuropsychological approach. *Journal of Neurolinguistics 6*: 103–137, 1991.

Mitchum CC, and Berndt RS. Verb retrieval and sentence construction: Effects of targeted intervention. In J Riddoch and G Humphreys (Eds.), *Cognitive neuropsychology and cognitive rehabilitation.* Hove, UK: Lawrence Erlbaum Associates, 1994, pp. 317–348.

Mitchum CC, Greenwald ML, and Berndt RS. Cognitive treatments of sentence processing disorders: What have we learned? *Neuropsychological Rehabilitation 10*: 311–336, 2000.

Mitchum CC, Haendiges AN, and Berndt RS. Model-guided treatment to improve written sentence production: A case study. *Aphasiology 7*: 71–109, 1993.

Moore WH, and Weidner W. Bilateral tachistoscopic word perception in aphasic and normal subjects. *Perceptual and Motor Skills 39*: 1001–1011, 1974.

Moore WH, and Weidner W. Dichotic word perception of aphasic and normal subjects. *Perceptual and Motor Skills 40*: 379–386, 1975.

Morris C. Foundations of the theory of signs. In: *International Encyclopedia of Unified Science*. Chicago: University of Chicago Press, 1938, pp. 77–138.

Moutier F. *L'aphasie de Broca*. Paris: Steinheil, 1908.

Naeser MA. A structured approach teaching aphasic basic sentence types. *British Journal of Disorders of Communication 10*: 70–76, 1975.

Naeser MA, Haas G, Mazurski P, and Laughlin S. Sentence level auditory comprehension treatment program for aphasic adults. *Archives of Physical Medicine and Rehabilitation 67*: 393–399, 1986.

Nettleton J, and Lesser R. Application of a cognitive neuropsychological model to therapy for naming difficulties. *Journal of Neurolinguistics 6*: 139–157, 1991.

Neuberger J. Do we need a new word for patients? *British Medical Journal 318*: 1756–1757, 1999.

Newcombe F, Oldfield C, Ratcliff GC, and Wingfield R. The recognition and naming of object-drawings by men with focal brain wounds. *Journal of Neurology, Neurosurgery and Psychiatry 34*: 329–340, 1971.

Nickels L. *Spoken word production and its breakdown in aphasia*. Hove, UK: Psychology Press, 1997.

Nickels L, and Best W. Therapy for naming disorders (Part I): Principles, puzzles and progress. *Aphasiology 10*: 21–47, 1996.

Nolan KA, and Caramazza A. An analysis of writing in a case of deep dyslexia. *Brain and Language 20*: 305–328, 1983.

Office of Technology Assessment. *Assessing the efficacy and safety of medical technologies*, OTA-H-75. Washington, DC: U.S. Government Printing Office, 1978.

Pachalska M. The concept of holistic rehabilitation of persons with aphasia. In AL Holland and MM Forbes (Eds.), *Aphasia treatment*.

World perspectives. San Diego, CA: Singular Publishing Group, 1993, pp. 145–174.

Panzeri M, Semenza C, Ferreri T, and Butterworth B. Free use of derivational morphology in an Italian jargonaphasic. In J-L Nespoulous and P Villiard (Eds.), *Morphology, phonology and aphasia*. New York: Springer Verlag, 1990, pp. 72–94.

Papagno C, and Basso A. Perseveration in two aphasic patients. *Cortex 32*: 67–82, 1996.

Papanicolaou AC, Levin HS, and Eisenberg HM. Evoked potential correlates of recovery from aphasia after focal left hemisphere injury in adults. *Neurosurgery 14*: 412–415, 1984.

Papanicolaou AC, Moore BD, Levin HS, and Eisenberg HM. Evoked potential correlates of right hemisphere involvement in language recovery following stroke. *Archives of Neurology 44*: 521–524, 1987.

Paradis M. *Foundations of aphasia rehabilitation*. Oxford: Pergamon Press, 1993.

Patterson KE, and Hodges JR. Deterioration of word meaning: Implications for reading. *Neuropsychologia 10*: 1025–1040, 1992.

Patterson KE, Purell C, and Morton J. Facilitation of word retrieval in aphasia. In C Code and D Müller (Eds.), *Aphasia therapy*. London: Edward Arnold, 1983, pp. 76–87.

Patterson KE, and Shewell CC. Speak and spell: Dissociations and word-class effect. In M Coltheart, G Sartori, and R Job (Eds.), *The cognitive neuropsychology of language*. Hove, UK: Lawrence Erlbaum Associates, 1987, pp. 273–294.

Pederson PM, Jorgensen HS, Nakayama H, Raaschou HO, and Olsen TS. Aphasia in acute stroke: Incidence, determinants, and recovery. *Annals of Neurology 38*: 659–666, 1995.

Pederson PM, Jorgensen HS, Nakayama H, Raaschou HO, and Olsen TS. Aphasia in acute stroke: Incidence, determinants, and recovery. Reply. *Annals of Neurology 40*: 130, 1996.

Penfield W, and Roberts L. *Speech and brain mechanisms*. Princeton, NJ: Princeton University Press, 1959.

Penn C. A profile of communicative appropriateness: A clinical tool for the assessment of pragmatics. *The South African Journal of Communication Disorders 32*: 18–23, 1985.

Penn C. Aphasia therapy in South Africa: Some pragmatic and personal perspectives. In AL Holland and MM Forbes (Eds.), *Aphasia treatment. World perspectives*. San Diego, CA: Singular Publishing Group, 1993, pp. 25–53.

Pickersgill MJ, and Lincoln NB. Prognostic indicators and the pattern of recovery of communication in aphasic stroke patients. *Journal of Neurology, Neurosurgery and Psychiatry 46*: 130–139, 1983.

Pizzamiglio L, Galati G, and Committeri G. The contribution of functional neuroimaging to recovery after brain damage: A review. *Cortex 37*: 11–31, 2001.

Pizzamiglio L, Mammucari A, and Razzano C. Evidence for sex differences in brain organization in recovery from aphasia. *Brain and Language 25*: 213–223, 1985.

Pizzamiglio L, and Roberts M. Writing in aphasia: Learning study. *Cortex 3*: 250–257, 1967.

Plaut DC, and Shallice T. *Connectionist modeling in cognitive neuropsychology: A case study*. Hillsdale, NJ: Lawrence Erlbaum Associates, 1994.

Poeck K. What do we mean by "aphasic syndromes"? A neurologist's view. *Brain and Language 20*: 79–89, 1983.

Poeck K, Huber W, and Willmes K. Outcome of intensive language treatment in aphasia. *Journal of Speech and Hearing Disorders 54*: 471–479, 1989.

Porch BE. *Porch index of communicative ability: Therapy and development*, Vol. 1. Palo Alto, CA: Psychologists Press, 1967.

Posteraro L, Zinelli P, and Mazzucchi A. Selective impairment of the graphemic buffer in acquired dysgraphia: A case study. *Brain and Language 35*: 274–286, 1988.

Pring TR. Speech therapists and volunteers: Some comments on recent investigation of their effectiveness in the treatment of aphasia. *British Journal of Disorders of Communication 18*: 65–73, 1983.

Pring TR. Evaluating the effects of speech therapy for aphasics: Developing the single case methodology. *British Journal of Disorders of Communication 21*: 103–115, 1986.

Pring TR. On choosing a methodology to assess the effectiveness of therapeutic interventions: A brief reply to Fitz-Gibbon. *British Journal of Disorder of Communication 22*: 163–166, 1987.

Prins RS, Schoonen R, and Vermeulen J. Efficacy of two different types of speech therapy for aphasic stroke patients. *Applied Psycholinguistics 10*: 85–123, 1989.

Prins RS, Snow CE, and Wagenaar R. Recovery from aphasia: Spontaneous speech versus language comprehension. *Brain and Language 6*: 192–211, 1978.

Prutting CA, and Kirschner DM. A clinical appraisal of pragmatic aspects of language. *Journal of Speech and Hearing Disorders 52*: 105–119, 1987.

Rapp B, Benzing L, and Caramazza A. The autonomy of lexical orthography. *Cognitive Neuropsychology 14*: 71–104, 1997.

Rapp B, and Caramazza A. On the distinction between deficits of access and deficits of storage: A question of theory. *Cognitive Neuropsychology 10*: 113–141, 1993.

Rapp B, and Caramazza A. The modality-specific organization of grammatical categories: Evidence from impaired spoken and written sentence production. *Brain and Language 56*: 248–286, 1997.

Rapp B, and Caramazza A. A case of selective difficulty in writing verbs. *Neurocase 4*: 127–140, 1998.

Rapp B, and Caramazza A. Selective difficulties with spoken nouns and written verbs: A single case study. *Journal of Neurolinguistics 15*: 373–402, 2002.

Rasmussen T, and Milner B. The role of early left-brain injury in determining lateralization of cerebral speech functions. *Annals of the New York Academy of Sciences 299*: 355–369, 1977.

Raven JC. *Guide to using the coloured progressive matrices sets A, Ab, B.* London: HK Lewis, 1965.

Raymer AM, Thompson CK, Jacobs B, and le Grand HR. Phonological treatment of naming deficits in aphasia: Model-based generalization analysis. *Aphasiology 7*: 27–53, 1993.

Reuter-Lorenz PA, and Brunn JL. A prelexical basis for letter-by-letter reading: A case study. *Cognitive Neuropsychology 7*: 1–20, 1990.

Riddoch MJ, and Humphreys GW (Eds.). *Cognitive neuropsychology and cognitive rehabilitation.* Hove, UK: Lawrence Erlbaum Associates, 1994.

Robertson IH, and Murre JMJ. Rehabilitation of brain damage: Brain plasticity and principles of guided recovery. *Psychological Bulletin 125*: 544–575, 1999.

Robey RR. The efficacy of treatment for aphasic persons: A meta-analysis. *Brain and Language 47*: 582–608, 1994.

Robey RR. A meta-analysis of clinical outcomes in the treatment of aphasia. *Journal of Speech, Language, and Hearing Research 41*: 172–187, 1998.

Robey RR, Schultz MC, Crawford AB, and Sinner CA. Single-subject clinical-outcome research: Designs, data, effect sizes, and analyses. *Aphasiology 13*: 445–473, 1999.

Roeltgen DP, and Heilman KM. Apractic agraphia in a patient with normal praxis. *Brain and Language 18*: 35–46, 1983.

Roeltgen DP, and Heilman KM. Lexical agraphia, further support for the two-strategy hypothesis of linguistic agraphia. *Brain 107*: 811–827, 1984.

Roeltgen DP, Sevush S, and Heilman KM. Phonological agraphia: Writing by the lexical-semantic route. *Neurology 33*: 755–765, 1983.

Rosati G, and De Bastiani P. Pure agraphia: A discrete form of aphasia. *Journal of Neurology, Neurosurgery and Psychiatry 42*: 266–269, 1979.

Rosenbek JC, Kent DR, and La Pointe LL. Apraxia of speech: An overview and some perspectives. In JC Rosenbeck, MR McNeil, and AE Aronson (Eds.), *Apraxia of speech*. San Diego, CA: College Hill Press, 1989, pp. 1–28.

Russell WR, and Espir MLE. *Traumatic aphasia*. London: Oxford University Press, 1961.

Sabbagh MA. Communicative intentions and language: Evidence from right-hemisphere damage and autism. *Brain and Language 70*: 29–69, 1999.

Sacchett C, and Humphreys GW. Calling a squirrel a squirrel but a canoe a wigwam: A category-specific deficit for artefactual objects and body parts. *Cognitive Neuropsychology 9*: 73–86, 1992.

Sands E, Sarno MT, and Shankweiler D. Long-term assessment of language function in aphasia due to stroke. *Archives of Physical Medicine and Rehabilitation 50*: 202–206, 1969.

Sarno MT. *The functional communication profile: Manual of directions*. New York: New York University Medical Center, 1969.

Sarno MT. Recovery and rehabilitation. In MT Sarno (Ed.), *Acquired aphasia*, 2nd ed. San Diego, CA: Academic Press, 1991, pp. 521–582.

Sarno MT, and Levita E. Natural course of recovery in severe aphasia. *Archives of Physical Medicine and Rehabilitation 52*: 175–178, 1971.

Sarno MT, and Levita E. Recovery in treated aphasia in the first year post-stroke. *Stroke 10*: 663–669, 1979.

Sarno MT, Silverman M, and Sands E. Speech therapy and language recovery in severe aphasia. *Journal of Speech and Hearing Research 13*: 607–623, 1970.

Saussure de F. *Cours de linguistique générale*. Paris: Payot, 1916.

Schoonen R. The internal validity of efficacy studies: Design and statistical power in studies of language therapy for aphasics. *Brain and Language 41*: 446–464, 1991.

Schuell H. *Minnesota Test for the Differential Diagnosis of Aphasia.*
Minneapolis: University of Minnesota Press, 1955.

Schuell H, Carroll V, and Street B. Clinical treatment of aphasia. *Journal
of Speech and Hearing Disorders 20*: 43–53, 1955.

Schuell H, Jenkins JJ, Carroll JB. A factor analysis of the Minnesota Test
for Differential Diagnosis of Aphasia. *Journal of Speech and Hearing
Research 5*: 349–369, 1962.

Schuell H, Jenkins JJ, and Jimenez-Pabon E. *Aphasia in Adults.* New York:
Harper & Row, 1964.

Schwartz M. What the classical aphasia categories can't do for us. *Brain
and Language 21*: 3–8, 1984.

Schwartz M, Fink RB, and Saffran E. The modular treatment of agrammatism. *Neuropsychological Rehabilitation 5*: 93–127, 1995.

Schwartz M, Linebarger M, Saffran E, and Paté D. Syntactic transparency and sentence interpretation in aphasia. *Language and Cognitive
Processes 2*: 85–113, 1987.

Schwartz M, Saffran ED, Fink RB, Myers JL, and Marin N. Mapping
therapy: A treatment programme for agrammatism. *Aphasiology 8*:
19–54, 1994.

Schwartz M, Saffran EM, and Marin OSM. Fractionating the reading
process in dementia: Evidence for word-specific print-to-sound
association. In M Coltheart, KE Patterson, and JC Marshall
(Eds.), *Deep dyslexia*. London: Routledge & Kegan Paul 1980a,
pp. 259–269.

Schwartz M, Saffran E, and Marin OSM. The word order problem in
agrammatism: 1 Comprehension. *Brain and Language 10*: 249–262,
1980b.

Seidenberg MS, and McClelland JL. A distributed developmental model
of visual word recognition and naming. *Psychological Review 96*:
523–568, 1989.

Seron X. *Aphasie et neuropsychologie.* Bruxelles: Pierre Mardaga, 1979.

Seron X, and Deloche G. (Eds.). *Cognitive approaches to neuropsychological
rehabilitation*, Hillsdale, NJ: Lawrence Erlbaum Associates, 1989.

Seron X, Deloche G, Moulard G, and Rouselle M. A computer-based
therapy for the treatment of aphasic subjects with writing disorders.
Journal of Speech and Hearing Disorders 45: 45–58, 1980.

Seron X, and De Partz M-P. The re-education of aphasics: Between
theory and practice. In AL Holland and MM Forbes (Eds.), *Aphasia
treatment. World perspectives.* San Diego, CA: Singular Publishing Group,
1993, pp. 131–144.

Shallice T. Phonological agraphia and the lexical route in writing. *Brain 104*: 413–429, 1981.

Shallice T. *From neuropsychology to mental structure.* Cambridge: Cambridge University Press, 1988.

Shallice T. Multiple semantics: Whose confusions? *Cognitive Neuropsychology 10*: 251–261, 1993.

Shallice T, and Coughlan AK. Modality specific word comprehension deficits in deep dyslexia. *Journal of Neurology, Neurosurgery and Psychiatry 43*: 866–872, 1980.

Shallice T, Rumiati R, and Zadini A. The selective impairment of the phonological buffer. *Cognitive Neuropsychology 17*: 517–546, 2000.

Shallice T, and Warrington E. The selective impairment of auditory verbal short-term memory. *Brain 92*: 885–896, 1969.

Shapiro K, Shelton J, and Caramazza A. Grammatical class in lexical production and morphological processing: Evidence from a case of fluent aphasia. *Cognitive Neuropsychology 17*: 665–682, 2000.

Shewan C. *The Auditory Comprehension Test for Sentences (ACTS).* Chicago: Biolinguistics, 1979

Shewan CM, and Bandur DL. *Treatment of aphasia: A language-oriented approach.* London: Taylor & Francis, 1986.

Shewan CM, and Kertesz A. Effects of speech and language treatment in recovery from aphasia. *Brain and Language 23*: 272–299, 1984.

Silveri C, and di Betta A. Noun–verb dissociation in brain-damaged patients. Further evidence. *Neurocase 3*: 477–488, 1997.

Skinner BF. *Verbal behavior.* New York: Appleton-Century Crofts, 1957.

Slamecka NJ, and Graf P. The generation effect: Delineation of a phenomenon. *Journal of Experimental Psychology: Human Learning and Memory 4*: 592–604, 1978.

Sparks R, Helm N, and Albert M. Aphasia rehabilitation resulting from Melodic Intonation Therapy. *Cortex 10*: 303–316, 1974.

Spreen O, and Benton A. *Neurosensory center comprehensive examination for aphasia,* rev. ed. Victoria, BC: University of Victoria, Department of Psychology, 1977.

Stemmer B, Giroux F, and Joanette Y. Production and evaluation of requests by right hemisphere brain damaged individuals. *Brain and Language 47*: 1–31, 1994.

Strauss Hough M, and Pierce RS. Pragmatics and treatment. In R. Chapey (Ed.), *Language intervention strategies in adult aphasia,* 3rd ed. Baltimore: Williams & Wilkins, 1994, pp. 246–268.

Subirana A. Handedness and cerebral dominance. In BJ Vinken and GW Bruyn (Eds.), *Handbook of clinical neurology*, Vol. 4. Amsterdam: North Holland Publishing Company 1969, pp. 248–272.

Thompson CK, Fix SC, Gitelman DR, Parrish TB, and Mesulam M-M. FMRI studies of agrammatic sentence comprehension before and after treatment. *Brain and Language 74*: 387–391, 2000.

Thompson CK, Shapiro LP, and Roberts M-M. Treatment of sentence production deficits in aphasia: A linguistic-specific approach to *wh*-interrogative training and generalization. *Aphasiology 7*: 111–133, 1993.

Thompson CK, Shapiro LP, Tait ME, Jacobs BJ, and Schneider SL. Training *wh*-question production in agrammatic aphasia: Analysis of argument and adjunct movement. *Brain and Language 52*: 175–228, 1996.

Thulborn KR, Carpenter PA, and Just MA. Plasticity of language-related brain function during recovery from stroke. *Stroke 30*: 749–754, 1999.

Tikofsky RS, and Reynolds GL. Preliminary study: Non-verbal learning and aphasia. *Journal of Speech and Hearing Research 5*: 133–143, 1962.

Tikofsky RS, and Reynolds GL. Further studies on non-verbal learning and aphasia. *Journal of Speech and Hearing Research 6*: 329–337, 1963.

Tsvetkova LS. Basic principles of a theory of reeducation of brain-injured patients. *The Journal of Special Education 6*: 135–144, 1972.

Ulatowska HK, Allard L, Reyes BA, Ford J, and Chapman S. Conversational discourse in aphasia. *Aphasiology 6*: 325–331, 1992.

Van Lanckner D, and Kempler D. Comprehension of familiar phrases by left- but not by right-hemisphere damaged patients. *Brain and Language 32*: 265–267, 1987.

Vignolo LA. Evolution of aphasia and language rehabilitation: A retrospective exploratory study. *Cortex 1*: 344–367, 1964.

Vignolo LA, Macario E, and Cappa S. Clinical–CT scan correlations in a prospective series of patients with acute left-hemisphere subcortical stroke. In G Vallar, S Cappa, and CW Wallesch (Eds.), *Neuropsychological disorders associated with subcortical lesions*. Oxford: Oxford University Press, 1992, pp. 334–343.

Visch-Brink EG, Bajema IM, and Van de Sandt-Koenderman ME. Lexical semantic therapy: BOX. *Aphasiology 11*: 1057–1115, 1997.

Von Monakov C. Diaschisis. (1914) In KH Pribram (Ed.), *Brain and behaviour I: Moods, states and mind* (Trans. G. Harris). Baltimore: Penguin, 1969, pp. 27–36.

Wada J. A new method of identifying the dominant hemisphere for language: Intracarotid sodium amytal injection in man. *Medical Biology 14*: 221–222, 1949.

Wade DT, Hewer RL, David RM, and Enderby PM. Aphasia after stroke: Natural history and associated deficits. *Journal of Neurology, Neurosurgery and Psychiatry 49*: 11–16, 1986.

Warrington EK, and McCarthy R. Category specific access dysphasia. *Brain 106*: 859–878, 1983.

Warrington EK, and Shallice T. Semantic access dyslexia. *Brain 102*: 43–63, 1979.

Warrington EK, and Shallice T. Category specific semantic impairments. *Brain 107*: 829–854, 1984.

Weidner WE, and Jinks AFG. The effect of single versus combined cue presentations on picture naming by aphasic adults. *Journal of Communication Disorders 16*: 111–121, 1983.

Weigl E. The phenomenon of temporary deblocking in aphasia. *Zeitschrift fur Phonetik, Sprachwissenschaft und Kommunikationsforschung 14*: 337–364, 1961.

Weigl E, and Bierwisch M. Neuropsychology and linguistics: Topics of common interest. *Foundations of Language 6*: 1–18, 1970.

Weisenburg TH, and McBride KE. *Aphasia: A clinical and psychological study.* New York: The Commonwealth Fund, 1935.

Weniger D, Huber W, Stachowiack F-J, and Poeck K. Treatment of aphasia on a linguistic basis. In MT Sarno and O Hook (Eds.), *Aphasia. Assessment and treatment.* Stockolm: Almqvist & Wiksell International, 1980, pp. 149–157.

Wepman JM. *Recovery from aphasia.* New York: Ronald Press, 1951.

Wepman JM. Aphasia therapy: A new look. *Journal of Speech and Hearing Disorders, 37*: 203–214, 1972.

Wepman JM. Aphasia: Language without thought or thought without language? *ASHA, 18*: 131–136, 1976

Wepman JM, and Jones LF. Five aphasias: A commentary on aphasia as a regressive linguistic problem. In D Rioch and EA Weinstein (Eds.), *Disorders of communication.* Baltimore: Williams & Wilkins, 1964, pp. 190–203.

Wernicke C. *Der aphasische Symptomenkomplex.* Breslau, Germany: Cohn & Weigart, 1874.

Wertz RT. Aphasia in acute stroke: Incidence, determinants, and recovery. Letter to the Editor. *Annals of Neurology 40*: 129–130, 1996.

Wertz RT, Collins MJ, Weiss D, Kurtzke JE, Friden T, Brookshire RH, Pierce J, Holtzapple P, Hubbard DJ, Porch BE, West JA, Davis L, Matovitch V, Morley GK, and Resurreccion E. Veterans Administration cooperative study on aphasia: A comparison of individual and group treatment. *Journal of Speech and Hearing Disorders 24*: 580–594, 1981.

Wertz RT, Weiss DG, Aten JL, Brookshire RH, Garcia-Bunuel L, Holland AL, Kurtzke JF, LaPointe LL, Milianti FJ, Brannegan R, Greenbaum H, Marshall RC, Vogel D, Carter J, Barnes NS, and Goodman R. Comparison of clinic, home, and deferred language treatment for aphasia: A Veterans Administration cooperative study. *Archives of Neurology 43*: 653–658, 1986.

Whitaker H. A case of the isolation of the language function. In H Withaker and HA Whitaker (Eds.), *Studies in neurolinguistics*, Vol. 2. New York: Academic Press, 1976, pp. 1–58.

Whurr R, Lorch MP, and Nye C. A meta-analysis of studies carried out between 1946 and 1988 concerned with the efficacy of speech and language therapy treatment for aphasic patients. *European Journal of Disorders of Communication 27*: 1–17, 1992.

Wiegel-Crump C, and Koenigsknecht RA. Tapping the lexical store of the adult aphasic: Analysis of the improvement made in word retrieval skill. *Cortex 9*: 411–418, 1973.

Wilcox MJ, Davis GA, and Leonard LB. Aphasics' comprehension of contextually conveyed meaning. *Brain and Language 6*: 362–377, 1978.

Wilk JJ, and Paradis M. Linguistic foundations of rehabilitation methods. In M Paradis (Ed.), *Foundations of aphasia rehabilitation*. Oxford: Pergamon Press, 1993, pp. 101–193.

Williams SE, and Canter CJ. Action-naming performance in four syndromes of aphasia. *Brain and Language 32*: 124–136, 1987.

Willmes K, and Poeck K. Ergebnisse einer multizentrischen Untersuchung über die Spontanprognose von Aphasien vaskulärer Aetiologie. *Nervenartz 55*: 62–71, 1984.

Wilson B, Baddeley A, Evans J, and Shiel A. Errorless learning in the rehabilitation of memory impaired people. *Neuropsychological Rehabilitation 4*: 307–326, 1994.

Wilson B, and Patterson K. Rehabilitation for cognitive impairment: Does cognitive psychology apply? *Applied Cognitive Psychology 4*: 247–260, 1990.

World Health Organization. *The international classification of impairments, disabilities and handicaps—a manual of classification relating to the consequences of disease.* Geneva: Author, 1980.

Zingeser L, and Berndt RS. Grammatical class and context effects in a case of pure anomia: Implications for models of language processing. *Cognitive Neuropsychology 5*: 473–516, 1988.

Zingeser L, and Berndt RS. Retrieval of nouns and verbs in agrammatism and anomia. *Brain and Language 39*: 14–32, 1990.

INDEX

Page numbers followed by *f* and *t* indicate figures and tables, respectively.